Elementary School Health Instruction

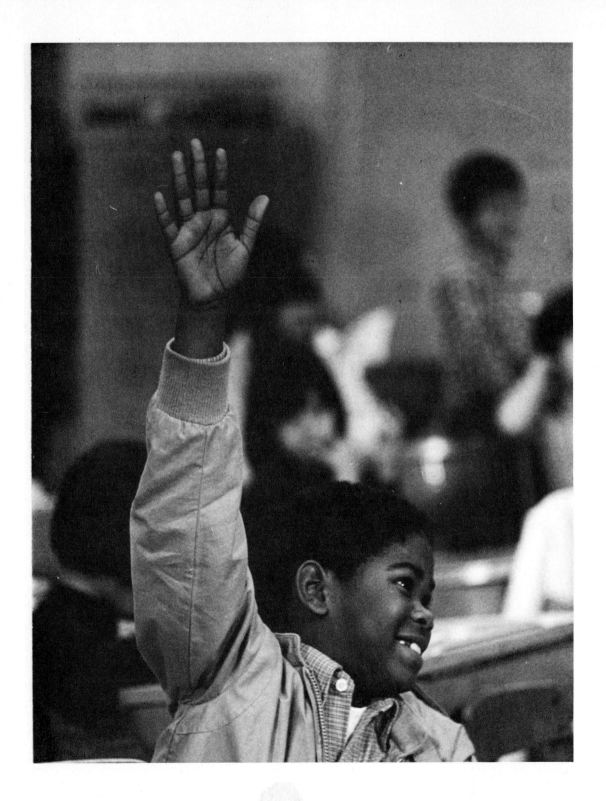

Elementary School Health Instruction

Marion B. Pollock, Ed.D.

Professor Emeritus
Department of Health Science
California State University
Long Beach, California

Kathleen Middleton, M.S.

Health Educator and Editor
ETR Associates
Santa Cruz, California

Second Edition

with 220 illustrations

TIMES MIRROR/MOSBY   COLLEGE PUBLISHING

ST. LOUIS · TORONTO · BOSTON · LOS ALTOS 1989

Editor: Pat Coryell
Editorial Assistant: Shannon Ruyle
Designer: Liz Fett
Project Manager: Kathleen L. Teal

Second Edition

Copyright © 1989 by Times Mirror/Mosby College Publishing
A division of The C.V. Mosby Company
11830 Westline Industrial Drive, St. Louis, Missouri 63146

Previous edition copyrighted 1984

Printed in the United States of America

Library of Congress Cataloging in Publication Data

Pollock, Marion B.
  Elementary school health instruction/Marion B. Pollock, Kathleen
Middleton.—2nd ed.
    p. cm.
  ISBN 0-8016-4039-3
  1. Health education (Elementary)   I. Middleton, Kathleen.
II. Title.
LB1587.A3P64 1989
372.3′7—dc19 88-20104 CIP

TS/DC/DC 9 8 7 6 5 4 3 2

This book is dedicated
To the healthy growth and development
of all elementary school children, and
to their teachers, whose efforts and
commitment contribute so greatly to
its protection and promotion.

MBP

To my son, *Kirby Owen,* who brings
new meaning to the concepts of
health and love; may he, and his
future teachers and classmates
benefit from the work within this
book.

KM

Preface

Health education during elementary school years can have a powerful influence on the quality of life each student will ultimately enjoy as an adult. That is because childhood years are those during which health enhancing habits and attitudes can be shaped or reinforced most easily. Whatever other forces impact children's beliefs and actions, elementary school teachers are potentially among the most influential. What an elementary school teacher does to foster development of a healthful life-style among students can be crucial not only to their present and future well-being but also potentially to that of their families and friends, and even, some day, to that of the total community.

Health education is not a luxury, it is a necessity. It cannot be delayed as it often is until the seventh or tenth grade. That is too late. Children do not wait until they are in their teens to set their values and habits relative to health behavior. They begin to do that almost at birth.

Audience

This second edition of ELEMENTARY SCHOOL HEALTH INSTRUCTION remains a textbook designed to help prospective elementary school teachers teach children what they need and want to know about health. At a minimum, elementary teachers should have a sound background of up-to-date information about personal health and health behavior. They need to have a clear understanding of the interrelationships among school health services, the quality of the school's environment, and the nature of the health instruction that is provided. Although the book is intended for use in college classrooms as the text in a course designed for undergraduate study, it can also be used by health-concerned professionals as a medium for independent study. Elementary teachers who have not had prior professional preparation for health teaching, as well as school nurses, school principals, school physicians, community health educators, and others involved in making decisions affecting the quality of school health programs and curricula will find it a valuable resource.

Although the book focuses primarily on instruction, the role of health services and provision of a safe and sanitary environment in protecting and promoting the health of both students and staff is emphasized throughout. The intent overall is to provide the reader with the concepts and skills needed to understand, plan, and carry out a curriculum that reflects modern concepts of comprehensive school health instruction.

Recent Developments

Most adults, whether teachers, administrators, or parents, think of health instruction as *Hygiene*. In schools where health instruction has been provided at elementary levels, the subject matter tends to focus on grooming standards of personal care, and watered-down study of the anatomy and physiology of certain body systems. In some schools, lessons are limited to practice in flossing and brushing teeth or meal planning based on the four food groups. There is nothing wrong with that except it is not enough, and the same material is apt to be repeated at every grade level. Even children know that there must be more to health instruction than that.

Most teaching activities emphasize acquisition of health facts as an end in itself rather than as a foundation to the ability to choose wisely among alternate actions affecting one's health. The focus has been almost entirely given to provision of bits of information about health, not on health promotion. Today there is a shift to experiential learning activities, which requires identification of measurable objectives before they can be planned or their success evaluated.

There has been a change in the primary goals of health teaching. Rather than focusing on disease prevention as before, the emphasis of health instruction is shifting instead to health *promotion*. No longer germs, nor heredity, nor environment, but one's life-style is recognized as the major cause of illness and early death. This change in direction is reflected in the content of new health school books, the trend toward providing youngsters with active participation in classroom investigations instead of time spent passively filling in the blanks in workbooks, and general acceptance of the fact that health has many dimensions rather than that of physical wellness alone.

An emerging approach to health instruction has evolved from recognition that facts are not enough, nor are they as much use to the student as health-related skills. In some pace-setting schools, telling children what to do and believe about their health and equating ability to recite these given with successful health instruction has been abandoned. Instead, the concepts and skills children are learning promote acceptance of responsibility for personal actions and choices as these affect their health and safety. They are participating effectively and competently in self-care procedures appropriate to existing and learnable skills and understandings. Self-reliance and thinking skills are fostered in vital school room health instruction today. Ways to plan and implement curricula of that kind are explained in this edition.

Historically, when certain health problems have seemed uncontrollable by medical means, health education begins to be recognized for its potential in preventing disease and promoting health. Now the swiftly growing incidence of AIDS has done it again. AIDS education is being promoted at every level of society, even among children at third grade levels. Drug and alcohol abuse, and tobacco use by young children have for some time motivated development of teaching materials designed to cope with these problems. Many of these materials have been created by outside organizations and sold to schools wishing to do something about this aspect of health education, but whose teachers do not feel qualified to develop and teach their own curriculum plans. Study of the chapters in this book should equip any teacher, at the very least, to ask the right questions about packaged learning guides for health education offered for their use.

Basis for Revision

Reviews of the first edition were elicited from professors of health education representing several colleges and universities offering courses in health instruction for prospective elementary teachers. Other current textbooks on elementary level health instruction were closely analyzed. Instructors, both users or non-users of the first edition, gave detailed remarks about the book. Students in university classes currently enrolled in courses, such as that for which the book was designed, reviewed its content, made suggestions for changes, and participated in pre-tests of some of its materials. A careful synthesis of all of these comments formed the basis for the decisions made to add new sections or ideas or delete some discussions and to reorganize chapters or parts of chapters.

New To This Edition:

1. As now arranged, the text is divided into two distinct sections. These are inextricably integrated because of the adherence of the second part to the theories set forth in the first.

    Part One, THEORETICAL FOUNDATIONS, has been almost completely revised. The sequence of topics addressed in each chapter has been re-ordered, and most of the material has been rewritten. The content has been strengthened and updated by the incorporation of ideas and facts gleaned from a wide range of references not limited to those directly concerned with school health education or with health education for children. Some of these references have been drawn from other disciplines such as education, social education, teacher education, childhood education, community health education and currently published research findings. Current university level textbooks concerned with health education, educational evaluation, measurement, psychology, and other professional fields germane to curriculum development have been studied and important areas have been integrated into each chapter.

    Part Two, CONTENT AND PRACTICE, has been revised by Kathleen Middleton. Dr. Betty Hubbard, from the University of Central Arkansas, assisted in the development of three additional chapters (Chapters 10, 12, and 14), which present content appropriate for health instruction at the Primary, Intermediate, or Middle school levels of education. This section of the book was revised after study of the opinions and suggestions resulting from reviews obtained and offered by health education professionals, both university faculty and practicing elementary teachers. In addition, the content suggestions provided in Chapter 14 and the activities in Chapter 15 represent curriculum adjustments responsive to the need for a stronger emphasis on middle school curriculum.

2. Many of the illustrations are new and feature children at school in natural settings.

3. Tables of information, once placed in the appendices, have been moved to Chapter 2 where they more logically support the discussion.

4. Each chapter now begins with a set of measurable objectives which specify what the reader should know and be able to do when the chapter has been completed.

5. Boxed information features principles, case studies, summaries, lists references, and annotated suggested readings.

6. Questions, problems, and exercises at the close of chapters have been completely revised or replaced with new items. These questions require the reader to use the concepts and information just acquired in new ways, and to encourage dialogue and cooperation among students.

7. Chapter 1 has been extensively revised in order to reflect the changing focus and content of the discipline as it appears today. Key terminology is defined early in the chapter in order to facilitate the reader's quick grasp of the language of health education before getting into the complexities of a total school health program as explored in the next chapter. Chapter 2, with the pretest included as a motivating device, has been even more carefully developed. The chapter formerly titled ''Evaluating Health Teaching and Learning'' has been reorganized, augmented with additional content,

so now it is presented in two chapters, one focusing on evaluation (Chapter 6), and the other on measurement and testing (Chapter 7).

8. A number of changes in format and content have been made. A new Chapter 8, "Preventing Criticism and Controversy in Health Teaching," is more appropriately now included in Part Two. Chapter 9, "A Scope and Sequence Plan for Elementary School Health Instruction," is followed by six chapters, two each developed for primary, intermediate, and middle school students. The first of each pair provides content summaries for each of the ten content areas defined in the scope and sequence chart and the second details ten suggested learning opportunities which implement ten of the objectives developed for health instruction at the specified level of progression.

9. Chapter 8 has been significantly revised to deal more broadly with controversial areas in health education, now including specific information and techniques for planning AIDS education and drug abuse prevention. Selected excerpts from Federal guidelines on AIDS education and prevention of drug abuse are featured.

10. Chapter 9 lists the objectives for all students K through 8 as well as those selected for development here.

11. All of the material originally included in the learning opportunities for, or in Chapter 9 on content for the primary level student will be found in the new Chapter 10. Similarly, Chapters 12 and 14 encompass much of the content specified in former Chapter 8 as appropriate for intermediate and middle school students, along with some of the material outlined in the related learning opportunities. The result is that the learning opportunities are more concise, and all of the related subject matter is grouped together.

12. Subheadings for each of the subordinate activities included in each of the learning opportunities facilitate selection of those most suited to the needs and abilities of specific students or groups.

13. A new lesson specifically designed to help younger students understand AIDS has been added in Chapter 13. More information on AIDS infection and methods for its prevention is found in Chapter 14.

Readability and Student Involvement

Through the second edition of this book, the reader is addressed directly as "you" and encouraged to think about and reply or resolve the answer to a posed query relative to what has just been said or explained. The intent is to involve the reader as an active participant in a dialogue and motivate greater interest and attention to the message.

As in the first edition, we've included many marginal and full-page illustrative sketches to be used as examples of suggested student materials. This makes it much easier to develop lesson plans and lightens the look of the pages. The drawings are simple and easy to reproduce and students will enjoy working with them.

The activity chapters (Chapters 10, 12, and 14), require neither the usual pedagogy nor reference lists because they are unique to the author and the book. However, a single objective has been provided which applies equally well to all three of these chapters.

Format of the Learning Opportunities

Most texts offered for use by elementary school teachers cover much the same subject matter, the school health program in its entirety, and sometimes quite a lot about growth and development and the kinds of health problems experienced by elementary school children. What is very different about this book is the style in which the learning opportunities are developed. Typically most such texts focus on ideas and give suggestions for lessons that engage children in activities which amplify pieces of the recommended subject matter. Few texts, however, offer rationales that go beyond the "one-liner" style, for example, "Use a testing kit with children to demonstrate the taste centers in their tongues." This text stands alone in offering discussion of the worth and functionality of measurable objectives.

Part Three has been deleted as a section of the second edition. Many of the tables and listings in the final chapter of the first edition, "Resources for Elementary School Health Education" have been deleted, either because they were judged too difficult to use, or too infrequently needed by teachers. Tables 12-2, 12-3, and 12-4 will be found now in Chapter Two of the second edition; Table 12-1 and 12-5, the section on selected health education curriculum projects, the glossary of terms, and bibliography area are listed among the appendices. An index of the total book is its final element.

Acknowledgments

We wish to acknowledge the contributions of the following people whose thoughtful reviews of the first edition were valuable aids in making the revision just described. These were Bryan E.M. Cooks, Ph.D., M.P.H. of Colorado State University, and the following others:

Mary Bonstrom
University of Minnesota-Minneapolis

Karen Douglas
West Virginia University

Larry Harrison
University of Northern Colorado

Patrick Tow
Old Dominion University

Cindy Wolford
Kent State University

The many others whose contributions merit special thanks include our good friend and colleague, Don A. Beegle, M.S., M.P.H. Professor of Health Science at California State University Long Beach who ferreted out all the references cited in Part One, and updated the Bibliography making it more useful and usable for those who might wish to find further information relative to any content area. Ric Loya, M.S. health teaching specialist at Huntington Park High School and lecturer at CSULB, who allowed his students to participate in reviewing the first edition and pretesting some of the materials. Judith K. Scheer Ed.S. Lecturer at San Francisco State University, for her review and assistance with lessons in Part Two, and her continual support of the project. Armi Lizardi and Helen Cease who together photographed children at an elementary school in Pasadena for use in the book. Jolly Urner, Lower School Director at Polytechnical School in Pasadena, and Glenny Cameron who cooperated in securing the necessary consents for use of the pictures, Norma MacDonough, school nurse at Monterey Hills Elementary school in South Pasadena who gave her time for advice and counsel regarding school health problems of children, and Helen Cease, Ph.D. elementary school principal who shared her experiences relative to teacher's curriculum skills at entry level, to Beverly Bradley, Ph.D., AIDS education consultant, California State Department of Education for her valued assistance in supplying copies of the health service reporting forms reproduced in the book.

Finally, we wish to acknowledge our obligation and gratitude to the Editors and Editorial Staff of Times Mirror/Mosby. Most particularly to Nancy K. Roberson, Publisher, Pat Coryell, Editor, Shannon Ruyle, Editorial Assistant, and Kathleen Teal, Project Manager whose calm competence and friendly support were greatly appreciated.

Marion B. Pollock
Kathleen Middleton

To the instructor

AN INSTRUCTOR'S MANUAL is available that provides recommendations for using the manual in combination with the text to effectively maximize the teaching and learning process. Designed to correspond with each chapter of the text, the manual contains:

1. Brief chapter overviews
2. Key terms relevant to the health content of each chapter
3. Learning opportunities that provide teaching suggestions for the college classroom, including analyses of related literature, case studies, and classroom exercises that extend information in the text
4. A selection of possible solutions keyed to the discussion questions, problems, and exercises contained within the text
5. Multiple-choice, true-false, short-response, and essay test questions with answer keys

The manual includes full-size pages of the worksheets, patterns, and transparencies, perforated and ready for immediate use, for convenience of reproduction in developing learning opportunities.

Contents

PART ONE   Theoretical Foundations

1   Health Instruction: Promoting Positive Life Styles, 3

2   The Comprehensive School Health Program, 22

3   Planning and Organizing the Curriculum, 68

4   Defining Goals and Objectives for Health Teaching, 96

5   Developing Effective Teaching and Learning Plans, 116

6   Health Education Evaluation, 147

7   Designing Classroom Tests and Evaluation Activities, 172

PART TWO   Content and Practice

8   Preventing Criticism or Controversy in Health Teaching, 203

9   A Scope and Sequence Plan for Elementary School Health Instruction, 221

10   Content Appropriate for Primary Level Students, 232

11   Primary Level Teaching Activity Ideas, 249

12   Content Appropriate for Intermediate Level Students, 309

13   Intermediate Level Teaching Activity Ideas, 327

14   Content Appropriate for Middle School Students, 403

15   Middle School Teaching Activity Ideas, 427

Appendixes, A-1

Glossary, G-1

Bibliography, B-1

PART ONE

Theoretical Foundations

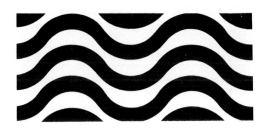

Chapter 1. Health Instruction: Promoting Positive
Life Styles

Chapter 2. The Comprehensive School Health
Program

Chapter 3. Planning and Organizing the Health
Curriculum

Chapter 4. Defining Goals and Objectives for
Health Teaching

Chapter 5. Developing Effective Teaching and
Learning Plans

Chapter 6. Health Education Evaluation

Chapter 7. Designing Classroom Tests and
Evaluation Activities

Health Instruction: Promoting Positive Life Styles

When you finish this chapter you should be able to:

- **Define the meanings of key terms concerned with health promotion through health instruction.**

- **Describe the basic components of the total school health program.**

- **Explain the relevance of Piagetian and health belief model theories to the development of age-appropriate health teaching plans.**

- **Evaluate the influence of social, legislative, economic, educational, and other community influences in determining the quality of a school health program.**

- **Describe the unique role of the elementary school teacher in promoting the health of children and ultimately the community.**

Elementary teachers can be the most effective health educators a child will ever encounter during his or her entire school experience. That is because childhood years are those during which most health practices and attitudes are being learned and established. Lewis and Lewis (1980, p. 148) conclude that the principal determinants of health status in adulthood are formed very early, and these can be influenced for the better by those who care about the health of children.

Health behaviors begin to be shaped almost at birth. From then on, virtually everything we do affects health—and not just our own. Health information and a child do not wait to be introduced by a teacher, however. Long before children start school they have learned a great many aspects of health behavior. They have learned food likes and dislikes and ways of getting along with family and friends. They have well-established attitudes and value systems, based on a host of health-related experiences at home and in the neighborhood. They have accumulated a growing number of beliefs about health and the cause of illness.

The primary source of health training has always been the parents. It still is, but today another "parent"—the television set—has become the favored babysitter and largest source of information about everything in life, including health. The average child between the ages of 6 and 11 spends 25 hours per week, roughly one-third of nonschool hours, watching TV. By high school graduation, a student has been exposed to some 350,000 commercials (Bennett, 1986, p. 14). An example of the efficacy of this bombardment of sales pitches is illustrated by the following. Over a period of 5 years a study of viewers aged 6 to 17 found that TV viewing is the most powerful predictor of whether a child becomes obese. The more hours spent watching TV, the more apt it is that a child will be overweight. This is attributed to the fact that

foods are the most heavily advertised product on television.

The fact that children learn by imitation is well established, and television shows offer many examples of behaviors that no one would describe as ideal. The implications of this for promoting eventual alcohol abuse, violence and aggressive behaviors, premature sexual activities, teenage pregnancy, use of tobacco products, and other harmful habits should be obvious (Grzelka, 1987, p. 27). The commercial television programs that children watch most are designed to sell a product. Often such programs seem to be advertisements interrupted by entertainment, rather than the other way around. The products that are promoted are almost always ones that affect health. Educational programs such as Sesame Street, although great fun to watch, do teach fundamental concepts and cognitive skills. However, Postman (1985, p. 144) believes that another outcome is that what children learn to love is television, not education or schooling.

In short, education in school about health, even if it begins in kindergarten, must be carefully planned if it is to reinforce or counteract what children have already learned that affects their healthy growth and development. Direct health teaching cannot be safely postponed, as it sometimes is, until grade 7 or 10 without being too late as well as too little.

What should be taught about health during elementary school years? What does a child need to know about it after completing each of the grades? Clearly there are no specific bits of information, however true today, that can be prescribed as adequate for solving health problems common among youngsters of any given age. Even if there were, their usefulness can only be judged according to today's best sources. By the time a child reaches adulthood, there will be new information making some of what has been learned obsolete.

What can a very young child comprehend according to Piagetian theory? What methods are most appropriate based on what is known about levels of learning in terms of readiness? What skills and knowledge have the greatest potential for transfer?

If schools are to be effective in helping today's child survive in the twenty-first century, health teaching limited to study of the structure and functioning of the body systems will not suffice. The study of *hygiene* as conducted in the past (i.e., the focus on care of the body and grooming standards and practices) is much less relevant to the solution of space-age health problems than it was to those health problems of even 20 years ago.

Health instruction that begins and continues throughout elementary school years has the advantage of timeliness. Decisions and actions that affect an individual's health do not wait for physical, social, or legal maturity. They are needed and happen during early childhood. What an elementary school teacher does to foster the development of a healthful life style among students can be crucial not only to their own well-being but also to that of their families and even the total community some day.

THE LANGUAGE OF HEALTH EDUCATION

Notice how many words or word combinations related to health have already been used in the preceding pages. Rather than assume that certain key terms will be interpreted as intended, brief explanations and discussion will be presented to clarify these terms.

Health

Many definitions of health have been proposed over the years. Today, the one with widest official acceptance is "a state of complete physical, mental, and social well being and not merely the absence of disease or infirmity" (World Health Organization, 1947). This was a significant shift toward a holistic view of health as a quality of life having several dimensions, even though such a condition is impossible to achieve. No one is entirely well in all three dimensions at once. Callahan (1979) has said "It is a dangerous definition and it desperately needs replacement by something more modest." He argues that this definition is so vague that it puts both medicine and society in the impossible position of having to attain what is unattainable.

Dunn's (1980) concept of health as *high level wellness* expresses the notion of a continuum rather than a set state. He perceived wellness as a "direction of progress" and health as "an integrated method of functioning which is oriented toward maximizing the potential of which the individual is capable."

The School Health Education Study (SHES, 1967) defined health as a "*quality of life* (ital. added) involving dynamic interaction and interdependence among the individual's physical well being, his mental and emotional reactions, and the social complex in which he exists."

Health, as a state of being, can range from very good to very poor. Perhaps health can better be described as an *index* that measures function rather than status.

The perspectives of these definitions of health may vary, but together they illustrate its complexity and marvel. Hochbaum (1979) defined health most simply but no less effectively as "what helps me to be what I want to be, and to do what I want to do . . . what helps me live the way I would like to live."

Healthy/Healthful

There are few people who do not value health, although actual behavior is often inconsistent with that fact. In the United States, the consumer is constantly being urged to buy products or services because it is "healthy" or "healthful" to use them. Most often it is the former term that is used to describe anything that is supposed to be good for you. Is there any difference in the meaning of those two words? Healthy refers to an optimum state or quality. Healthful refers to some thing or action that promotes well-being. For example, a healthy rattlesnake can be very unhealthful for the victim of its bite. The more healthy the growth of pathogenic bacteria, the less healthful is the effect on the host. Vigorous exercise is healthful only if the individual is healthy enough to tolerate its physical expenditures. Viewed in this way, should a bowl of bran flakes be referred to as ''healthy'' or ''healthful'' food? (The latter is correct.) Watch for the use of these two words in advertising claims. How often are they misused? Resultant misconceptions may be the basis of decisions that can adversely affect health.

Health Behavior

McAlister (1981) defines health behavior as ''any action that influences the probability of immediate and long term physical and physiological consequences affecting physical well being and longevity.'' It may also be defined as the pattern of choices and actions representative of all of the decisions that affect one's total health.

Gochman (1982) proposed that ''health behavior be considered substantively to denote personal attributes such as beliefs, expectations, motives, values, and other cognitive elements; personality characteristics, including affective and emotional states and traits; and overt behavior patterns, actions, and habits that relate to health maintenance and wellness, to health restoration, and to health improvement'' (p. 169).

Health Promotion

Health promotion is a term that is often used interchangeably with disease prevention, although the former has many other interpretations. The logic seems to be that whatever prevents disease is also health promoting. Carlyon (1984, p. 20) says that the key element that distinguishes wellness (i.e., health) promotion from disease prevention is that it is not the purpose of wellness promotion to reduce or prevent risk factors for particular diseases; it is to help people develop life styles that can maintain or enhance health. Green and Anderson (1986, p. 516) define health promotion as ''any combination of health education and related organizational, economic, and environmental supports for behavior of individuals, groups, or communities conducive to health.'' Duncan and Gold (1986, p. 47) define the term as ''all of the means by which healthy behavior may be encouraged.''

Disease Prevention

Disease prevention requires anticipatory action based on knowledge of disease causation and progression. Related actions may be primary, secondary, or tertiary in nature. Primary prevention is practiced before the disease occurs by taking measures to maintain health and taking specific actions to protect against disease (e.g., routine physical examinations, good nutrition, immunizations, use of seat belts, etc.). Secondary prevention depends on early diagnosis and prompt treatment of a disease. Tertiary prevention has to do with rehabilitation, i.e., helping people disabled or handicapped by disease, accident, stroke, or other health problem to adjust as well as possible so as to resume normal life activities or employment (Green, K., 1985, p. 9).

Life Style

The concept of ''life style'' covers the decisions made and actions taken by individuals that affect their health. Lalonde (1974, p. 32) was one of the first to identify life style as a major cause of illness and early death. He described it as "the aggregate of decisions by individuals which affect their health, and over which they more or less have control," and he noted that such personal decisions and habits that are bad, from a health point of view, create self-imposed risks. When these risks result in illness or death, the victim's life style can be said to have contributed to or caused his or her own illness or death. Among such self-imposed risks, Lalonde listed destructive habits concerned with drug use, faulty dietary choices, lack of appropriate exercise, careless driving, failure to wear seat belts, and promiscuity and carelessness leading to syphilis and gonorrhea.

Green and Anderson (1986, p. 255) categorize four kinds of behavior, or health-related habits, as potentially harmful. These are alcohol abuse, smoking, eating patterns, and drug use. Those four patterns of behavior, together with physical activity or exercise, stress management or recreation, and safety practices, constitute the set of personal actions that are termed "life style." All of them are amenable to prevention as an outcome of comprehensive school health education programs. Although they are health related, they are not necessarily health directed.

Life style is responsible for over half of the years prematurely lost in the more developed nations of the world. The children in your classes will not yet have built the set of habits that will constitute their life style as an adult. However, the life styles of those they are observing and beginning to copy may be harmful or healthful. What you teach and how you teach it can make a difference.

Risk Factors

Risk factors are the characteristics or behavioral patterns that increase a person's risk of disease or disorders (in particular, heart disease, stroke,

and cancer). Risk factors can be divided into those that cannot be modified (e.g., age, sex, family history, personality type) and those that can be modified (e.g., blood serum cholesterol level, high blood pressure, and cigarette smoking).

Self-Care

The active involvement of ordinary lay persons, on their own behalf, in health promotion and decision making and disease detection and treatment is called "self-care" or "medical self-care." It is not a substitute for professional care, but a partnership with it (Keever and Lelm, 1984, p. 20). Even small children can participate effectively in self-care activities. Experimental programs carried out by Lewis and Lewis (1980) led them to conclude that children are far more competent than adults believe them to be and that given the opportunity to practice self-care skills they might grow up to do "that which we as adults do very poorly"—that is, take care of themselves.

Ferguson (1980) successfully taught medical skills (e.g., use of the stethoscope, thermometer, pressure cuff, pulse recording, etc.) to a group of first and second graders. The teaching focused on things that the children said they would like to know about. It was discovered that one of the most important self-care skills was the ability to ask good questions and then figure out how to find the answers.

Prior to conducting a similar experimental course, Sehnert (1980) asked a group of sixth-grade children to indicate the person most responsible for maintaining their health among these: "mother, doctor, teacher, or myself." Only 21 percent chose "myself" before completing the course. Asked the same question after the course, the figure had increased to 85 percent. Clearly, as a corollary to learning self-care skills, these youngsters had also learned *self-reliance.* Brown (1986) argues that instead of trying to stuff as much knowledge, skills, and values into their heads as possible, we need to motivate children to manage their own lives. They need to learn self-reliance, not dependence, which is what teachers tend to do when they do things *for* children, telling them what to do, exerting control over them for their own good. He suggests that the rule should be "Do not do for children what they can do for themselves." Three methods effective for making children self-reliant, independent thinkers are proposed:

1. Behavioral patterning—Arrange for children to behave in appropriate ways and they will become what they do. Children who act responsibly, become responsible.
2. Expectation—Expect children to think, feel, and behave as self-reliant people do, and they will.
3. Modeling—The most powerful way children learn self-reliant behavior is by seeing that kind of behavior exhibited by parents, teachers, and other adults significant in their lives.

Admittedly, children cannot be completely independent of their families. The issue is whether we can find ways to help them grow into self-reliant individuals. Comprehensive school health education is the discipline whose subject matter and goals are most closely allied with and conducive to developing self-reliance.

WHAT IS HEALTH EDUCATION?

Generally speaking, the term refers to any health-related educational activities, whether in schools, community, clinical, or work settings. The same term is applied as descriptive of the discipline itself, the profession of its specialists, the outcome of its successful activities, any program designed to change health behaviors in some desirable way, and the special processes employed in effecting favorable changes in knowledge, attitudes, or practices.

Green et al. (1980) define health education, whatever the setting, as "any designed combinations of methods to facilitate voluntary adaptations of behavior conducive to health." That certainly fits all the settings and is probably the most often cited definition in the literature. But schools are in some ways different from those other settings. The fundamental assumption of the definition is that changing behavior is the primary goal, if not the only goal, of health education. Whether all of the health behaviors a child has learned need to be changed is debatable and certainly a question of importance for health instruction in schools.

Carlyon and Cook (1981) define health education as "any activity with clear goals planned for the purpose of improving health-related knowledge, attitudes, or behavior." They say that "the prevalent notion that the sole purpose of health education is to change behavior is erroneous. It may be used to prevent, initiate, and sustain behavior as well." This would seem more appropriate as description of health education in schools.

Inasmuch as this textbook will focus almost exclusively on health education in elementary and middle schools, the term will be used to refer to the total school health program, its purposes, procedures, and strategies. The school health program has three interrelated components: (1) health services, (2) environmental health (the provisions taken to ensure students a safe and sanitary place in which to study and play), and (3) health instruction. The overall purposes of the school health program are to protect, maintain, and promote the health of the children and adults who live and work together every day of the school year.

Although planned and sometimes unplanned teaching and learning experiences occur as an outcome of the first two program components, only those people involved in health instruction are directly concerned and responsible for planning the curriculum and providing the instruction designed to fulfill its goals.

Health education, or Health as it is sometimes termed, is seldom if ever listed among the courses elementary students are required to study every year. But it is there. Goodlad's nation-wide survey (1984) identified specific health education topics included in the curricula of science (nutrition and drugs/alcohol), social studies (themes of understanding self, family, and friends), and physical education (typically "wet days" emphasis on health and safety topics including nutrition) during both primary and upper–elementary school years.

WHAT HEALTH EDUCATION IS NOT

Sometimes it helps to define a term or activity by describing what it is not. Too often what is offered students in elementary schools is best described as one of those things that it is not. Health education is not simply a minor aspect of physical education, nor is it hygiene with another name. It is not a program focused on promoting physical fitness, although fitness is surely a parallel goal of health education. It is not simplified information about the anatomy and physiology of the body and its systems. It is not biology as it applies to human functioning. It is not sex education. It is not one or two short units specific to current health concerns, such as AIDS and drug abuse, temporarily hosted by another course as a means of meeting state requirements or satisfying community pressure. It most certainly is not simply an assembly lecture topic, a physical education rainy day

activity or incidental teaching in response to momentary health-related problems or happenings. Most emphatically it is not a dreary set of "do's" and "don'ts" applied to food selection, sexuality, or the satisfaction or denial of any other human need. It is education for healthful living—individual, family, and community.

SOURCES OF MISPERCEPTIONS OF HEALTH EDUCATION

If that is the case, why is health instruction often misinterpreted or confused with other related courses or disciplines, as we have just shown? There are several reasons. First, the professional preparation of school administrators, who make most of the decisions regarding what will be taught and how much time it will be allotted, seldom includes study of either the content or the methodology of health education. Second, many of the teachers, parents, and other adults involved in curriculum planning have confused impressions of health education based upon their own school experiences. As Kolbe and Gilbert (1984) point out, "Perceptions of health education are usually drawn from remembrances of relatively unsophisticated school lectures about 'personal hygiene' that administrators, parents, and influential community members experienced during their own schooling" (p. 63). Third, health seems logically linked to physical education inasmuch as the purposes of both focus on the maintenance and promotion of health. Fourth, health teaching historically had its genesis in early state legislation mandating the teaching of "health and physical education"; the title has stuck despite the now firmly established independence of health education as its own discipline. Although there are few today that attempt to provide a joint major, many colleges and universities still title the department or division as before, although offering separate majors in health education, physical education, and sports. The result is that the media, and authorities in education outside the field of health education, continue to speak of "health and physical education" as if they were one discipline rather than two. For example, the Paideia Proposal (Adler, 1982)[1] recommends that 12 years of physical education, sports, and athletic exercises be accompanied by instruction about health as part of the general education of all students in public schools.

In Bennett's recent (1986) report on elementary education, "Health and Physical Education" is listed among the disciplines essential to the education of all elementary-age school children (p. 36). Most of the related discussion focuses on the need for exercise, the ability to do a desirable number of pull-ups, and participation in sports and fitness. Later, it is specified that health and nutrition education should be included as part of this aspect of the elementary curriculum.

So, if you are confused by the fact that health is so often linked with physical education, remember that what you are seeing is what we call the "missing comma syndrome." Think "health" (comma) and "physical education" because that is what it's supposed to mean.

WHY HEALTH TEACHING IN ELEMENTARY SCHOOLS?

The early years of a child's life are those during which important health-related attitudes and practices are established. A life style begins to take shape virtually at birth; and health educa-

tion begins just as early, as soon as an infant begins to react to the environment, both human and physical. Within the limits of their experience and understanding, even preschool children have already accumulated a set of attitudes and habits that will be the basis of their life styles as adults. Adult life styles do not suddenly emerge sometime after one's twenties to direct future behavior that may lead to chronic illnesses or early death. A life style is learned, every bit of it, and it happens day by day.

For these reasons and many others, health teaching cannot be neglected until the seventh or tenth grade, as is the case in some school districts.

Education for health is so universally accepted as a primary objective of education that its place among the basic subjects is virtually unquestioned. Nearly every statement of the goals of education since the 1917 "Cardinal Principles of Education" has placed health high on the list of its priorities. The National Education Association (NEA) Project on Instruction (1963) reaffirmed this commitment to the value of and need for health education in these words: "The schools, as the only social institution that reaches all children and youth, has responsibility for teaching the basic information, and for helping young people develop the habits and attitudes essential for healthful living."

Elementary children at every grade are highly interested in information about their body and its parts, about safe living/first aid, and prevention of health problems. Asked whether they thought studying about health is important, 88 percent of those queried in a survey of over 5,000 Washington State students in grades 4 through 12 agreed that it is (Trucano, 1984).

Nearly every one of the states has education codes or legislation either mandating, encouraging, or supporting the provision of health instruction in schools. In 38 of the states, health

---

[1]Paideia signifies the general learning that should be the possession of all human beings.

is specifically mandated. Nearly half of the states also have a State Board of Education or Department of Education policy statement supporting health education programs. For example, the New Mexico State Board of Education has established 11 goals that all school systems are to pursue, including the following related to school health. "Districts are to design and implement programs which will ensure that students: (1) maintain a positive self image, and (2) practice good health habits and develop an awareness of environmental conditions for the maintenance of mental, physical, and emotional well being" (ASHA, 1987, p. 5). Sixteen states require a specific number of health instruction hours during one or more years in grades K through 6. The average number of hours required per year was 40.64 (ASHA, 1987, p. 6).

Although compulsory immunizations have nearly eliminated the incidence of certain communicable childhood diseases, children do suffer colds and the flu, infestations of head lice, and other acute conditions that can be prevented or controlled by the services and instruction provided through the school health programs.

Today specific health-related behavioral problems have become worrisome. For example, some youngsters are experimenting with alcohol. It is reported that the average age of first use of alcohol is 12.3. By age 13, 30 percent of boys and 22 percent of girls drink on a regular basis (The PULSE, 1987, p. 1). Obviously the best time to start teaching children to say "no" to alcohol or other drugs is in the preteen years.

About 25 to 30 percent of 10 year olds have at least tried smoking cigarettes. Many children claim first use as young as age 5 or 6. While development of the habit usually does not occur until late childhood or adolescence, it is recommended that tobacco education programs be initiated while children are in elementary school, preferably during kindergarten or first grade (Tucker, 1987, p. 25).

Use of smokeless tobacco is growing rapidly, helped along by advertising promoting its use as an alternative to smoking and showing famous professional athletes spitting what is obviously tobacco juice. At present, the largest population of smokeless tobacco users are young adult males. However, a recent survey of Oklahoma school children indicated that about 13 percent of third-grade boys and 22 percent of fifth-grade boys were already users (Christen and Glover, 1987, p. 11).

Hypertension is being found among children and adolescents in numbers large enough to suggest that intervention in the form of comprehensive health instruction will be necessary so those children will be less likely to develop hypertension as adults. The condition is associated with obesity, which is linked to poor nutrition and excessive TV watching, overconsumption of foods high in fats and sodium, cigarette smoking, and lack of exercise. The implications of all of this for health instruction should be clear as it relates to the development of a life style that will help children make choices during their lives that may prevent coronary heart disease or other complications that could develop from hypertension (Harris, 1987, pp. 31-33).

Table 1-1 lists the 15 national health problem priority areas defined in *Healthy People: The Surgeon-General's Report on Health Promotion and Disease Prevention* (U.S. Dept. of HEW, 1979). Of the 227 national health objectives developed as targets for success in alleviating these problems, 67 or fully 30 percent could be attained directly or indirectly by the schools through appropriate school health services, through procedures taken to ensure a healthful school environment, through health instruction, and through physical education programs that promote cardiovascular and physical fitness.

TABLE 1-1: Fifteen priority areas: 1990 health objectives for the nation

Preventive health services
1. High blood pressure control
2. Family planning
3. Pregnancy and infant health
4. Immunization
5. Sexually transmitted diseases

Health protection
6. Toxic agent control
7. Occupational safety and health
8. Accident prevention and injury control
9. Fluoridation and dental health
10. Surveillance and control of infectious diseases

Health promotion
11. Smoking and health
12. Misuse of alcohol and drugs
13. Nutrition
14. Physical fitness and exercise
15. Control of stress and violent behavior

Source: As presented in *Prospects for a Healthier America: Achieving the Nation's Health Promotion Objectives,* Washington, D.C.: 1984, p. 59.

During the critical elementary school years, the elementary teachers in our nation can have a tremendous influence on the health of the adults these children will some day be. Curricula designed to promote positive life styles need to be offered to children before they have developed patterns of behavior that need to be changed. Perhaps it is too optimistic to think that in the few hours available to teach about health (estimated average of 40 hours per year) much could be done to counter the persuasions of advertisers, the pressures of peers, and misconceptions derived from the conventional wisdom. But good teaching can make a difference, particularly if the instruction is mindful of the fact that life styles are learned, not born, and

that many health problems can be prevented or controlled if you know how.

As evidence, there are the results of a recent three-year study of several different health instruction programs recently conducted under the aegis of the Centers for Disease Control and the Office of Disease Prevention and Health Promotion. In general, it showed that health education does work, that it works better when there is more of it, and that it works best when it is carried out with broad administrative support and teacher training programs and when continuity across grades is planned for and implemented. It works best when there is attention to the building of foundations of basic health knowledge rather than starting with categorical health problems at secondary levels of education and beyond (Journal of School Health, Oct. 1985). Elementary health instruction needs to provide that sound foundation of basic health knowledge, but always as means of promoting positive health behaviors.

WHO TEACHES HEALTH?

The answer to this question is everybody. Although responsibility for health education of the young is shared by the home, school, and community, there is no one who does not in some way influence the health of children. In that sense everybody is a health teacher, although often not in the positive sense.

Home

Primary responsibility for health education rests with the family, which usually includes more than the parents and a child. Often there are brothers and sisters, aunts and uncles, cousins, grandparents, and sometimes sets of step relatives, in-laws, and other close kith and kin. Every family member with whom a child has contact is teaching that child something about health. Whether this instruction is done consciously or unconsciously, children's health beliefs, attitudes, and practices are most powerfully derived from those communicated by word or behavior by family members. It is not solely the outcome of specific training, nor just the result of observing and adopting family practices. A family's religious beliefs and ceremonies, the emotional climate of the home (whether serene and pleasant or the reverse), the quality of family relationships (based on mutual respect and love versus dominated by fear or neglect), and many other social factors have a tremendous influence on the health and health behavior of small children. When they enter kindergarten, children bring with them an already well-established system of beliefs, attitudes, values, and habits associated with health.

School

Children are required to attend school for 5 or 6 hours a day, 5 days a week, over 30 weeks a year for up to 13 years. The school is the social institution legally responsible for educating the children and youth of the United States, and health has long ranked high among the primary goals of education. But health instruction is only one part of the school health program. **Health services** (e.g., health counseling and guidance, communicable disease control, and emergency care) and a **healthful school environment** (e.g., regulated, healthful temperature levels, ventilation, sanitary food services, and provision of safety devices and procedures) are just as important. (These two program elements are described in more detail in Chapter 2.)

Every member of the faculty and staff of a school in some way adds to whatever formal health teaching is provided at any one grade. This is because every adult in the school serves as a model for the children by virtue of his or her

role. The harmful health habits that adults exhibit or whose effects are evident (e.g., poor grooming, tobacco breath and nicotine-stained fingers, or obesity) do not go unnoticed by children. It is difficult to persuade youngsters that smoking is harmful when they know that their parents and teachers are often smokers. Because personal beliefs and attitudes underlie almost everything that adults say and do, children can not fail to be influenced by teachers' statements and actions in situations outside the classroom.

Community

Health teaching is as communitywide as it is Schoolwide. Commercial organizations spend billions of dollars annually in the attempt to influence the health habits and choices of children. Sometimes this is done directly and constructively, as in the production and dissemination of useful instructional materials. More often it is done less directly through sponsorship of television shows whose advertisements are designed to convince the viewer to buy a product. That product is nearly always health related, whether for good or for bad, but the motive for promoting its use is profit not health.

Individuals in the community whom children hold in awe or admire, powerfully influence their beliefs and practices. Police officers, fire fighters, physicians, musicians (particularly popular singers), television and film stars, and athletes are role models whether they wish to be or not. What is taught by their examples can be beneficial or harmful. Campaigns against drug abuse, cigarette smoking, sexually transmitted diseases (STDs), and other life style risk factors often feature messages delivered by well-known community figures for this reason. Celebrities, professional athletic stars, and authority figures need to be aware that their personal health habits are copied by children, who try to act like those whom they admire.

Not least among community influences are those exerted by a child's peers and older children. Children teach children, sometimes more effectively than adults can. Health concerns are high on the list of topics about which youngsters want to know. They tend to seek information from other young people more readily than from parents, teachers, or any other adults. The problem is that when peers do not know the answers, rather than lose face by admitting that they don't know, they often provide misconceptions or misinformation. Yet, if effective health instruction were a part of general education at every grade, the reliance of younger children on older ones might result in desirable reinforcement for the instruction provided by elementary teachers.

ANALYSES OF CHILDREN'S BELIEFS ABOUT HEALTH AND ILLNESS

We know that what children and adults believe about health and illness influences the day-to-day actions and the choices they make, which together constitute a life style. However, children have not yet formulated the rigid pattern of behaviors typical of adults, hence they are more responsive to instruction and accepting of change. The effectiveness of health instruction during elementary school years is critical to the quality and even to the length of life those children will later enjoy as adults.

Effective health teaching cannot be based on adult views of the value of healthful behavior or on assumptions about children's health beliefs and attitudes. What is needed is health instruction that is age appropriate in content and in stage of cognitive development at every grade.

Most of the research devoted to investigating the origin and development of the health beliefs and attitudes held by children has employed two theoretical models: (1) the Health Behavior Model (HBM), an expectancy theory derived from social psychology, and (2) Piaget's cognitive development theory (Mickalide, 1986). It is not possible to discuss these two theories adequately here, but the concepts behind each will be outlined briefly.

The Health Behavior Model

The HBM provides information about what children believe relative to (1) their personal susceptibility to illness, (2) how serious the related health risks are, (3) the probable benefits of an action taken to reduce that susceptibility and seriousness, and (4) the barriers to undertaking or continuing actions recommended to reduce them (expense, fear, pain, embarrassment, etc.). Susceptibility and seriousness have strong cognitive components and are partially dependent on knowledge. The model is sensitive to the individual's value system as well (Rosenstock, 1974, pp. 328-335).

Piaget's Cognitive Development Theory

Application of Piaget's theory bridges the gap between *what* children believe and *why* they believe what they do. Four major stages of cognitive development are described, each of which is characterized by qualitatively different schemes and all of which are experienced in order by every child. These four invariant stages include: (1) the sensori-motor stage (birth to age 2); (2) the preoperational stage (age 2 to age 7); (3) the concrete operational stage (age 7 to age 11); and (4) the formal operational stage (age 11 to adulthood).

Preoperational children tend to view illness as punishment for some transgression and to confuse cause and effects of illness. They perceive health and illness as two separate happenings rather than as opposite ends of a continuum. Circular reasoning is prominent and they lack the ability to generalize between similar experiences (Mickalide, 1986, p. 7). Their definition of health is general and undifferentiated (Kalnins and Love, 1982). They reason egocentrically, relating each health-related experience to themselves (Green and Bird, 1986).

Children at the concrete operational level tend to see health as the ability to perform desired activities. In third or fourth grade they blame germs for disease and begin to grasp the concept of causal sequencing. This age group only gradually becomes future oriented as they mature, hence behaviors promising rewards of future health are not relevant to them (Natapoff, 1982).

Children at the formal operational stage consider mental health as integral to global health status. They understand linkages between behavior and health outcomes and recognize individual susceptibility in the onset of disease (Mickalide, 1986). Only these oldest children, with a good grasp of reversibility in their judgments can see health and sickness as reciprocal components of the larger aspect of "health."

It is easy to find out what the children in your own class believe about health and illness. Just ask them. Their answers should not be too different from those given by most youngsters in American schools. For example, as part of the Connecticut study Byler et al. (1969) asked students in grades K through 6 "What is health?" Their answers are as delightful to read as they are informative. Some answers from grades K through 2 include "You brush the dirt off your teeth" and "You don't have measles or mumps." In grades 3 and 4, comments made included "Smells clean" and "Eats only a cup of sugar." When students in grade 5 were asked

"What is a healthy person?" some said, "He eats right and drinks milk" and "He doesn't smoke or drink." Sixth graders said, "Health is germs,""Health is whether you are alive," and "Health is not getting bored which brings on bad health."

All these children viewed health as a state arising from regular observance of certain practices or rules related to exercising, eating good food, not being sick, and keeping clean.

Selected Generalizations and Recommendations

Some observations and recommendations made by researchers who have studied children's beliefs about health include:

Young children commonly view health as a long-term state and illness as a short-term condition.

Across all grades, health was attributed to "foods I eat," and the causes of illness were attributed to germs and bad weather.

Younger children differ more among themselves in their beliefs about health than do older children (Dielman et al., 1980, p. 235).

School health educators and health-care professionals run the risk of confusing and frightening children if their messages are too sophisticated. Conversely, information that is too simplistic for a given cognitive developmental stage may bore or insult the child and may be ignored (Mickalide, 1986, p. 19).

Teaching young children principles of health maintenance to prevent illness is meaningless to them (Natapoff, 1982, p. 38).

Health as a motive for acting wisely does not play a prominent part in most children's cognitive worlds, nor do they often perceive themselves as vulnerable to health problems (Dielman et al., 1980, p. 235).

The differences between the adult at 35 and the adult at 40 are insignificant in comparison to the tremendous differences between a child of 5 and a child of 10 in the ability to understand causal relationships (Mickalide, 1986, p. 19).

Educational interventions designed to develop or modify health beliefs will have greater success if they are introduced to 6 through 8 year olds rather than to older groups (Dielman et al., 1980, p. 236).

Health education that centers on a young child's desires and current goals will be more effective than programs that emphasize future health. The more health teaching is related to everyday activities, the more effective it will be (Natapoff, 1982, p. 42).

Children's concepts of health and illness change qualitatively with cognitive development that affects the progression from preoperational to concrete to formal thought as proposed by Piaget (Kalnins and Love, 1982, p. 9).

Health-oriented educational programs that are consistent with the child's ability to process information may be more effective than traditional disease-oriented programs (Natapoff, 1982, p. 34).

THE GOALS OF HEALTH EDUCATION

The goals of health education support those of general education. The first goal is to help each child develop a pattern of health behavior that tends to maintain or enhance rather than to diminish wellness; second, to look beyond personal wants to the general well-being of the community, family, and friends when taking actions that can affect the health of others; and third, to consider not only the needs of those alive today, but those of the generations to come. To achieve these ends, health teaching seeks to equip children with fundamental health concepts and problem-solving skills that will be as basic to sound decision making in the future as they are today. Perhaps the ultimate goal is the development of an individual who is self-reliant, comfortable with her or his weaknesses and strengths, and humane and sensitive to the rights and needs of others. This requires building a meaningful and worthy system of values to serve as personal behavioral guidelines. Admittedly, such ideal development is not easily attained if it must depend on formal education alone. Nonetheless, it is the goal of the total school health program and of health teaching in particular.

THE SPECIAL ROLE OF THE ELEMENTARY TEACHER

The school's responsibility for the total school health program is based on four fundamental beliefs: (1) the school must help maintain the health of the students in its charge as a means of ensuring their continued fitness to learn; (2) the school should maintain an environment that contributes to rather than detracts in any way from social, emotional, mental, or physical health; (3) the school should do its best to ensure the optimum health of each child through appropriate health services designed to appraise, protect, and promote well-being; and (4) the school should educate young people to make sound decisions about matters affecting their health and that of their family and friends. All school personnel contribute to these goals, but the role of the elementary teacher is unique.

The elementary teacher is the key person in every instance. Although in some school districts health education may be assigned to "floating" health specialists or school nurses, most commonly the classroom teacher is responsible for all health teaching, along with teaching the other basic subjects. In most elementary schools a teacher works with the same group of boys and girls throughout the school year. All the health instruction a child receives, as well as the daily monitoring and adjusting of the classroom environment, is the primary responsibility of that one teacher. Even though school health services are provided by health-care professionals, the teacher's observations and prompt referrals provide the link between each child and any health care that may be needed during the school day.

Mayshark et al. (1977) acknowledged the significance of the elementary school teacher's contribution to the health of the school child in these words:

If we were told that only one category of school personnel would be permitted to work for student health and that we had the authority to select this category, it would have to be the elementary teachers. Such a choice does not depreciate the important contributions of other school personnel, but it does recognize the immense responsibility that falls to this dedicated group. (p. 128)

Only the elementary school teacher works every school day, all day, with the same children. As a consequence, each child's total performance is well known, not only in terms of that youngster's usual appearance and behavior but also as compared with the others in the room of the same age and level of development. Even small changes from the usual or expected behaviors are more quickly apparent to the classroom teacher than to any other observer. In fact the elementary school's first line of defense against an epidemic of communicable disease is the alert teacher's ability to spot signs of illness and to see to it that a sick child is quickly separated from the others and sent home. In addition to visual perceptions, teacher observation includes the sense of smell in detecting the use of substances such as smokeless tobacco, cigarettes, alcohol, marijuana, or any other mind-altering substance. Touch may be important, as in the case of noting possible fever. Hearing also could be a source of information about a child's well-being (sounds of hoarseness, coughing, sniffling, wheezing). A more subtle but no less profound influence on health can be traced to the daily close relationship between teacher and students. Teachers are role models for impressionable young children. Particularly in the primary grades, but also during the intermediate school years, youngsters tend to love, admire, and emulate their teachers' behaviors. Brown (1986, p. 28) suggests that "adults can promote self-reliance by showing an awareness of their own identity and autonomy, by defining for themselves appropriate values and behavior standards, by acting responsibly and by providing children with experiences that help them grow into self-reliant adults."

Elementary teachers shape a child's concept of health and health education as powerfully by what they do as by what they say. Thus a teacher's personal health behavior can enhance or counteract the message intended by health instruction. The very *way* a teacher presents health information, even the topics selected and the method employed, can reveal her or his attitude toward the importance or worth of that material and thus influence students' acceptance and use of it in their daily lives.

Comprehensive health education in elementary schools has the potential to promote and protect the health of children, not just while they are in school but also during adolescence and adulthood. However important the contributions of other school personnel, family, and community, the classroom teacher's role is special and often pivotal in shaping children's attitudes and beliefs about self-reliance and the value of self-care in promoting their own health. Health teaching is not *telling* children about health and illness. It is giving them the concepts and intellectual tools they need in order to build and maintain a healthful life style.

SUMMARY

The purpose of health instruction is to foster the development of healthful life styles among children and youth during their public school education, K through 12. Elementary teachers have limited time available for health teaching and typically little background in health coursework. Nevertheless, they are potentially the most influential health instructors any child will ever encounter. To compensate for the above-mentioned limitations, there are several advantages that go with an elementary-level assignment. First, there is the element of timeliness. These teachers are working with youngsters who are eager to learn about their bodies, how each part works, and what they can do to help themselves grow to be like grown-ups whom they admire. Second, elementary school children and their teachers live and work together all day, every day in the school year. Health teaching can be integrated throughout the curriculum as enrichment, rather than set apart as topics unrelated to the other studies. There is an opportunity to provide incidental teaching responsive to everyday, real-life health concerns and interests as they occur, rather than as tied to the chapters in a textbook or topics in a curriculum guide. Third, young children tend to regard their teacher with admiration, affection, and respect; more than anything they want to please him or her. Hence they are far more readily motivated

to change any behaviors that might need modification or to accept new ideas or practices presented to them.

It takes more than that, of course. Because health education is a discipline as basic to the general education of children as are reading, writing, and arithmetic, there is a certain irreducible minimum of information about it that elementary teachers need to know. Most importantly, they need to be comfortable in their understanding of the language and the goals of health education. They must know what health education is, which means that they must also be clear about what it is not.

The term "health education" as used in this text refers to the total school health program, which includes formal health instruction and required health services, procedures, and facilities designed to provide a safe and healthful environment for students and staff. Children are learning about healthful living as an outcome of the total program, and every member of the staff plays a part in that education. But planning and implementing health instruction is the responsibility of the teaching staff.

Teachers need to have some experience with the stuff of health instruction, its content areas, supporting concepts and facts, and the experiential teaching strategies that bring it alive, whether gained in preservice or inservice study. They need to be able to apply what they have learned about learning theory and readiness to the selection of the health content and teaching activities appropriate for specified age groups of children. They must be able to identify children's existing health beliefs and attitudes and to infer what learning opportunities would effectively reinforce those that reflect good practice or motivate new or improved behaviors.

Most importantly, perhaps, they need to know that health instruction places less emphasis on personal hygiene and the prevention of common communicable diseases, and instead seeks to promote self-reliance, self-responsibility, and the development of a healthful life style. The goal is never memorization of health-related facts or rules to live by; it is to give children the chance to discover how to find the answers to their own questions and health problems within the limits of their ability to think and act upon those answers.

QUESTIONS AND EXERCISES

Discussion questions

1. In what ways do the purposes of health promotion differ from those of disease prevention programs? How would those differences influence the focus of health instruction expected to promote health?

2. Interpret the meaning of the following statement: "Health teaching in the elementary school has the advantage of timeliness over that done at any other level of education."

3. Describe the unique role of the elementary teacher in preparing children to be effective health consumers and eventual self-reliant adults.

4. In what ways do the goals of health education support and overlap those of general education?

Problems and exercises

1. Differentiate between *healthy* and *healthful.* Which would you use to describe: (a) a daily regimen of exercise planned for a young office worker; (b) regular patterns of adequate rest and sleep for everyone; (c) a state of optimum physical fitness; (d) the ability to get along well with friends, family, and neighbors; and (e) flossing and brushing one's teeth as recommended by dental authorities.

2. Assume that you are invited to appear before a parent group to answer questions about the health curriculum in your school. One parent asks, "Aren't parents responsible for teaching -their children to practice good health habits? Why do we need health teaching taking up important time in the elementary school curriculum?" How would

you answer this query? How could you synthesize what you have learned here about community influences and possible negative health teaching to justify the importance of school health instruction. In a short paper, outline all of the principal reasons why school health programs are essential to maintain and protect the health of children while they are in school and to support and complement the goals of general education.

3. Consider these two definitions of health.
   1. Good health is a process of continuous adaptation to the many microbes, irritants, pressures, and problems that challenge humans daily.
   2. Health is a quality of life involving dynamic interaction and interdependence between the individual's physical well-being, mental and emotional reactions, and the social complex in which he or she exists.
   Which of them seems to be a better description of health? How might acceptance of either one over the other influence (a) the emphasis of health instruction given to support it, (b) the comprehensiveness of a resulting curriculum plan, and (c) the relevance of that health teaching to the stated goals of health education? Prepare a written set of answers to these questions for use in class discussions.

4. Make an informal survey of five or six young children in your immediate neighborhood. Having determined their age and grade in school, record their answers to the question, "What is health?" Analyze the answers you obtain relative to the age of the children surveyed and see if you can identify patterns of beliefs corresponding to Piaget's levels of cognition. If possible, compile the survey results of your entire class and draw some conclusions regarding the results.

5. From the moment you get up in the morning until you fall asleep at night, you are making decisions and taking actions based on those decisions. Of the actions common to those in our society, how many can you name that do not affect health in some way? Can decisions of this kind depend on conventional wisdom ("everybody knows that so and so is what one should do")? Should there be a planned curriculum for health teaching at every grade, K through 12? Why or why not?

6. In your opinion, should the 15 priority areas upon which the 1990 health objectives for the nation have been based (see Table 1-1) define the curriculum for health teaching for all school children? Name those that you would recommend for elementary-level consideration as well as any you would add that are not among those listed. Write a short paragraph justifying your selection of topics based on what you have learned about children's beliefs and abilities.

7. Looking ahead to your first job as an elementary teacher, what other courses might you elect now to help you fulfill your future responsibilities for health teaching? Would you look for health content courses? If so, which ones and for what reasons?

REFERENCES

Adler M: The Paideia proposal, New York, 1982, Macmillan.

American School Health Association: School health in America ed 4, Kent, Ohio, 1987, ASHA.

Bennett W: First lessons: a report on elementary education in America, Washington, DC, 1986, US Department of Education.

Brown B: We can help children to be self-reliant, Children Today 15:1, Jan/Feb 1986.

Byler R et al: Teach us what we want to know, 1968, Connecticut State Board of Education.

Callahan D: For Health and society: some ethical imperatives. In Knowles, J ed: Doing better and feeling worse, New York, 1979, W Norton.

Carlyon W: Disease prevention/health promotion: bridging the gap to wellness, Health Values 8:3, May/June 1984.

Carlyon W and Cook D: Science education and health instruction, BSCS, 4:1 1981.

Christen A and Glover E: History of smokeless tobacco use in the United States, Health Educ 18:3, June/July 1987.

Dielman TE et al: Dimensions of children's health beliefs, Health Educ Q 7:3, Fall 1980.

Duncan D and Gold R: Health promotion—what is it? Health Values 10:3, May/June 1986.

Dunn H: High level wellness, Thorofare, NJ, 1980, Slack.

Ferguson T: Teaching medicine to kids: medical self-care, New York, 1980, Summit Books.

Gochman D: Labels, systems and motives: some perspectives for future research and programs, children's health beliefs and health behaviors, Health Educ Q 9:2, 3, Summer/Fall 1982.

Goodlad J: A place called school, New York, 1984, McGraw-Hill.

Green K: Health promotion: its terminology, concepts, and modes of practice, Health Values 9:3, May/June 1985.

Green K and Bird J: The structure of children's beliefs about health and illness, J Sch Health 56(8):325-328, 1986.

Green L and Anderson C: Community health, St Louis, 1986, Times Mirror/Mosby.

Grzelka C: Children and television, Health Links 3:(2), July 1987.

Harris J: High blood pressure in children and adolescents, Health Educ 18:3 June/July 1987.

Healthy people: the surgeon general's report on health promotion and disease prevention, Washington, DC, 1979, Department of Health, Education and Welfare.

Hochbaum G: An alternative approach to health education, Health Values 3:4, July-August 1979.

Kalnins I and Love R: Children's concepts of health and illness: implications for health education: an overview, Health Educ Q 9:2,3, Summer/Fall 1982.

Keever B and Lelm K: Introducing medical self-care in the curriculum, Health Educ 15:3, May/June 1984.

Kolbe L and Gilbert G: Involving the schools in the national strategy to improve the health of Americans, Prospects for a healthier America: achieving the nation's health promotion objectives, Washington, DC, 1984, Department of Health and Human Services.

Lalonde M: A new perspective on the health of Canadians, Ottawa, 1974, Information Canada.

Lewis C and Lewis M: Child-initiated health care, Sch Health 50:3, March 1980.

Mayshark C et al: Administration of school health programs, St Louis, 1977, The CV Mosby Co.

McAlister A: Social and environmental influences on health behavior, Health Educ Q 8:1, Spring 1981.

Mickalide A: Children's understanding of health and illness: implications for health promotion, Health Values 10:3, May/June 1986.

Natapoff J: A developmental analysis of children's ideas of health, Health Educ Q 9:2, 3, Summer/Fall 1982.

National Education Association: Project on instruction: schools for the sixties, New York, 1963, McGraw-Hill.

National Education Association, Committee on the reorganization of secondary education: Cardinal principles of secondary education, U.S. Bureau of Educ. Bulletin **35**:32, 1918. In Vredevoe, LE: An introduction and outline of secondary education, Ann Arbor, Mich., 1957, Edwards Bros., pp. 36-37.

Postman N: Amusing ourselves to death, New York, 1985, Viking Penguin.

Results of the school health education evaluation, J Sch Health 55:8, Oct 1985, entire issue.

Rosenstock Irwin: Historical origins of the health belief model. In Becker, Marshall (ed.): The Health belief model and personal health behavior, Health Education Monographs **2**:4, Winter 1974, pp. 328-335.

School Health Education Study: Health education: a conceptual approach to curriculum design, St Paul, 1967, 3M Education Press.

Sehnert K: On teaching self-care to children, Medical Self-Care, New York, 1980, Summit Books, pp 199-202.

The PULSE, July 1987, American School Health Association, p 1.

Trucano L: Students speak, Seattle, 1984, Comprehensive Health Education Foundation.

Tucker A: Elementary school children and cigarette smoking, a review of the literature, Health Educ 18:3, June/July 1987.

World Health Organization: Chronicle of the WHO, New York, 1947.

SUGGESTED READINGS

Brown B: We can help children to be self-reliant, Children Today 15(1):2, 6-29, 1986. Identifies major areas of competence needed by individuals if optimum development of self-reliance is to be achieved. Suggests 28 specific steps parents and teachers can take to help youngsters develop self-reliance with reference to those competencies. Well worth reading and applying throughout the general education of children.

Green K and Bird J: The structure of children's beliefs about health and illness, J Sch Health 56(8):325-328, 1986. Reports research exploring what children know about health and illness, what affects them, and what the relationship between them appears to be. Eighty-two children in grades 1, 3, 5, and 7-8 ranked self-initiated behaviors highest among causes of health but only second to germs and bad weather as causes of illness. Only the oldest of the children in the study could understand that health and illness were reciprocal aspects of "health."

Green L and Anderson C: Community health, chapter 11, St Louis, 1986, Times Mirror/Mosby. pp 254-282. Discusses epidemiology of the principal health-related life style risk factors (i.e., alcohol misuse, cigarette smoking, nutrition, obesity, malnutrition, and drug abuse). Emphasizes preventive strategies (educational, protective, and coercive). School health education and immunization requirements for children in school are listed among primary interventions.

Petosa R: Enhancing the health competence of school-age children through behavioral self-management skills, J Sch Health 56(6):211-214, A 1986. Defines self-management skills as "techniques used by individuals to elicit or reinforce actions they consciously have chosen to adopt." Describes such skills (e.g., self-monitoring, goal setting, tailoring). Recommends use of behavioral contracts between students and teachers as an effective way to teach self-management strategies to children.

Pratt C et al: The effects of a preschool health education program upon children's health knowledge and reactions to health exams, Health Educ 18(1): 12-15, 1987. Reports results of research conducted with 53 children, mean age 4.6 years, applying three separate interventions. Using a packaged curriculum, Preschool Health Education Project (PHEP), one group received instruction at school and at home, another received only the home instruction, and the third received no instruction at all. Both the groups receiving instruction learned significant amounts of information about their bodies and self-care, showing that preschool children can learn much that can serve as the basis for future learning about health during primary and later years.

CHAPTER 2

The Comprehensive School Health Program

When you finish this chapter you should be able to:

- Explain the purposes and functions of a comprehensive school health program.

- Analyze the interrelationships among the basic components of such a program.

- Appraise the quality of an existing school health program.

- Interpret student cumulative health records.

- Develop a feasible system for the orderly emergency care of injured or ill school children.

- Identify available community resources appropriate for use in solving school health problems.

- Describe appearances and behaviors symptomatic of hearing and vision problems as well as common illnesses of children.

- Distinguish among mandatory, permissive, and tort laws affecting the school health program.

What do we mean when we speak of a school health program? Generally it is the composite activities, procedures, facilities, and services provided by a school, in collaboration with parents and community organizations, to protect the safety and health of its students. Such programs usually encompass three interdependent components. These are health instruction, health services, and provisions for a healthful school environment. The purposes of each of these program elements complement and are complemented by the procedures and activities of the others.

A program of some kind can be found in every school in the nation. Not all of them can be described as comprehensive if the term is intended to reflect the best practice possible. Usually health instruction is the least well-developed aspect of a program. Education in this country has always been subject to local control, hence the quality and quantity of health instruction vary widely among districts and even among schools. At the elementary level, health teaching is seldom given top priority except in the case of topics temporarily viewed as crucial by the community. Yet although elementary teachers' attention to planned health teaching may often be fractional, legally and professionally they are responsible for certain activities associated with health services and the quality of the school environment. A complete description of the many aspects of these two important components of the total program is not possible in a book focused primarily on health instruction; however, it is the intention of this chapter to give you an overview of the potential for health teaching and learning implicit in those other areas.

No child should be admitted to the public schools unless his or her health has been certi-

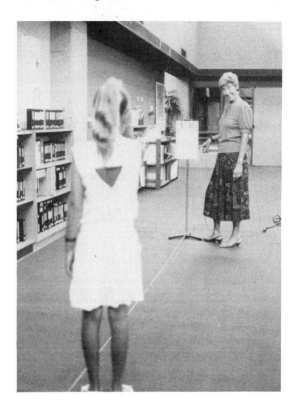

fied by medical examination, and all required immunizations have been completed or formally waived. Once admitted, it is a school's responsibility to maintain, protect, and so far as possible promote the health of that well child. That is the purpose of every school health program.

Johns' chart "A Concept of a Comprehensive School Health Program" (see Fig. 2-1) graphically presents an ideal program, illustrating its interrelationships. At the center is the individual student surrounded by a world consisting of the school, the family, and the community. Below that central focus, all of the elements shown are school based. Above it, all of them are community based. Two special kinds of organizations (youth groups and parent-

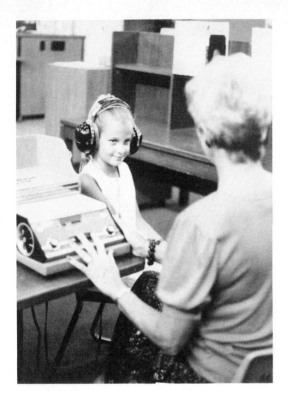

among states as well. In general, the laws governing health services and the school environment are far more restrictive and comprehensive than those concerning health instruction. Public health laws usually are enforced more rigorously than those of state education codes. Most schools are inspected regularly (especially food services areas) to see that they are complying with state laws governing sanitation and safe maintenance of buildings and grounds. In addition, state health and safety codes spell out requirements for the design of school facilities, for fire protection, disaster control, asbestos removal, and other environmental safety provisions.

Currently 38 (75%) of the states have laws mandating comprehensive school health education (Kolbe, and others 1987). However, this

teacher organizations) are set to the sides, since they are both school and community based. Liaison bodies, the Community Health Council and the School Health Committee, facilitate effective coordination and cooperation between school and community. As the concerns and principal activities of the individuals, groups, or primary divisions are explained, take time to refer back to the chart and note how each fits into and contributes to the total program (Journal of School Health, 1984).

LEGAL ASPECTS OF THE SCHOOL HEALTH PROGRAM

Because every aspect of public school education is regulated by the individual states, legislation affecting the school health program varies

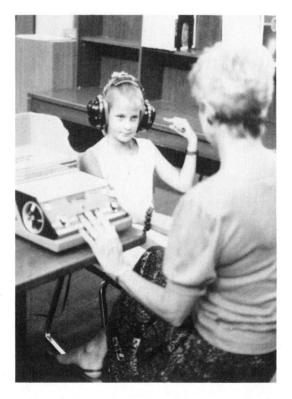

FIG. 2-1

A Concept of A Comprehensive School Health Program*

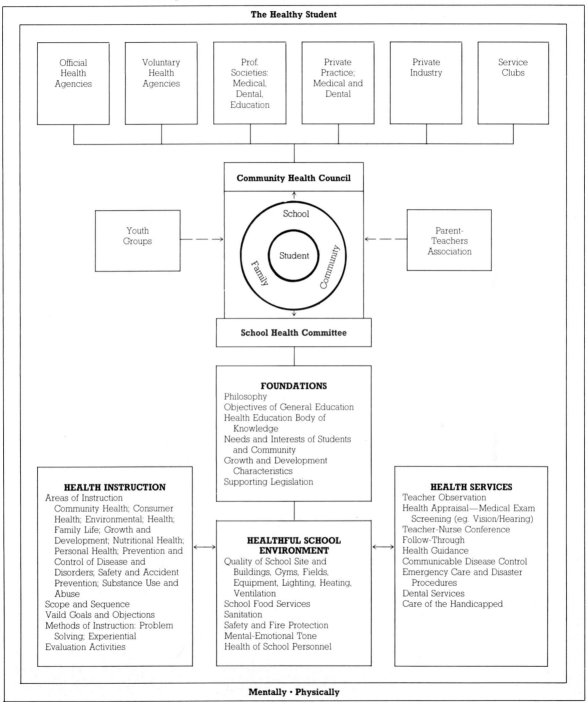

*Adapted with permission from Edward B. Johns.

does not mean that implementation is always monitored or enforced. Essentially the kind and amount of health instruction a child receives depends on decisions made at the local level (Noak, 1982). It is largely state law, however, as expressed in its health and safety codes, that accounts for the fact that basic health services and provisions for a safe and sanitary school environment are universally provided by schools. Variations in the number and quality of those afforded students in a school can be attributed to the difference between mandated and permissive legislation. Cost and budget are also factors, of course.

Mandated Versus Permissive Legislation

The difference between **mandated** and **permissive** legislation is that the first says that something *shall* be done, and the second usually says that something *may* be done. In the latter case, the school is not required to do what is specified, but it can if it wishes. With mandated procedures, those who are charged with implementing the law can be held accountable if its provisions are not carried out. Ignorance of the law does not protect the individual from blame if for that reason alone it was not obeyed. Do you know if there are mandates currently defining the scope of health instruction in elementary schools in your state? If so, what are the requirements?

Legislation Affecting Teachers Directly: Tort Law

The laws discussed so far are concerned with the total school health program. Other laws are related to specific responsibilities of teachers and other school personnel with respect to the health and safety of students. Every teacher needs to be aware of these **tort** (civil liability) laws.

A tort is an act, or absence of an act, by which someone either directly or indirectly causes an injury to a person, property, or reputation. In every state, the teacher is liable for his or her own tort. A few states, such as California, New York, and Washington, have enacted laws making the district liable also; however, in other states, under common law, the district can do no wrong. Thus in most states, the teacher is the only one who can be sued for damages when a student is injured or a reputation is damaged.

In general, a tort is considered to be the result of negligence. **Negligence** is defined as either *failure* to do something that a reasonable person would do, or *doing* something that a reasonable or prudent person would *not* do. So negligence can be an act either of omission or commission. For instance, California law mandates that a first-aid kit be taken along whenever students are to be away from school on a field trip. If an accident occurred and no first-aid equipment was available, the teacher would be liable to a suit for negligence. Find out what your state laws stipulate as essential equipment to be taken along or procedures to be followed on field trips.

It is not uncommon for parents or guardians of children injured in school to bring suit for damages against school personnel. (About 60% of the accidents among children of school age occur on school grounds, in the building, or between school and home). Teachers are responsible for the children in the classroom, and on the playground. Whether they can be held liable for damages in case of an accident on school grounds depends on the circumstances. The difference between responsibility and liability is significant. **Responsibility** is established by school and community policy. **Liability** is established by law and is decided by the courts. Liability can be established only if the teacher or other school personnel being sued can be proven either negligent in the performance of duties ordinarily associated with the position or imprudent in the discharge of those responsibilities.

In the event of an accident, a teacher may be held liable if she or he has (1) failed to warn children of danger or to provide adequate supervision; (2) knowingly conducted a class under unsafe conditions; or (3) committed any other imprudent act. Failure to provide first-aid treatment or provision of the wrong kind of first aid can be interpreted as negligence and therefore grounds for a liability judgment. All schools should have a clearly stated first-aid policy, and all teachers should be required to obtain and maintain certification in first-aid procedures.

Mandatory Reporting Law: Child Abuse

All, or nearly all states require that suspected child abuse be reported, although definitions of that crime differ somewhat. Most states require that a report be made immediately. A teacher or school worker is not obligated to investigate child abuse, but it must be reported. Failure to do so is deemed negligence. Those required by law to report suspected abuse include teachers, principals, school superintendents, physicians, nurses, dentists, and other professionals who are concerned with the health care of children. These persons are not liable for either civil damage or criminal prosecution as a result of a report, even if it turns out to be unfounded, unless it is proved that the report was made falsely and with malice.

One or more of the following categories of injury is included in the definitions of child abuse in all states.

1. Physical injury, as evidenced by injuries on several body surfaces; different colored bruises indicating similar blows over time; injuries hidden by clothing; glove or socklike appearance of burns indicating scalding by immersion; fear of adults; and fear of speaking in front of parents.

2. Emotional assault or deprivation, as evidenced by the child being withdrawn, depressed, or considered a behavior problem; displaying signs of emotional turmoil such as repetitive movements, giving inordinate attention to small details, and displaying antisocial behavior such as drug abuse, aggressiveness, or vandalism.

3. Physical neglect, as evidenced by the child's always being dirty, sleepy, hungry, or left alone and unsupervised for long periods; clothes inadequate or inappropriate for the weather; and a cold or unsanitary home.

4. Sexual exploitation, as evidenced by urogenital or rectal injuries or pain or irritation in those areas; a child walking with the knees bowed in because of such irritation or pain; a diagnosis of sexually transmitted disease; a report by the child that an adult ''bothers'' him or her when the parents are away; and actual incest, seduction, or forced sexual contact, including rape.

Every educator should know her or his state's mandatory reporting statute, how child abuse is defined in that state, and what the indications are for possible abuse. This information can be obtained from several sources such as a district attorney's office, a state attorney general's office, or a local superintendent's office.

School Health Policy

Policy statements should specify how far school personnel may and should go in providing first aid, how and under what circumstances parents (or their designees) will be notified in the event of illness or other emergency, and how and under what circumstances injured children will be removed from school for treatment. A signed statement establishing parental responsibility for the expense of any such treatment should be obtained and kept on file.

As a teacher you will be responsible for protecting the health and safety of the children while in your classroom and on the school grounds. Be certain that you know what your responsibilities are and that you take appropriate action to fulfill them at all times. For example, most elementary teachers are assigned specific play yard supervision times. If for any reason an assigned teacher was late in getting to the playground and in the interim a child was injured, that teacher would be guilty of negligence and liable for damages.

If you plan any out-of-the-ordinary school activities, be certain that state laws and school policy permit their being carried out and that you know what safety procedures will be required and are ready to implement them if necessary.

HEALTH SERVICES

Health services include the procedures carried out by members of the school health team (physicians, nurses, dentists, psychologists, counselors, teachers, custodians, dietitians, pupil personnel specialists, and others) to appraise, promote, and protect the health of every child in the school. The total well-being of the child—physical, social, emotional, and intellectual—is the primary concern (Joint Committee on Health Problems in Education 1964). Certain activities usually provided to accomplish this goal include the following.

Continuous Observation

Observation must be carried out by every teacher almost without conscious effort. Although a simple form of appraisal, observation is extremely important as a means of detecting any deviation from expected patterns of growth and development. Comparisons are based on established norms and also on past observations of a particular child's body build, health status, and behavior. During each year of a child's grade-school experience, these observations depend on the experienced eye and perceptions of the teacher. The teacher is the only one who sees the child every day and in the company of numbers of other children who are of the same age and required to fulfill the same educational assignments. For this reason a teacher is in some ways better able than parents to observe small but significant changes in appearance or behavior. A parent does not have the same opportunity for comparisons and may lack the time for it as well.

Observation can enable a teacher to detect signs and symptoms of common childhood diseases and of physical and emotional problems that if uncorrected could interfere with learning. Every teacher must be alert to signs of ill health or disability linked to alterations in a student's appearance or performance. Obvious signs such as a pale or flushed face, noticeable weight loss or gain, or physical or emotional distress signal problems. More subtle signs such as inattention or straining to see or hear should not be overlooked. Sudden negative personality changes or changes in standards of work provide clues to health status problems as well. Some of the conditions that can easily be noted by a classroom teacher are the following:*

General appearance—very thin or obese; sudden change in weight; unusually pale or flushed; poor posture; unkempt hair; change in gait; lethargic or hyperactive.

Eyes—crossed, inflamed, or watery eyes; squinting to see; frowning or scowling; holding book very close or unusually far away from the eyes; frequent sties; unnecessary wearing of dark glasses.

Ears—noticeable discharge; turning head to one side when listening; failure to hear well as revealed by irrelevant replies to questions or lack of response.

Nose and throat—persistent mouth breathing; enlarged glands in neck; frequent colds; persistent runny nose or sniffling; odor from mouth or nose.

Skin or scalp—rash on face or body; sores on face or body; numerous pimples; excessively dry skin; nits on hair; visible lice; scratching; bald spots.

Teeth and mouth—irregular teeth; stained or eroded teeth; cracking of lips; pale or blue lips; puffy or bleeding gums.

Behavior when playing—tiring easily; shortness of breath after moderate exercise; lack of interest in games or activities; unusual clumsiness; poor coordination; unusual excitability.

General behavior—docile and withdrawn; drowsy; aggressiveness; depression; day dreaming excessively; inability to work well with other children; excessive thirst; frequent need to use the toilet; unusual tenseness.

---

*Adapted from Dukelow, D.A., editor: Health appraisal of school children, Washington, D.C., 1969, Joint Committee on Health Problems in Education, National Education Association and American Medical Association.

In addition watch for behaviors such as inattention in class, irritability, acting out, stammering or other speech abnormality, or too frequent absences especially when any of these is unusual for a child.

Depending on the criticality of a problem and its persistence, a teacher should make note of symptoms needing further investigation or make an immediate referral to the school nurse or other designated person. For example, inattention displayed by a normally eager student might be remarkable but would not be a cause for concern unless noted for more than a few days. On the other hand, a child who is watery eyed and feverish and complains of a sore throat or stomachache should be referred at once. Immediate action in the latter situation protects not just the health of the sick child but also that of the others.

Always pay close attention to a pupil's complaints about pain or illness. Even when not accompanied by other signs of illness, the child should be referred to the appropriate school person for further diagnosis and action.

Child abuse prevention. Teacher observation has been described as the first line of defense against child abuse, because the teacher is in such close and continuing contact with children older than five years (Fraser, 1979). Child abuse is not limited to physical acts of aggression against a child; it includes any act of either omission or commission that endangers or hinders a child's physical or emotional growth and development. Child abuse is more readily apparent when physical injury rather than emotional deprivation is the source. Fortunately a teacher has the child's health record and the cooperation of the school nurse for evidence of past incidents that may provide further clues to the problem.

Health Appraisals

Medical examinations. At least four physical examinations during the school life of a child are recommended by every professional group concerned with the well-being of children. Some states (33%), require such examinations as a condition of admission and attendance. Twenty states (39%) require them for acceptance to organized sports activities (Kolbe, and others, 1987). Examination by the family physician, with parents present, is the best procedure for the small child about to enter school. If a problem is detected, its solution can begin at once. Most school districts have an established health history form that is sent to parents for appropriate notations by the physician and returned to the school files. Frequently physicians are employed by school districts or assigned to schools by the public health department to provide at least minimum examinations in cases where parents are unable or unwilling to pay for private health care.

Screening. Screening tests are preliminary appraisal techniques used by teachers, nurses, or trained volunteers to identify children who appear to need diagnosis by health-care specialists. Of those performed in schools, the most common are the vision and hearing tests.

Vision screening tests. Teacher observation of symptoms of eye disease is a reliable kind of vision screening. In fact, it may be more meaningful than the results of a rapid screening procedure (California Association of Ophthalmology, 1985). Swollen eyelids, sties, redness, discharges, squinting, and the need to hold a book close to or unusually far from the eyes when reading are clues to a need for a professional eye examination.

The Snellen test is that most often used in schools to test visual acuity (sharpness of vision). Eye specialists use this method in their offices almost universally. It is inexpensive, easily administered, and needs no particular electrical equipment, although the chart must be well lighted. No special training is needed for its use other than familiarity with the procedures, and only about one minute per child is needed for its completion. Elementary teachers frequently are expected to administer the test, but if there is a school nurse, it is the latter's responsibility. A teacher does need to know how to interpret the resulting scores, however.

The test involves the correct identification of simple objects or letters, often the "tumbling E" of progressively smaller sizes. Each letter size is numbered according to the standard distance at which a person with average vision should be able to read it easily. The numerator represents the distance from the student to the chart, so it is always the same (usually 20 feet). The denominator represents the lowest line in the chart that the child can read (i.e., the smallest symbols that were identified correctly). Average visual acuity is recorded as 20/20, meaning that at a distance of 20 feet, the eye reads the 20-foot line on the chart. A test score of 20/30 means that the child reads at 20 feet the line that should be readable at a distance of 30 feet. What would a score of 20/40 mean? Interpret a score of 20/10.

All children who consistently show any signs of visual difficulty, regardless of their visual acuity scores, should be referred for further examination (see Fig. 2-2). In addition, children 4 years old through grade 3 with 20/40 or less visual acuity (i.e., 20/50, 20/60, etc.), and all children in grade 4 and above with visual acuity of 20/30 or less, should be referred for complete professional examination. Scores are interpreted differently for younger children because as they mature the shape of the eyeball changes, and visual acuity usually increases as a result. In every case, however, when test scores indicate below-average vision (i.e., the

FIG. 2-2

Date _____

UNIFIED SCHOOL DISTRICT
REPORT OF VISION SCREENING

Name _____ School _____ Grade _____

The above student has received a routine vision screening test during which the following observations were made:

Visual Acuity on Snellen Chart   R.E. _____   L.E. _____   Both _____
Appearance

Frowns to see	_____	Headache	_____
Eyelids crusted, swollen	_____	Dizziness	_____
Sensitive to light	_____	Blurring Vision	_____
Watery eyes	_____	Burning eyes	_____
Discharge	_____	Trouble reading	_____
Eye wanders	_____	Other	_____
Frequent styes	_____		

It is urged that you consult an eye specialist in regard to these observations to see what action, if any, should be taken. (C.A.C., Title V, Section 594, defines test failure.)

Please have the examiner complete the bottom portion of this form and return the entire form to the principal, teacher or nurse of this school.

_____   _____   _____
Principal or Nurse   Address   City

Eye Examiner's Report to the School

Visual acuity: without lenses   R.E. _____   L.E. _____   Both _____
                  with lenses   R.E. _____   L.E. _____   Both _____

Diagnosis: _____

Prognosis: _____

Recommendations:
   Glasses prescribed: Yes _____   No _____
   Glasses to be worn constantly ____ for class only ____ reading ____ other ____
   Preferential seating _____ Child should return for further care _____
                                                                    (when)
   Other recommendations _____

Signed _____ Date _____
Address _____ City _____ Phone_____

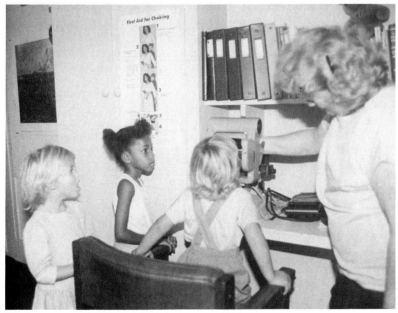

Armi Lizardi

second number is greater than 20), those individuals are retested at a later time to be certain that the findings are not just a result of a temporary reaction to an unusual circumstance. The importance of periodic screening is also justified by many studies that show that the incidence of visual defects increases with age and that visual acuity can never be assumed to be constant (Appleboom, 1985).

This is illustrated by an actual case. A school nurse, whose responsibility it was to check the eyesight of children in an elementary school district periodically, discovered that her own child's visual acuity had gone from 20/30 to 20/200 in one year. Ordinarily he would not have been reexamined for another two years. Since she never saw her child at work in his classroom, but only at home, his reading problems were not apparent. It was his teacher who noticed that he was having a great deal of difficulty and sent word to his parents. With professional diagnosis and provision of appropriate glasses, the boy's reading and schoolwork were soon back to normal. What might have been the outcome if the biennial school vision examinations had been the only means of detecting any changes in his vision?

Hearing screening tests. Here again, the classroom teacher can note behaviors indicative of hearing loss even before it can be verified by screening tests. Inattention or failure to carry out assignments sometimes can be traced to the fact that the child simply does not hear well. Cocking the head to one side, faulty pronunciation of certain words, and frequent requests for repetition of directions or words are other symptoms. When a child seems slow to understand, a hearing problem may be the cause.

In such a case, consult the child's health record to see if a hearing problem has already been identified. Check with the school nurse in any case. Just moving such a youngster to a seat nearer the teacher might do a lot to solve the problem.

FIG. 2-3

UNIFIED SCHOOL DISTRICT

HEARING SCREENING REPORT

Student's Name ___Robert Olson___ Age _6_ Date _5/10/87_

School _____ School Address _____

Dear Parents: A series of hearing tests have been completed on your child. The results indicate a possible hearing problem in the

Right Ear [ ]   Left Ear [ ]   Both Ears [X]

This audiogram is enclosed for your doctor's interpretation. It is suggested that you ask your physician to complete this form and return it to the school named above.

_____
School Nurse

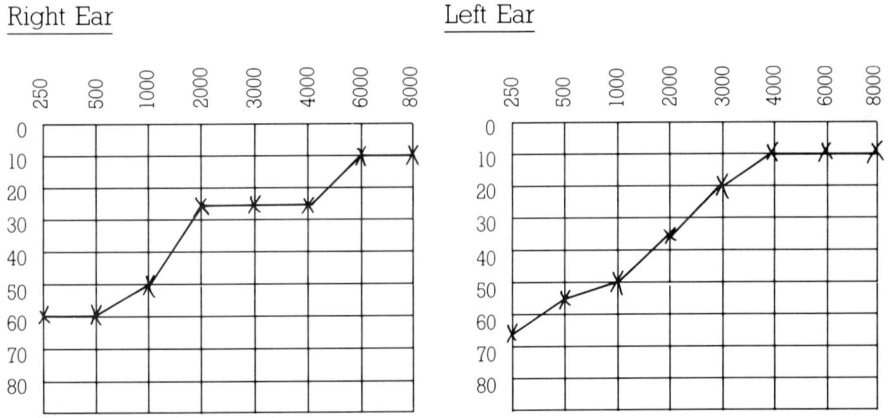

Right Ear   Left Ear

ISO 1964 Standard
Date of Test ___5/10___

Dear Doctor: The school seeks the advice and cooperation of parents and physicians in maintaining the student's health and making the best plans for his school program.

Physician's Report to the School

Audiometric Findings

Right Ear

250	500	1000	2000	3000	4000	6000	8000
60	60	50	25	25	25	10	10

Left Ear

250	500	1000	2000	3000	4000	6000	8000
65	55	50	35	20	10	10	10

Date: ___5/25___

Results of other hearing tests:
   Otitis media - acute
Date of examination: ___5/25/87___
[X] Child is under medical treatment   [ ] No further medical treatment is needed

___Joseph Otto, M.D.___   _____
Signature of Physician   Date

FIG. 2-4

UNIFIED SCHOOL DISTRICT

Report of Hearing Test

_____   _____   _____
School   Address   Telephone

To Parent or Guardian:

As a result of a recent hearing testing program at school, we believe that your child, _____, should have further examination, to determine whether or not there is an actual hearing loss. An audiometer was used for these tests, and your child did not pass within normal limits. Other observations which make us believe that there may be a hearing loss are:

_____
_____
_____
_____
_____
_____
_____

We feel that you should bring this to the attention of your family doctor. Please take this form to your doctor, and ask him to complete it and return it to us. If you would like to discuss this with our school nurse, do not hesitate to call. We urge your prompt attention to this matter.

_____   _____   _____
Date   School Nurse   Principal

Examiner's Report of Ear and Hearing Examination

Hearing Acuity: Right ear: _____   Left ear: _____
Other Findings: _____
_____
_____
_____

Recommendations: _____
_____
_____
_____

_____   _____   _____
Date   Telephone   Signature of Examiner

Hearing screening is the task of a trained audiometrist, although school nurses very often hold credentials for this work (see Figs. 2-3 and 2-4). In most school districts, hearing screening is conducted at intervals of two to three years. Referral to a physician normally would depend on the results of a pure-tone audiometry threshold test showing some amount of hearing loss or on any significant teacher observation or history of hearing disorders.

The kind of hearing loss most common among elementary school children is called *conductive* loss. The cause may be impacted ear wax, foreign objects in the ear, otitis media (inflammation of the middle ear), or severe ear infections.

The need for instruction about hearing and its protection is attested to by the high incidence of hearing loss in our society. Noise pollution is a major problem in industry and in the community. Studies show that although elementary school teachers report that they teach about hearing health, most of that instruction is based on show and tell. Frager (1986) urges that more time be given to providing hands-on activities to help youngsters understand why and how noise threatens hearing. For example, students could be allowed to examine sound measurement devices and to use them in actual noisy environments. Experiments with a marble dropped from a given distance onto surfaces such as wood, tile, foam, and carpet could be arranged to help them understand the role of sound insulation in protecting hearing.

Teacher-nurse conference. A school nurse often is given responsibility for the health of the children in a number of schools. In small districts there may be just one nurse who visits all of the schools. In any case, the nurse sees a child infrequently except in unusual cases. A referral may be the first time a particular child visits the nurse's office. The child's teacher may know far better how atypical a child's behavior or appearance is. It is impossible for a nurse to

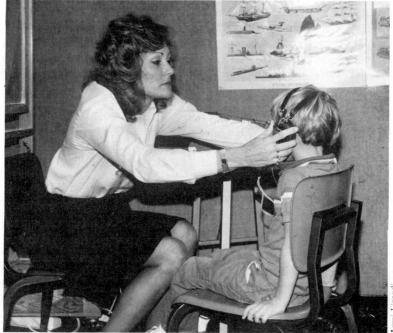

Armi Lizardi

know every child in even one school as well as does that child's teacher. Therefore, the most important link between school-provided health care and the individual child is the conference between the nurse and the teacher. Health records can only provide an index of status and history up to the last date of entry. The nurse depends on the teacher to refer a child who appears to have a health problem at present. Similarly, a teacher often can solve a child's learning problem through consultation with the nurse. The nurse has more experience in interpreting medical histories as recorded in a child's health folder and in evaluating present symptoms in light of that record. Consultations are sometimes scheduled annually so that each of them can better understand the needs of the children whose health and education are their mutual concern.

A teacher-nurse collaboration is much more than just a team approach to the solution of a suspected student health problem. A case history vividly illustrates this point. An eight-year-old child, normally high spirited, self-assured, and outgoing visibly changed between one day and the next. She coughed weakly from time to time and looked half frightened, half puzzled. She told the teacher that she had a funny feeling in her stomach. The nurse talked to her but could get no more information, nor was there anything in the health record that might help to explain the problem. She sent the youngster back to class. The teacher, not satisfied, persisted and urged that the child's parents be contacted and advised. This was done, the family physician was consulted, and before the day was over the child was in surgery. An x-ray examination and other tests had revealed that a tumor pressing on the child's heart was the cause of her distress. This is an unusual case, but it happened and it shows that you should never hesitate to refer a child a second time if you believe that there is a chance that some-

thing has been missed. Sometimes a child will feel better for a little while just because of the referral. Trust your wider experience with a student if you see changes that signal a possible problem.

Follow-through procedures. Follow-through procedures are intended to provide a check on what is done for a child once a condition needing treatment or correction has been called to the attention of parents. When there is no nurse assigned to a school, the teacher or school administrator must assume this responsibility. The essential aspect of the activity of the follow-through procedures is the communication of what has happened in the case to the person who made the original appraisal. If a teacher requests that the nurse evaluate a child's hearing acuity, for example, and the test shows that more elaborate examinations are needed, the parents would be notified. In follow-through procedures, the nurse would contact the parents after a week or so to find out what has been done about the problem. This information would be entered in the child's health record and also reported to the teacher. If nothing has been done about it, further referrals are made until some action is taken to remedy the problem. If you make a referral but never receive any report of its outcome, don't forget about it. Follow through yourself. Contact the person to whom you made the referral and find out what, if anything, was done about it. If necessary, make another referral.

Health records. Most, if not all, school districts maintain some sort of cumulative health folders as a means of storing and organizing all the data accumulated for each child during school years. A health record typically contains information from every relevant health examination or treatment and all important information related to the health history of the individual: for example, height and weight at specified intervals, dates and types of immunizations

FIG. 2-5

HEALTH RECORD - UNIFIED SCHOOL DISTRICT

Name _____ Address _____ Phone _____
Last   First   M.I.

Parent _____ Sex _____ School _____

Grade	K	I	2	3	4	5	6
Date							
Height							
Weight							
Eyes: R - L							
Color Test							
Ears: R - L							
Skin							
Teeth — Cavities							
Teeth — Prophylaxis							
Teeth — Occlusion							
Tonsils							
Chest							
Heart							
Nutrition							
Blood Pressure							
Posture							

CODE: Normal N   Slight Defect SD   Marked Defect MD   Defect Corrected DC   Non-remedial Defect ND

Name _____ Date of Birth _____
Last   First   Middle   Month   Day   Year

PERSONAL HISTORY: (Check if applicable to your child. Enter year of occurrence if known.)

✓ HEALTH PROBLEMS	Yr.	✓ COMMUNICABLE DISEASES	Yr.	IMMUNIZATIONS (Required by law)
Allergies		Chicken Pox		*Diphtheria, Tetanus, Pertussis
Asthma		Diphtheria		or Dates: 1. 2. 3. 4.
Colds, frequent		Measles, German (3 Day, Rubella)		*Diphtheria, Tetanus (7-18 years)
Diabetes		Measles (10 Day, Rubeola)		Dates: 1. 2. 3. 4.
Emotional Problem(s)		Meningitis		*Measles Vaccine (10 Day, Rubeola)
Hay Fever		Mononucleosis		Date:
Headaches		Mumps		*Polio Vaccine — Sabin (Oral) TOPV
Head Injury		Pertussis (Whooping Cough)		or Dates: 1. 2. 3. 4.
Hearing Problem		Scarlet Fever		*Polio Vaccine — Salk IPV
Heart Condition		Strep Throat		Dates: 1. 2. 3.
Nervous Problem		Tetanus		Measles Vaccine, German (3 Day)
Nose Bleeds		Tuberculosis - Child		Date:
Rheumatic Fever		Tuberculosis - Family		Mumps Vaccine - Date:
Seizures		Other serious conditions:		Smallpox Vaccine - Date:
Stomach aches		CHDP Physical Yes No		Tuberculin Test, Negative - Date:
Vision Problem		Continuing Medication		Tuberculin Test, Positive - Date:
Wears Glasses		Yes No		Scoliosis Screening Pass / Fail

Parent's or Guardian's Signature: _____ Date: _____

CONTRARY TO BELIEF STATEMENT
This statement in accordance with Sec. 3384, Chapter 7, Health and Safety Code, State of California
I certify that the following immunizations are against my beliefs: (Please circle)
Polio   Measles (10 Day)   Diphtheria   Tetanus   Whooping Cough

received, anecdotal records of significant teacher observations, dental records, parental information, records of illnesses, results of any psychometric procedures, and nurse's reports (see Fig. 2-5).

Confidentiality. The record should be started when the child enters school and be accumulated from grade to grade. Ordinarily, if a child transfers to another school, whether in the same city or another, the record goes with him or her. It is an indispensable resource for understanding a child's special needs and thereby contributing to his or her optimum health and achievement.

Such a comprehensive record must be used with discretion. An important rule to be obeyed is maintenance of confidentiality. Only specified personnel should have access to these folders. Student office aids should *never* be allowed to file or retrieve data from these records. They should not be combined with academic records, disciplinary records, or any other data that may be open to individuals not directly concerned with health and medical matters. In addition, possible liability for libel and slander should be considered. Teachers and others must not make subjective statements in a health folder reflecting judgments about a child's character or personal habits. At best these can only be personal opinions or unconscious biases and could harm the child's future achievement and life (AAP, 1987, pp. 118-19).

Health guidance. Some kind of planned health guidance must be included for a school health program to be fully effective. All teachers have a role in guidance. Elementary school teachers have both the responsibility and a unique opportunity to guide because they usually work closely with the same small group of children all day.

The major guidance problem areas include physical and emotional health, home and family relationships, and peer group or boy-girl relationships. One of the tools of guidance is counseling—the procedures by which nurses, teachers, physicians, and others interpret a problem to students and parents, and help them to work out their own plan for its solution. Teachers and nurses can only assist them in the process.

Health counseling and follow-through activities do more to promote health than any other school activity. Sometimes parents, not aware or convinced of its seriousness, allow a health problem to go uncorrected. Health guidance is essential as a means of motivating appropriate action to treat any potentially handicapping conditions. In essence, the process is a problem-solving activity, and the steps are the same whatever the problem. The teacher or nurse helps the student and family understand the problem and identify ways to obtain information needed to solve it; they discuss tentative solutions and help the student and family choose the one best suited to their circumstances. The final step in guidance, as in referrals, is follow-through action.

Communicable disease control. Control of communicable diseases is a responsibility shared by the home, school, and community. Primarily it is the responsibility of parents to keep a sick child at home and in bed. The practice of rewarding continuous attendance is not compatible with best protection against disease or epidemic. Absences should be encouraged when children have even minor cold symptoms, since most childhood diseases have those same signs in the early stages.

The teacher is responsible for detecting and excluding any child from the classroom who has symptoms of a communicable disease. Each day's first task must be to look at each arriving child for signs such as the flushed cheeks of fever, watery or red eyes, skin rash or eruptions, persistent coughing, sniffles, hoarseness, frequent head scratching, or unusual pallor. Chil-

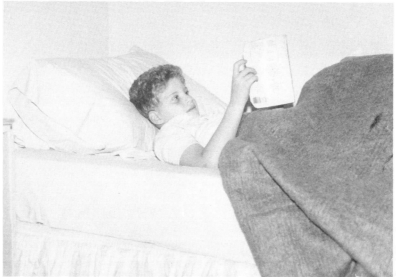

Armi Luzardi

dren exhibiting such conditions should be taken at once to the nurse or person designated as the excluding authority in the event of a child's illness.

If it is decided that a child may have a communicable disease and should be sent home, the next step is the responsibility of the nurse or school administrator. Policies should be established in accordance with local public health regulations. They must be thoroughly understood and complied with by all those concerned. These policies usually contain provisions for follow-through procedures to ascertain the diagnosis, provisions for reaching and notifying the parents and safely transporting the child home, and specified means of verifying total recovery as a condition of readmission to school.

Procedures must be established to determine if it is safe for a child to return to class, not only for the sake of the affected youngster, but also to protect the health of every other person in the school. In the case of a minor illness, such as an upset stomach, a note from a parent and inspection by the school nurse are usually ade-

quate. In case of a more severe illness such as chicken pox or mumps, a statement from a physician may be required. With certain diseases, where isolation is mandated by public health law, a certificate from a health department is required. In any case, the person whose responsibility it is to admit a child after an illness should be competent by training to make such a judgment.

Control of communicable diseases in the community is legally the responsibility of the board of health, but there are basic rules concerning the control and prevention of these diseases that must be obeyed by parents and school personnel. No communicable disease control program can be fully effective without the cooperation of parents. Therefore, schools must make every effort to acquaint parents with their role in disease prevention and control. Even the children should be aware of the necessity for strict adherence to public health rules (see Table 2-1).

Principals and superintendents must have accurate information concerning the legal sta-

Ex, health rules

TABLE 2-1 Teacher resource: communicable diseases

Disease	Type of pathogen	Source	Transmission	Entry	Period of communicability	Prevention	Control
Head lice (pediculosis)	Louse	Humans	Use of borrowed combs, brushes; close contact with infected humans	Hair or head	As long as lice and nits remain	Nonuse of borrowed combs, etc.; inspection	Application of medications to hair and scalp; frequent inspection
Impetigo	Bacteria	Humans	Contact	Skin	2 to 7 days	Isolate any infected children	Medical attention and readmission only with medical advice
Rubeola	Virus	Human	Respiratory discharge		1 to 2 weeks	Immunization	Isolation and treatment
Scabies	Mites	Humans	Infected skin and clothing worn by infected person		As long as skin is affected	Isolation of infected invididuals; cleanliness of body and bedding	Medical treatment and personal hygiene
Ringworm	Fungi	Humans, animals	Direct contact; indirect contact with clothing, hair	On skin	As long as lesions are present	No vaccine; avoid contact with infected person	Cleanse infected areas daily; disinfect articles in contact with infected area; apply antibacterial agent topically
Influenza ("flu")*	Virus	Humans, some animals suspected	Direct contact; indirect contact through droplet spread; discharge from nose and throat, possibly airborne	Mouth, nose	3 days from onset of symptoms	Vaccination dependent on viral strain; avoid enclosed crowded places during epidemic	Isolate infected person; disinfect bedding or clothing in contact with discharges

Disease	Agent	Reservoir	Mode of transmission	Portal	Period of communicability	Prevention	Control
Mumps*	Virus	Humans	Direct contact; indirect contact by droplet spread or articles freshly soiled with saliva	Mouth, nose	48 hours before swelling occurs to 9 days after	Vaccination lasts about 4 years; life-long immunity after infection	Isolate infected person during period of communicability
Chicken-pox	Virus	Humans	Direct contact; indirect contact by droplet spread or articles freshly soiled by discharges	Mouth, nose	5 days before eruptions first occur to 6 days after	Long immunity after infection; immune globulin may lessen severity of attack	Isolate infected person for 1 week after eruptions occur; disinfect contact articles
Conjunctivitis ("pink eye")	Bacteria	Humans	Contact with discharge from eyes or upper respiratory tract, usually through fingers or clothing	Eyes	During the course of active infection	Good personal hygiene	Infected person should not attend school during acute stage; disinfect soiled articles
Pinworm disease (enterobiasis)	Intestinal roundworm	Infected humans, particularly children	Direct transfer of eggs (same host); indirect transfer of eggs through clothes or bedding	Mouth	2 to 8 weeks if untreated	Frequent bathing; good personal hygiene; daily bedding and clothing changes	Disinfect soiled articles (eggs killed at temperatures of 132° F or higher)
Hepatitis (viral)	Virus	Humans	Person to person; contaminated needles and syringes; transfusions from an infected person	Mouth, skin puncture	Latter half of incubation period (30 to 35 days) to 3 to 5 days after onset of jaundice	Good personal hygiene; sanitary disposal of feces; sterilization of needles and syringes; careful screening of blood donors	Isolate infected person first 2 weeks of illness and 1 week after onset of jaundice
Common cold	Virus	Humans	Direct contact, indirect contact through droplet spread or soiled articles	Nose, mouth	First 24 hours of symptoms to 5 days	None known; however, adequate nutrition and rest may increase resistance	Rest; avoid contact with infected person; treat symptoms

Continued.

TABLE 2-1 Teacher resource: communicable diseases—cont'd

Disease	Type of pathogen	Source	Transmission	Entry	Period of communicability	Prevention	Control
German measles (rubella)*	Virus	Humans	Direct contact with secretions from an infected person; indirect contact through droplet spread	Nose, mouth	2 to 4 days before rash until 2 to 5 days thereafter	Vaccination, natural immunity	Isolate infected person
Scarlet fever	Bacteria (streptococci)	Humans	Direct contact; indirect contact	Nose, mouth	Approximately 10 days from onset of infection	Some immunity from first infection	Isolate infected person; disinfect contaminated articles
Tetanus*	Bacteria	Intestinal canal of animals and humans	Puncture wounds, scratches, burns	Skin puncture	Not directly communicable among humans	Repeated vaccinations	Thoroughly clean all wounds; update immunization
Diphtheria*	Bacteria	Humans	Direct contact; indirect contact with articles soiled with discharges from infected person; ingestion of infected raw milk	Mouth, skin wounds	Usually 2 weeks or less	Vaccinations with booster	Isolate infected person; disinfect soiled articles; contacts immunized, antibiotics prescribed
Pertussis (whooping cough)*	Bacteria	Humans	Direct contact with mucous membrane discharges; indirect contact through droplet spread or contact with articles freshly soiled with discharges	Mouth, nose	7 days after exposure to 3 weeks after onset of cough	Vaccinations with booster	Isolate infected person, disinfect soiled articles; antibiotics prescribed

Modified from School health curriculum project, grade 7, San Bruno, Calif, 1981, U.S. Center for Health Promotion and Education.
*Diseases best controlled through use of vaccine.

tus of immunization in their state. State laws vary, and they are revised often. Administrators must require that immunizations have been obtained, but they can only go as far as state law permits. If a school board wants to require immunization against specified diseases as a condition of entrance to school, the right to do so must be established by law.

Emergency care and disaster procedures. The school has three responsibilities for emergency care and disaster control: (1) to prevent accidents from happening in school, (2) to provide safety education, and (3) to develop a plan for handling emergencies. The last of these is sometimes neglected because it is assumed either that accidents will not happen or that what should be done in such an event can be left to common sense. Yet accidents do happen in schools and on the playground, and they are not always handled wisely because of excitement, forgetfulness, lack of knowledge, or panic on the part of one or more school personnel. The unexpected must always be expected; every contingency must be anticipated and a plan ready and practiced to meet it.

Several steps are necessary to develop effective plans for emergency situations. The faculty must be made aware of the possibility of accidents and emergencies and must be responsive to the suggestion that they think through plans to cope with any eventuality in their classrooms. These individual plans should be correlated to form a written master plan and thoroughly studied and understood by all school personnel.

A filing system of data related to every student and staff member should be quickly accessible to the main office. It should include information such as name, parents' names (or names of nearest relative) and their address and home and business telephone numbers, name and telephone of the family physician or physician of

choice, hospital of choice, special directions for dealing with an accident involving that person, any known allergies or special conditions (e.g., hemophilia), and the person's religion. In case of an accident the school is responsible for providing immediate care and should do so in accordance with previously agreed to practices and instructions from the parents or stipulated relative.

Parents should be informed of every plan made by the school in anticipation of emergencies and given the opportunity to state the kind of care they want their children to receive. Informing parents of plans in advance gives them the chance to suggest modifications and helps prevent any criticism or litigation that might occur later if a parent did not approve of some action taken.

First-aid kits or cabinets must be provided and placed in strategic spots around the school. Their contents should be fresh and in accordance with accepted standards for first-aid needs. Every teacher should be qualified to administer first-aid procedures. A school nurse with first-aid status could make an important contribution to the school health program by giving instruction to new teachers.

At the first indication of an emergency, code signals should be sounded throughout the school, calling specified school personnel, as established by plan, or calling for a general exodus from the building as in a fire drill.

Parents or relatives should be notified calmly, and as soon as possible, and every needed assistance given them in caring for their children.

The school medical adviser should prepare detailed instructions for the guidance of teachers and the school nurse with reference to the immediate treatment of common emergencies such as abdominal pain, menstrual problems, and headaches, as well as less frequent emergencies such as epileptic attacks or insulin shock. The school nurse is responsible for making certain that accident provisions and plans for immediate treatment are known by all school personnel. When no nurse is assigned to the school, the principal or other designee must fulfill this responsibility.

A report of each accident or other emergency should be prepared and kept on file. This report should include names of persons concerned, date, time, location, nature of the accident, names of witnesses, and the manner in which the case was handled. Such records are frequently of great importance in later discussions of additional preventive measures or of liability. Frequently, forms for reporting serious accidents are supplied to schools by the liability insurance company with which they are insured.

Plans for transporting injured or ill children to home or hospital must be made. The school should provide private cars, school buses, ambulances, or other dependable means, as well as a method of summoning a driver and paying for such a trip. Nothing should be left for an after-the-accident argument. If private cars are used at times of accidents, the insurance covering those cars and their drivers should be adequate and up to date. It is advisable to establish in advance which exits to use in taking injured children from the building to a car. In short, every possible detail needs to be thought about and planned for. Moreover, each teacher must be a part of the school health team—informed, practiced, and ready to handle emergencies if they occur. The best-written plans are only words. You must translate them into action if need be.

Dental services. Dental disease begins in childhood. Until very recently it has not been uncommon to see nearly two-thirds of the school population affected to some degree by dental caries. This, despite the fact that now, as reported by the National Institute of Dental Research, about half of all children up to the age of 17 are free from any tooth decay. (*LA Times*, 1988). This dramatic change is attributed to the early training children are receiving in brushing and flossing techniques, and to the increased use of fluorides as decay prevention. Nearly half the children have never seen a dentist. Nearly half (45%) of the rest of the population has infrequent dental care (less than one visit per year), usually sought only for emergency conditions. Dental health is the responsibility of the individual, family, and community, in that order. The schools, as part of the community, are in a particularly strategic position to promote the dental health of children. As a part of its program, school health education should motivate children to practice good oral hygiene, especially correct use of dental floss, and seek dental consultation on a regular basis.

Undoubtedly the best place to teach children good oral health practices is in the home. Classroom teaching provides reinforcement and sometimes more effective instruction in specific dental hygiene techniques, particularly if it is provided over time. Studies show that a well-designed, ongoing curriculum based on specified cognitive and behavioral objectives can result in better skill development as well as increased knowledge about oral hygiene (Houle, 1982). Not only should information concerning nutrition and dental hygiene be provided, but arrangements should be made to allow students to practice basic dental care procedures in school.

Access to running water for toothbrushing practice for 25 or more students at a time is not likely to be possible in schools. However, students can be taught to clean their teeth by dry brushing. This method of toothbrushing requires neither toothpaste nor sinks. It involves the use of a dry, soft toothbrush to sweep and stimulate the oral cavity and tongue. Studies

**DRY BRUSHING
ANYTIME, ANYPLACE: DO IT RIGHT!**

The "Dry Brushing" technique is a method of toothbrushing suggested for classroom use. No toothpaste is required; it is not necessary to spit; no sinks are needed. This method supplements the dental care practiced by the student at home.

The technique reduces the incidence of tooth decay and gum disease by removing plaque, a sticky layer of harmful bacteria that continually forms on teeth, and eliminates a major cause of bad breath. It should be remembered, however, that once dental problems are present, the technique cannot cure them. Therefore, it is important to see your dentist periodically to make sure that your mouth is free from disease.

The suggested technique for dry brushing is as follows:

1. Wipe all soft tissue in the mouth, including cheeks, roof, inside the lips and gums with a dry, soft and small toothbrush. Do not brush the tongue yet. This step will stimulate the flow of fresh saliva and help remove debris.
2. Work bristle tips now wet with saliva between the gum margin and the tooth and vibrate the brush with bristles in place. This technique will remove plaque, stimulate circulation and work saliva around the gums.
3. Direct the bristles between the teeth and toward the biting surfaces. Vibrate the bristles in place. Brush biting surfaces.
4. Polish and brush your teeth in your usual manner, but do not damage the tissues.
5. Now, brush your tongue as thoroughly as possible.
6. The use of dental floss is introduced as soon as properly supervised teaching and monitoring is available, and adequate manual dexterity is demonstrated. To use floss, work it gently between the teeth. Curve it around the tooth and under the gum line. Move floss up and down across the tooth to remove the plaque.
7. When water is available after brushing and flossing, thoroughly rinse your mouth.

Endorsed by the California Dental Association, State Department of Health, Dental Division.

have demonstrated that the technique reduces the incidence of tooth decay and results in improved oral cleanliness even among children as young as kindergarten age (Lee, 1980).

Annual dental examinations and direct fluoride applications to the teeth, when needed, are recommended dental procedures. Those who urge provision of dental examinations at school believe that this supports dental health instruction, brings children's dental problems to the attention of school personnel, provides the children experience with a dentist in a familiar setting, thus relieving fears about dental treatment, and provides data for the assessment of the overall school dental health status (Rabich, and others, 1982). Others believe that examinations made in dental offices or clinics have the advantage of better equipment, the feeling of security provided by parental presence, and a better chance that needed dental treatment will be obtained. Either way, the educational value of the experience is more apt to motivate good dental hygiene than any amount of teacher talk. The provision of a lesson in advance of an actual examination both prepares the students for what is to happen and enhances the total learning outcome (Horowitz, and others, 1987).

Controls should be maintained over vending machines at school so that they are stocked with noncariogenic (caries-causing) snacks. It probably is nearly impossible to provide nutritious foods that are totally devoid of any sugars; however, there is evidence that it is the frequency with which snack foods are consumed that may be the greater hazard. The length of time they stay in the mouth and their physical form increase the potential for harm. Most hazardous to oral health are snacks such as confections, hard candies, and sticky dried fruit (Hinkle, 1982). The following are reasonable choices: milk, nuts, cheese, plain yogurt, popcorn, and unsugared gum (ADA, 1986). In general, eating between meals should be limited and followed by brushing the teeth as soon as possible.

There are many variations possible in developing a school dental health program. Whatever the plan, three basic forms of activity should be included: (1) dental health education, (2) preventive measures, and (3) referral with follow-through procedures in cases of discovered dental problems. Neglect of one of these aspects diminishes the effectiveness of the others.

Care of the handicapped: special education. Every child has the right to an education, and handicapped children are no exception. For many years schools were allowed to exclude certain children who were judged ineducable because of some disability. Some of these children simply stayed home, others were sent to expensive private schools, some were admitted to state institutions, and a select few in some school districts were admitted to special schools such as those for children who are multiply handicapped but educable. Today that picture has changed dramatically because of new strong federal laws and accompanying funds to assist in the education of such physically, mentally, or emotionally handicapped children. Special education has become a separate career choice for prospective teachers.

Handicapping conditions include mental retardation, speech impairment, visual impairment, learning disability, emotional disturbance, orthopedic problems, deaf-blindness, or health impairments from other problems such as autism. To qualify for special education, a child must have one or more such handicaps and also have need of special teaching because that condition limits her or his mobility, strength, or well-being.

The Education for All Handicapped Children Act (Public Law 94-142) went into effect in September 1978. Five principles of special education summarize key provisions of this act:

1. *Zero reject:* No handicapped child may be excluded from free appropriate public education.
2. *Nondiscriminatory evaluation:* Every handicapped child must be fairly assessed so that he or she may be properly placed and served.
3. *Appropriate education:* Every handicapped child must be given an education that is meaningful to him or her, taking the handicap into account.
4. *Least restrictive placement:* A handicapped child may not be segregated inappropriately from his or her nonhandicapped peers.
5. *Procedural due process:* Each handicapped child has the right to protest a school's decision about his or her placement (Scheiber, 1981).

Additional provisions stipulate structural

changes that must be made where necessary to ensure wheelchair access to buildings, free movement in the halls, and entrance to restrooms and classrooms. All buildings constructed after June 1977 are required to provide such access to restrooms and classrooms.

The schools have embraced the philosophy that every child has the right to learn to the extent possible, to be prepared for useful employment, and to be as independent as possible. Programs have been set up in most schools for the purpose. In 1981 it was reported that fully 98% of those requiring this sort of education appeared to be participating in some sort of special education program (Condition of Education, 1981). As of 1984, the estimated number of children being served in this way was over 4 million, or 11% of all those then in elementary and secondary schools in the United States (Condition of Education, 1987).

HEALTHFUL SCHOOL ENVIRONMENT

Inasmuch as the school health program is a composite of three interrelated areas of activity, obviously none of these exists in isolation from the others. Thus the activities of health services contribute to the quality of the school's environment, and health instruction is reinforced by learning gained through health services and participation in a safe and sanitary school environment (Newman, 1982). The key components of healthful school living include not only the physical aspects, but also the social and emotional currents in which the school's inhabitants live and work.

School Site and Plant

Most states have carefully prescribed requirements defining the acreage needed for a school, size of its rooms, type of construction, kind and number of sanitary facilities, number and location of fire hoses, and other health and safety features. Although standards vary from state to state, usually 5 acres, plus an additional acre for every 100 students enrolled, is the minimum land allocation for an elementary school.

Playgrounds

Recommendations for the number of acres needed for elementary schools are based on the need for playgrounds. Children, especially in the primary grades, need time to relax and play during school hours. Play not only enables the youngster to return to the classroom refreshed and ready to work, but it provides other kinds of learning experiences. Muscle coordination, teamwork, sportsmanship, and a host of game skills are practiced and learned during play.

Lighting

Most provisions for the quantity and quality of lighting are made by those responsible for designing and constructing the school building. The teacher's responsibility is to see that the lighting remains constant, and conditions, sources, and seating adjusted as necessary. Students should be allowed to arrange or change seats whenever this improves their ability to see their work. Activities involving close work such as reading should be alternated with other tasks for which vision is not as critical a factor. Failed lighting equipment should be reported at once. Observe the students as they read what is written on the chalkboard from their seats. Do they appear to read easily, or must they squint to see it? If they are having difficulty, check the light levels in the room with a light meter. The recommended illumination for chalkboard reading is 150 **footcandles** (a footcandle is the amount of light on a surface one foot from a standard lighted candle.)

Heating and Ventilation

Studies show that children react to temperature more directly and in some ways differently than do adults. Elementary school children have a higher metabolism rate than adults do. What will be comfortable for one age group may not be for the other. But anyone becomes sluggish when it is too warm, and too cold temperatures make people restless in the natural urge to get warm. The primary consideration must be the child's comfort. With more and more schools moving to year-around attendance patterns, extremes of temperature become more critical as threats to learning potential.

School Food Services

Food services have been an integral part of the school health program since the National School Lunch Act was signed by President Truman in 1946. Since then the Special Milk Program (1954) and School Breakfast Programs (1966, 1972) have been added. In 1980 it was reported that 26 million children in more than 94,000 schools were being provided free or low-cost lunches. Another 13 million were receiving nutritious breakfasts at school. Federal subsidies in support of these programs rose from the initial $100 million in 1946 to more than $2.7 billion in 1980.

The need for school food services is supported by studies revealing that not just the poor or neglected children but also those from well-to-do families come to school unfed or poorly fed. Good nutrition promotes health, builds energy, and enhances both the ability and desire to participate in the activities and demands of the day. Learning is hindered when the student is hungry.

However, lunches and other nourishment provided by the school are not intended solely to satisfy hunger and build energy. Concurrently, children learn about social and sanitary aspects of foods and eating patterns. Concepts of good nutrition are given practical application in the menus provided them, thus reinforcing lessons experienced in health classes. The Dairy Council of California has developed a foods guide for teachers to help them teach food classifications to children of seven Asian cultures in their own languages with phonetic translation in English (1981). Lists of common foods translated into Spanish can be obtained (Hernandez and others, 1972). It seems likely that whatever the extent of federal influence and subsidization of such programs, school food services will continue to be a priority of a good school health program.

Certain principles concerning the operation of school food services have been suggested as basic guidelines to their operation.

Balanced meals. Every lunch should be nutritionally balanced in accordance with the recommendations of nutrition authorities. Millions of children depend on the provision of school food services to meet their total nutrition requirements. A nutritious lunch at least five days a week is as important a school enterprise as special education for handicapped children.

School lunch menus. To receive federal aid, schools must serve nutritious lunches that meet the requirements for a type-A lunch as established by the Secretary of Agriculture (California State Education Administration Code, 1987). These lunches must meet one-third of the National Research Council's recommended daily nutritional allowance for school-age children. A type-A lunch consists of a meat or meat alternate, two or more vegetables or fruits, bread, and milk. A home-packed lunch can be well balanced, nutritious, and hot if thermos bottles are used. Health instruction might focus on identifying the kinds and amounts of foods that can be used to prepare such a meal at home. Aspects of sanitary food preservation can be emphasized as well.

Sanitation. Serving food in school requires perfect food-sanitation procedures. Essentials require good refrigeration, nonporous and undamaged dishes, tables and counters without cracks that are scrubbed clean after every use, and effective sterilization equipment for all eating and cooking utensils. Cooking and serving personnel must be free of communicable diseases and must comply with state, county, and city sanitation codes governing the handling of food.

Personal sanitation. Handwashing and toilet facilities should be adequately supplied with soap and hot water and convenient for users of the lunchroom.

Instruction. The school lunch programs should go beyond the function of feeding hungry children. If those in charge give time and planning to the educational possibilities, not only the nutritional aspects of diet choices but also courtesy, table manners, and polite dining-room behavior can be learned or reinforced.

Administration. Most school food service programs are controlled and administered by the school itself. In large school districts it is necessary to hire full-time food specialists. The educational authorities should be responsible for selecting the school lunch manager and other personnel. The manager is responsible for carrying out a program that is an integral part of the school health program and operates efficiently, providing an adequate and nutritious lunch under sanitary, attractive, and pleasant conditions. The training and supervision of the other food service workers is a parallel responsibility. Therefore the manager needs an understanding of nutrition, food buying, food preparation and care, and personnel management.

Enough time should be scheduled for lunch to allow food selection and eating at a leisurely pace. At least 20 minutes at the table should be allotted for elementary school children, with another 10 minutes for handwashing and passing from room to room. The earliest lunch hour should be 11:30 A.M. and the latest 12:30 P.M., with the youngest children served first.

Safety and Fire Prevention

More accidents involving children occur on school grounds or between school and home than anywhere else in the community. Safety precautions should be spelled out carefully and responsibility assigned for each specified procedure (Sorenson, 1985).

A school safety program should involve the identification of hazards, development of measures to prevent accidents, and regular inspection of such measures to check their continuing effectiveness and usage. Fire drills must be held regularly, and every member of the school staff must be thoroughly familiar with the location of fire exits and equipment, as well as being practiced in whatever responsibility has been assigned.

General recommendations for the development of a school safety program include an all-school safety council composed of teachers, students, and administrators to continually examine the school for hazardous situations and devise ways of preventing accidents.

A thorough plan for traffic safety, both inside and outside the school, must be worked out. Cooperation of the police can be obtained easily for installing traffic lights, marked crosswalks, and even for discussing with the children how to cross streets safely. Traffic inside the school must be regulated to ensure efficient movement where this is a pattern in a school (usually in middle schools only).

All school personnel should be required to study local laws and ordinances pertaining to school safety and fire prevention as well as those concerning liability for accidents. Subcommittees on safety might be appointed from among the students in upper elementary and middle school grades. Such committees could help direct the orderly response to a fire drill and could be given responsibility for monitoring safe practices in classrooms as appropriate.

Mental and Emotional Tone

The school health program depends on the willing cooperation of everyone concerned. Unless all teachers, administrators, and members of the staff do their work responsibly, competently, and with enthusiasm, the total program is diminished in effectiveness. The mental and emotional tone, or quality of the interpersonal environment, is crucial to every aspect of the program.

A good mental and emotional climate is one in which the morale of the teachers is high. They are relaxed and confident and enjoy their work, just as their students enjoy being in school. The classroom environment is conducive to learning. The room is orderly, and everyone cheerfully takes part in keeping it so. Pupils feel that they are accepted and respected as individuals by their teachers and by classmates. Both teachers and students are involved in setting standards for behavior and in finding solutions for school health problems. There is an active and welcome interest in the school on the part of the children's parents.

We've been describing the ideal environment. That some classrooms in some places fall short of that description (Mills, 1987) does not mean that it should not be continually sought as the goal.

Health of School Personnel

The health of the men and women who carry out the school's program is a crucial aspect of a school's environment. The primary consideration is, as always, protection of the child's health. Only persons should be employed in a school who are shown through medical and psychological tests to be free of emotional and physical disorders.

A teacher's health affects a student in many ways. Emotional health, and especially lack of it, can have a profound effect on the happiness and achievement of the children. An unhappy, frustrated, or emotionally disturbed teacher can create an atmosphere so full of hostility and tension that children fear coming to school (Sauls & Fuller, 1986).

A teacher's personal health behavior can be a more powerful influence than any lesson. For example, a teacher who is obese may be uncomfortable about teaching good nutrition habits or figure control and either avoid it or give little time to the topic. A teacher who comes to school obviously suffering from a severe case of common cold is teaching irresponsible behavior, at least by example, and at the same time endangering the health of everyone in the room.

The provision of facilities for rest, conferences, and sanitation promotes the health of faculty and staff. Work loads must be fair and equal. Arrangements for some free time each day are essential, particularly in the case of elementary school teachers, who in most schools work closely with the same students in one room for the entire day. The health of school personnel is not limited to the control of communicable diseases. It includes careful attention to the economic, social, and emotional well-being of teachers, as well as of every other school employee.

HEALTH INSTRUCTION

As health services are provided and the many aspects of a safe and sanitary school environment are experienced and enjoyed, learning something that relates to one's own health interests is an inevitable and concurrent happening. People learn by experience, and there is a wealth of health-related experiences in the two components of a school health program just described. Formal health instruction, involving curriculum development, lesson planning, classroom teaching techniques, and evaluation will be the focus of the remainder of this text. These elements of the teaching-learning tasks are common to all teaching, but health teaching is in many ways different, even unique. Its purposes are concerned with life style choices, not health information as an end in itself.

The aim of health instruction is to help students learn how to satisfy health-related urges and needs in ways that are constructive and responsible. Those are the more immediate, every-day actions that typically are taken without conscious thought. The important decisions, and there are few of those that do not affect health in some way, require problem-solving skills. These must be practiced and learned if the individual is not to be limited to choices based on trial and error or the conventional wisdom.

Health education is not accomplished through memorization and recitation of descriptions of diseases, body functions, and anatomy. Neither is it the outcome of single units of teaching focused on the health problems of the moment or year. In short, health instruction is not learning to say "no" to potentially life-threatening behaviors. It is learning to say "yes" to the choice of a life style that can enhance the quality of life and facilitate achievement of one's goals.

COMMUNITY HEALTH RESOURCES

The community resources available to help the health teacher are rich in quantity and available for the asking. Generally, community resource groups are categorized as (1) official, (2) voluntary, (3) professional, (4) private physicians and dentists, (5) industrial, (6) service clubs, (7) youth groups, (8) parent-teacher groups. Whatever the agency, group, or organization, their

interest in health makes them willing allies for health teaching. Find out what services and materials are easily available to you in your community. Pick those that complement the textbook you are using and use them in ways that will add to and broaden the scope of your students' health instruction.

Official health agencies are tax supported and responsible under law for the protection of the people within their jurisdiction. A public health agency may be local, state, or national in scope. A wide range of services, which vary to some degree depending on the budget, is available to all members of the community. A teacher might contact the health educator of a local public health office for a list of available films or other audiovisual aids or for consultation. A letter to the state health department asking for a catalogue of visual or written materials may open avenues to resources not available from the local office. At the national level the various health institutes, such as the National Cancer Institute, National Institute of Allergy and Infectious Diseases, and other branches of the U.S. Department of Health and Human Services, have large catalogues of pamphlets, booklets, and printed materials concerning health statistics and health problems in all age groups. Send a request for lists of available materials on school stationery, since a copy of such publications is usually free to teachers. You can also call one of the national clearinghouses for information (see Table 2-2).

Voluntary health agencies typically are concerned with a specific health problem or disease. They are supported by donations and organized and controlled by volunteers. A key purpose of such agencies is education about the health problem of their interest. Therefore certain amounts of the budget are allocated to the development and dissemination of educational materials. The American Cancer Society, American Heart Association, and National Society for

TABLE 2-2. Governmental agencies

Agency	Type of materials	Health topics	Levels
Environmental Protection Agency Forms and Publications Center Research Triangle Park, NC 27711 919/541-2111	Printed materials	Environmental health	General and adult
High Blood Pressure Information Center 1501 Wilson Blvd. Arlington, VA 22209 703/558-4880	Booklets	Disease prevention and control	General and adult
National Archives and Records Service General Services Administration National Audiovisual Center Washington, D.C. 20409 301/763-1896	Information lists Catalogues	Consumer health Drug use and abuse Environmental health Health careers Safety and first aid	General and adult
National Clearinghouse on Drug Abuse Information Room 10A56, Parklawn Building 5600 Fishers Lane Rockville, MD 20857 301/443-6500	Pamphlets Films	Drug use and abuse	General and adult
National Health Information Clearinghouse PO Box 1133 Washington, D.C. 20013 800/336-4797	Publications Pamphlets Answers specific questions on telephone	Alcohol and smoking Consumer health Disease prevention and control Drug use and abuse Family life Mental health Physical fitness Personal health Safety	General and adult
National Heart, Lung and Blood Institute 9000 Rockville Pike National Institutes of Health Bldg. 31/4 A24 Bethesda, MD 20205 301/496-1051	Printed materials	Disease prevention and control Nutrition	General and adult
National Highway Traffic Safety Administration U.S. Department of Transportation Washington, D.C. 20590 202/426-1828	Printed materials	Alcohol Safety	General and adult

TABLE 2-2. Governmental agencies—cont'd

Agency	Type of materials	Health topics	Levels
National Institute on Alcohol Abuse and Alcoholism National Institutes of Mental Health 5600 Fishers Lane Rockville, MD 20857 301/468-2600	Pamphlets Reprints	Alcohol	General and adult
National Institute of Dental Research National Institutes of Health Bldg. 31/2 C34 Bethesda, MD 20205 301/496-4261	Pamphlets	Nutrition Personal health	J J General and adult
Office on Smoking and Health Room 1-10, Park Building 5600 Fishers Lane Rockville, MD 20857 301/443-1690	Technical information center	Smoking	General and adult
Public Documents Distribution Center Department 20 Pueblo, CO 81009	Pamphlets		General and adult
Public Health Service Environmental Health Service U.S. Department of Health, Education, and Welfare Rockville, MD 20857 301/881-1870	Pamphlets Reprints	Environmental health	General and adult
Superintendent of Documents U.S. Government Printing Office Washington, D.C. 20402 202/783-3238	Pamphlets Posters	Alcohol Community health Disease prevention and control Drug use and abuse Environmental health Growth and development Nutrition Personal health (dental) Safety and first aid Smoking	J I,J I,J I J P,I K,P,I,J
U.S. Center for Health Promotion and Education Centers for Disease Control 1600 Clifton Atlanta, GA 30333 404/633-3311	Printed materials	General health education	General and adult
U.S. Office of Health Information and Health Promotion Hubert Humphrey Building 200 Independence Ave. S.W. Washington, D.C. 20201 202/655-4000	Printed materials	General health education	General and adult

Crippled Children and Adults are some of those that commonly have offices in major cities. Materials such as films, posters, pamphlets, charts, and student workbooks and worksheets often are printed in several languages. Speakers bureaus are another frequently available service. All these aids are readily obtainable, often with no more effort than a telephone call to the nearest office. If a voluntary agency has no local listing, write to the national office and ask for the address of the chapter or office nearest your home or school (see Table 2-3).

Professional health organizations include local medical, dental, nursing, or educational associations and, at the national level, the American Medical Association (AMA), the National Education Association (NEA), the American Dental Association (ADA), and the American Nurse's Association (ANA). The AMA, in association with the NEA, for many years produced a host of significant references and resources for school health. *Health Services* (1964) and *Healthful School Living* (1969) remain the classic references regarding these two aspects of the school health program.

Several national professional organizations specifically focus on health education in schools. These are the Association for the Advancement of Health Education (AAHE), the American School Health Association (ASHA), and the School Health Education and Services section of the American Public Health Association (SHES/APHA). The membership of these organizations includes health teachers, school physicians and nurses, and other individuals whose primary concern is the health and health education of children and youth. Teachers can benefit in many ways through affiliation with one or more of these groups. Some of the advantages include the potential for keeping up to date through the articles in the journals, as well as through meetings with teachers with similar

interests at regional and national meetings. In addition, position papers, curriculum guides, and other resource materials are regularly developed or updated and made available.

Locally, a teacher might obtain classroom subscriptions to health-related magazines and journals through the cooperation of the medical society. A teacher might interest a dental group in promoting a dental hygiene campaign by classroom demonstrations and examinations. Nursing groups might be persuaded to provide volunteers for schools in which such services are limited or to provide resource persons for the school health instruction program.

Private physicians and dentists and other local health advisers are a potential source of information, as well as service in special situations. Private practitioners who are parents of children in a school often are willing to serve as resource persons, to explain health problems to children, or to provide a field trip experience for a class. For instance, a dentist might allow a group of children to visit the office to view the equipment used in that work and to explain its function in the maintenance and promotion of oral health. Children would be far more likely to develop positive attitudes toward dentists and dental services after such an experience (Smardo, 1986).

These are but a few of the ways community resources can be used in health teaching. The public library and reference librarian are also community resources. The familiar *Yellow Pages* directory supplies the addresses and telephone numbers of most health-related organizations. A classroom without walls can be a reality if a teacher will just open the door to the abundance of community resources available for use in the classroom and outside the school.

Industrial organizations, either individually or with others, have developed a great number of instructional aids specifically for use in

Text continued on p. 60.

TABLE 2-3. Voluntary and nonprofit health agencies

Agency	Type of materials	Health topics	Levels	Comments
Agency for Instructional Television 1111 W. 17th St. Bloomington, IN 47401 812/339-2203	Films Videocassettes	Mental and emotional health Safety Social health	General and adult	
American Cancer Society, Inc. (national headquarters) 777 Third Ave. New York, NY 10017 212/371-2900	Program packages: *Early Start to Good Health* (K-3); *Health Network* (4-6) Other instructional kits Films and guides Pamphlets Posters	Community health Consumer health Disease prevention and control Drugs, alcohol, and to-bacco Family life Growth and development Mental and emotional health Nutrition Personal health	K,P,I,J J P,I,J P,I,J K,P,I K,P,I,J K,P,I,J I K,P,I,J	Contact local chapter
American Heart Association (national headquarters) The National Center 7320 Greenville Ave. Dallas, TX 75231 214/750-5300	Program packages: *Take Care of Your Heart; One Heart for Life* Brochures Pamphlets Films and filmstrips Cassettes Games Posters Photographic slides	Consumer health Disease prevention and control Drug use and abuse First aid Growth and development Nutrition Personal health	J J K,P,I J K,P,I,J K,P,I,J K,P,I	Contact local chapter
American Lung Association (national headquarters) 1740 Broadway New York, NY 10019 212/245-8000	Program packages: *Lung Health Module* Films Literature and periodi-cals Posters Buttons and stickers Slides and cassettes	Community health Disease prevention and control Growth and development Environmental health	J P J	Contact local supplier

Continued.

TABLE 2-3. Voluntary and nonprofit health agencies—cont'd

Agency	Type of materials	Health topics	Levels	Comments
American Red Cross National Head-quarters 17th and E Sts. N.W. Washington, D.C. 20006 202/737-8300	Educational series on blood and circulatory system Films and filmstrips Pamphlets and leaflets Textbooks Posters	Community health Consumer health Family life Growth and development Mental and emotional health Personal health Safety and first aid	K,P J I,J K,P,I,J P,I I,J K,P,I,J	Contact local chapter
Arthritis Foundation (national head-quarters) 3400 Peachtree Rd. N.E., suite 1101 Atlanta, GA 30326 404/266-0795	Pamphlets Reprints	Disease prevention and control	P,I,J	
Asthma and Allergy Foundation of America 9604 Wisconsin Ave., suite 100 Bethesda, MD 20814 301/493-6552	Pamphlets Films	Disease prevention and control Growth and development	General and adult	
Cystic Fibrosis Foundation (national headquarters) 6000 Executive Blvd., suite 309 Rockville, MD 20852 301/881-9130	Leaflets and pamphlets Films	Disease prevention and control Growth and development	General and adult	
Epilepsy Foundation of America 1828 L St. N.W., suite 406 Washington, D.C. 20036 202/293-2930	Pamphlets Paperback books Films Cassettes Slides	Disease prevention and control	General and adult	

Organization	Materials	Content areas	Grade level	Notes
Health Education Service, Inc. PO Box 7126 Albany, NY 12224 518/392-3951	Pamphlets Posters Videotapes	Family life Personal health (dental) Safety and first aid	J K,P I	Some materials available in Spanish
March of Dimes—Birth Defects Foundation 1275 Mamaroneck Ave. PO Box 2000 White Plains, NY 10602 914/428-7100	Program packages: *Starting a Healthy Family* (Units I, II, III); *Preparenthood Education Program (PEP)* Films and filmstrips Pamphlets	Consumer health Disease prevention and control Drug use and abuse First aid Growth and development Nutrition Personal health	J J K,P,I J K,P,I,J K,P,I,J K,P,I	Contact local office
Mental Health Materials Center 30 E. 29th St. New York, NY 10016 212/889-5760	Pamphlets Films	Family life Growth and development Mental and emotional health Personal health	General and adult	
Muscular Dystrophy Association (national headquarters) 810 Seventh Ave., 27th floor New York, NY 10019 212/586-0808	Pamphlets Films	Disease prevention and control	P	
National Association for Sickle Cell Disease, Inc. 3460 Wilshire Blvd., suite 1012 Los Angeles, CA 90010 212/731-1166	Fact sheets Brochures	Disease prevention and control	I	

Continued.

TABLE 2-3. Voluntary and nonprofit health agencies—cont'd

Agency	Type of materials	Health topics	Levels	Comments
National Congress of Parents and Teachers (NCPT) 700 N. Rush St. Chicago, IL 60611 312/787-0977	Program package: *Alcohol Alley* Health education curricula Pamphlets	Consumer health Community health Disease prevention and control Drug use and abuse Environmental health Family life Growth and development Mental and emotional health Nutrition Personal health Safety and first aid	General and adult	
National Council on Alcoholism, Inc. Publications Department 733 Third Ave., suite 1405 New York, NY 10017 212/986-4433	Pamphlets Books	Alcohol	General and adult	
National Easter Seal Society for Crippled Children and Adults 2023 W. Ogden Ave. Chicago, IL 60612 312/243-8400	Pamphlets	Dental health Disease prevention and control Growth and development Safety	General and adult	
National Health Council 70 W. 40th St. New York, NY 10018 212/869-8100	Pamphlets	Health careers	General and adult	
National Safety Council 425 N. Michigan Ave. Chicago, IL 60611 312/527-4800	Films Pamphlets Posters	Safety	General and adult	

Source	Materials	Topics	Level	Availability
National Society to Prevent Blindness (NSPB) (national headquarters) 79 Madison Ave. New York, NY 10016 212/684-3505	Pamphlet Films Charts	Disease prevention and control Growth and development Safety and first aid	P P P	Contact local affiliate
Public Affairs Committee, Inc. 381 Park Ave. S. New York, NY 10016 212/683-4331	Pamphlets Filmstrips	Alcohol Community health Dental health Disease prevention and control Drug use and abuse Family life Growth and development Health careers Mental health Nutrition Personal health Safety and first aid Smoking	General and adult	
United Cerebral Palsy Association, Inc. (national headquarters) 66 E. 34th St. New York, NY 10016 212/677-7400	Pamphlets	Disease prevention and control	General and adult	Contact local office
Wisconsin Clearinghouse for Alcohol and Other Drug Information 1954 E. Washington Ave. Madison, WI 53704-5271 608/263-2797	Pamphlets and booklets Fact sheets Posters	Drug use and abuse Family life Mental and emotional health Safety and first aid	J P,I,J I,J J	

schools. For example, the Metropolitan Life Insurance Company has materials for use at every level of health education, from kindergarten through grade 12. The National Dairy Council, representing the nation's milk industry, allocates a major portion of its budget to nutrition education. Their materials are not limited to the promotion of milk products but cover all aspects of nutrition. The teaching aids developed by this group are creative, dynamic, and educationally sound. National Dairy Council nutritionists frequently will assist with inservice education or even give demonstrations in some areas of the country. Other cooperative groups such as the Cereal Institute and the National Livestock and Meat Board also provide some teaching aids and student materials related to nutrition in general and their products in particular.

Most large industrial organizations are very concerned with safety, and many also are directing attention to alcoholism because of the impact this problem has on the performance of otherwise competent employees. It might be possible either to arrange a field trip to learn about their safety program or to persuade the safety or medical director to visit the school to describe such a program and its applications in a school or home. Toothpaste manufacturers often offer dental hygiene training kits or sound-assisted filmstrips designed to teach young children oral health-care techniques. Charts, booklets, and other materials useful in teaching about menstruation are free to the teacher who requests them from companies such as Kimberly-Clark and the Tambrand Corporation. The Kaiser Health Plan sponsors regional dramatic presentations titled "Professor Body-wise" on health topics for elementary students.

In short, there is no limit to the kinds of free or inexpensive teaching aids that can be obtained from commercial organizations. The main thing to be guarded against is the possi-

bility that some aspect of the material may not be acceptable in terms of district policy. It is prudent to preview any teaching aids obtained from resources outside the school to be certain that no objectionable advertising copy is included and that it is appropriate for use with the age group for which you are responsible.

Service clubs such as the Elks, Lions, Kiwanis, Shriners, Optimists, and others, although primarily social in purpose, always include community service as an integral part of their programs; hence the name *service* is used to describe them. Usually a specific health problem is chosen as the club's specific interest. For example, tiny white canes are given by the Lion's Club to those who donate money for service to the blind. Antidrug education is another project sponsored by the Lions. The Elks club raises money to fight cerebral palsy. The Shriners' annual charity football games or parades provide the money to support their hospitals for the care and treatment of burned or crippled children. A teacher should make a point of finding out what local service clubs can be called on to assist in solving a health problem that hinders or prevents a youngster from learning.

Youth groups, although composed of children and youth, are administered by community-based organizations and personnel. These include the Boy Scouts, Girl Scouts, Campfire Girls, Y-Guides, 4H Clubs, and church clubs. The programs of such groups are usually committed to the promotion of health in any way they can. A teacher might ask for their help in organizing fire prevention surveys, in participating or leading environmental clean-up projects, in serving as crossing guards, and in teaching younger children safety procedures or other positive health behaviors. The possibilities are limited only by the imagination and interest of the teacher.

Parent-teacher groups, such as the National Congress of Parents and Teachers

(NCPT), are another kind of organization whose members are derived from both community and school. The NCPT is dedicated to the health of school children. It has spearheaded the drive to secure national legislation supporting and promoting comprehensive school health education. On the local level, the chairperson of the health committee in particular is ready to help in any way possible. That person should be invited to serve as a regular member of the school health council. Parent members are often willing to assist with field trip arrangements and to help solve individual problems, such as a lack of adequate shoes, clothing, or health services of some kind. Parent members can be called on to provide materials that can be used for health teaching, such as discarded magazines for clipping pictures or health-related advertisements, to make costumes for school health dramatizations, or to raise money for needed teaching aids by selling fruit or other foods on school grounds as permitted by school policy or health laws.

School-Community Liaison Groups

Community health council. The eight kinds of community-based groups just discussed are possible sources of assistance for those administering a school health program. However, there are too many community-based organizations in most areas for a school to approach on a one-by-one basis. In these cases a cooperative body such as a community health council may be the answer. It ensures representation, at least on a rotating basis, of all eight kinds of agencies, and it provides a mechanism for mobilizing community resources to assist the school with problems that threaten the health or safety of teachers or students. Added community representation can be obtained by including religious leaders, interested and qualified civic leaders, and specialists from related fields such as law enforcement, social work, and recreation.

Whatever the problem or need brought to the council, each member can consult with the larger group that is represented and bring back suggestions or offers of assistance.

School health committee. Just as a community health council is a representative body of agencies and individuals interested in promoting community health, so a school health committee is a representative group of individuals interested in promoting and protecting the well-being of the child while at school.

In districts where a school health committee is in operation, it functions as a coordinating body. It has no regulatory powers but can only make recommendations to the administration. Membership is drawn from the administration, faculty, staff, student body, and parents. It may include the principal or a designee of the administration, school nurse, custodian, dietitian or food service manager, and selected teachers with expressed interest in health education. The most important aspect is the student representation. All people, including children, are better able to understand and accept new rules or requirements if they have had a voice in their development.

A school health committee functions as a data-gathering, problem-solving body. The problems are brought to it by administrators, teachers, crossing guards, bus drivers, parents, or staff. Its function is to analyze the problems and determine possible solutions. The kinds of problems that a school health committee might be asked to study are as varied as human behavior, including prevention of drug abuse among students, prevention of spray-can graffiti on school walls, control of a school wide epidemic of the flu, coping with vandalism of school property or facilities, and even establishment of a school dress code. Whatever the problem, a school health committee can be an effective mechanism for dealing with it.

A school health committee can be organized

informally, so that a member is always free to solve the problem individually but follows the agreed upon channels of communication when doing so. It can be an ad hoc committee that is disbanded once the problem has been solved. The third and best pattern is as a formal, continuing committee that functions as a problem-solving, recommending body when necessary and works to smooth any conflict that arises between school policy and shifts in community needs.

In some situations it may be advantageous to form a health council that represents both school and community. The school is part of the community, and many problems have aspects that need the expertise and knowledge available from both sources. Often the school's cooperation is essential to the solution of a problem that lies in the community, or a community crisis may lead to renewed emphasis on the school health program. The AIDS epidemic is an example of such a joint need and resulting educational effort. A drawback in combining two such bodies is that the resulting coalition may be so large that it is unwieldy. Perhaps a better solution would be to select an advisory group from the membership of each council to serve in that capacity whenever called on by the other.

In any case the development and implementation of a school health program never can be a unilateral task; it is a shared responsibility of the home, school, and community. Each has a role in the education of children, in promoting and protecting their health, and in shaping and protecting the environment in which they must live and learn.

SUMMARY

The comprehensiveness of a school health program is defined by the quality and quantity of the activities, procedures, facilities, and services provided by means of its three basic program components (i.e., health instruction, health services, and a healthful environment). Every school in the nation has some kind of a school health program; however, not all of them can be described as comprehensive. There are several reasons for the differences that exist. Briefly, these can be categorized as related to legal considerations, local school policies, budgetary constraints, community needs and concerns, and the philosophy of local decision makers regarding the worth or need for a given aspect of the program. Often more than one of these has influenced the nature of an existing program.

State and sometimes federal legislation have an impact on school health programs. For example, in order to receive federal financing for the school lunch program, the menus must include specified amounts and kinds of foods representative of the four food groups. Federal law and supporting funds are responsible for the establishment currently of nationwide special education programs for handicapped children. Health education curriculum projects have been funded and disseminated with the help of federal funds and supervision of federal agencies.

State requirements as spelled out in an education code and in a health and safety code affect school health programs significantly, depending on whether they specify health services, environmental protection or controls, or health instruction. Of the three, legislation concerning instruction is typically least restrictive, and even when instructional programs are mandated, their implementation is not often monitored or enforced. At the elementary level, recommendations for health instruction tend to be ambiguous and global. They speak of teaching "health habits" and promoting "good moral behavior." However, state health and safety code provisions are usually specific, and many of them are universally required among the states. This is because they deal with health problems that might either endanger the health and safety of students and school personnel or in some way hinder a child's potential for learning.

School policies, whether established at district level or specific to a particular school, have far more impact on health instruction than on health services and environmental aspects of the program. Education in this country has always been subject to local control; hence the quality and quantity of health instruction vary widely among districts and sometimes even among schools in the same district. Mandated health services and environmental standards usually are provided at least at required minimum levels. How much beyond those minimums a school goes in building its program depends on local school policy as a rule.

Budgetary constraints affect the quality of a program. However desirable it might be to employ enough qualified school nurses to carry out appraisal procedures, to be quickly available to meet emergency needs, to provide student counseling, and to supplement instructional services, many school districts have severely cut the number of such specialists. There is seldom enough money to support a nursing staff of that size. Similarly, purchase of materials and resources for health instruction or even the employment of health teaching specialists as district health coordinators or teachers is more often tied to cost considerations than to need or value.

Community needs and pressures can be a positive or a negative force when a school health program is being planned. When the incidence of some health problem becomes critical, typically a public clamor arises for education designed to alleviate that problem. If it is a new problem, then the schools try to respond to the public's concern by fitting the new topic into the existing curriculum. On the other hand, sometimes the public outcry focuses on removing some health topic from consideration by the schools. More often the vote is divided. Usually the fewer who urge a change, the louder their voices will be.

The school is required to meet community needs and interests. School administrators have the problem of deciding whose wishes should be satisfied. Whoever that may be, the change will have been wrought by the community. Sex education is a perennial case in point. Whether or not any education concerned with human sexuality should be provided young people is controversial even at the secondary level. But now AIDS is so terrifying a problem that the surgeon general has strongly urged that information on the mode of transmission and method of prevention be provided starting as early as third grade. Many adults will support this recommendation; many will not. Undoubtedly the decisions that will be made will vary from one school district to another.

Community health agencies interested in a specific health disorder or disability often devote time and money to devising educational materials devoted to teaching children what it is believed they need to know about their particular concern. Understandably, such agencies want to see those materials at work, and so they put pressure on school authorities to include them in the curriculum of some school discipline, usually health education if possible.

It is entirely appropriate that a school health program be based upon knowledge of student and community needs and, to the extent possible, represent the activities needed to meet them. But it takes a nice balance between what is possible and feasible and what is beyond the purview of the schools as the instrument of so great a responsibility.

The Edward B. Johns' chart depicted in Figure 2-1 graphically illustrates a model school health program. If a school provides those services competently, maintains the safety, sanitation, and comfort of the children and adults who live and work in its environment, provides health instruction appropriate to the needs and interests of its students, cooperates effectively with interested community agencies, and maintains positive relationships with parents and other community leaders, then it can be described as a comprehensive school health program. As a prospective teacher you should be able to describe a quality program and anticipate the very real contribution that you will be able to make in your new role.

QUESTIONS AND EXERCISES

Discussion questions

1. Elementary teachers are expected to teach a full curriculum specified for any given grade level. Why should they also be concerned with health services or the quality of the school's environment? What is the relevance of attention to these aspects of the school program to instruction?

2. Why is teacher observation so crucial a factor in the maintenance and promotion of student learning and health?

3. The principal purposes of the total school health program are to maintain, protect, and promote the health of the child. For each of the components of that program (health services, healthful environment, and health instruction) describe at least four specific functions with which teachers are directly involved or responsible.

4. If you suspected that a student was in need of protection from what appeared to be child abuse, the symptoms of which were more behavioral than physical, what would be the best thing to do, both professionally and legally?

5. Which is the more important service to students and their parents that a classroom teacher can provide: guidance or counseling? How might the nature of the problem affect your answer to that question?

6. Should the same nutritional standards required of a federally sponsored school lunch menu be applied to the selection of snack foods supplied by vending machines on school grounds? Why or why not? Defend your point of view with specific arguments.

7. If you were asked to recommend the ten most essential members of a school-community liaison group, whom would you list? What would be your rationale for those choices?

Exercises and problems

1. Prepare a bibliography of at least six key references on school health that could be used when setting up a functional school health program. Explain your choices on the basis of their authorship, subject matter, and potential long-term validity as resources.

2. Visit an elementary school and arrange to interview the principal or other school administrator on school policy relative to emergency care and disaster control. Is safety education provided, if so, what is the nature of that instruction and how is it carried out? Is there an established plan of action? Is every school worker familiar with his or her responsibilities in the event of an emergency? If possible, obtain a copy of the plan and check to see if it satisfies the suggestions made in this text or others dealing with safety in schools.

3. Familiarize yourself with the dry brushing technique for classroom practice. Write or call your nearest dental association for suggestions regarding sources of classroom sets of free brushes, disclosing wafers, or educational pamphlets. Then offer to instruct one or more elementary school classes in the procedure, and write a short report of the entire experience. What did you learn about teaching children how to do something as opposed to teaching them facts? Would you do anything differently another time?

4. Inspect an elementary school building or at least the building in which your education class is being held. Are public telephones, drinking fountains, toilets and wash basins, aisles between desks, cafeteria counters, or other facilities reachable by a person in a wheel chair? In a short paper, describe any problems you identify and list possible solutions.

5. As a second-grade teacher you have observed that one of your students often squints when looking at the chalkboard and soon loses interest when required to read at that distance. His health record shows that last year his eyes were tested and recorded as 20/40, but the most recent test showed visual acuity of 20/20. Should the child be referred for a more comprehensive examination at this time? Why or why not?

6. Consider the following health problems often encountered by a teacher of elementary school children, and name a community group who might assist in solving each.

   a. You have been asked to serve as the school coordinator of health instruction, and you want to obtain relevant and up-to-date films or other resource materials for use in setting up an inservice program.

   b. A school nurse is asked to present instruction regarding menstruation to fifth-grade classes and wants some pamphlets and charts appropriate for this purpose.

   c. A school wishes to set up a peer group–conducted street-crossing safety program.

   d. A class wishes to take a field trip and needs help with local transportation and supervision during the trip.

   e. The school nurse discovers that many of the children in a school have a great need for dental care. Many factors are involved in the problem such as economics, ignorance, and malnutrition.

   f. In order to comply with community pressure to begin some instruction in the elementary school relative to the prevention of AIDS, a school principal wishes to arrange appropriate instruction for all of the faculty as a first step in such an endeavor.

7. You are asked by your principal to serve as the convening chairperson of a new school health committee. There being no specialists on the school faculty, presumably every teacher is equally competent to serve. What criteria might you consider for use in choosing among the school teachers, and which members of the total staff would you select as most representative of the total school program?

REFERENCES

American Academy of Pediatrics, Committee on School Health: School health: a guide for health professionals, Elk Grove Village, Ill, 1987, AAP.

American Dental Association: Diet and dental health, Chicago 1986, ADA.

Appleboom T: A history of vision screening, J Sch Health 55(4):138-41, 1985.

California Association of Ophthalmology: The vision screening committee, as cited by Orange County Department of Education, California, 1985.

California State Education Administration Code (CFR) Title 5-15558, 1987 required school lunch menus for federal support.

Condition of education, statistical report, Washington, DC, 1981, National Center for Statistics, US Department of Education.

Condition of education, statistical report, Washington, DC, 1987, National Center for Statistics, US Department of Education, p 182.

Dairy Council of California: Asian foods guide for teachers, Fall 1981.

Frager A: Toward improved instruction in hearing health at the elementary level, J of Sch Health 56(5):166-169, 1986.

Fraser B: The educator and child abuse, Chicago, 1979, National Committee for Prevention of Child Abuse.

Hernandez M and others: Valor nutritivo de les alimentes Mexicanos, Mexico City, DF, 1972, Instituto Nacional de la Nutricion.

Hinkle M: A mixed message: the school vending machine, J Sch Health 52:1 1982.

Horowitz L and others: Self-care motivation: a model for primary preventive oral health behavior change, J Sch Health 57(3):114-118, 1987.

Houle B: The impact of long-term dental health education on oral hygiene behavior, J Sch Health 52(4):256-261, 1982.

Joint Committee on Health Problems in Education: Healthful school environment, Washington, DC, 1969, NEA-AMA.

Joint Committee on Health Problems in Education: School health services, Washington, DC, 1964, NEA-AMA.

Kolbe L and others: School health in America, ed. 4, Kent, Ohio, 1987, ASHA.

Lee J: Daily dry toothbrushing in kindergarten, J Sch Health 50(9):506-509, 1980.

Los Angeles Times: Where the ouch went, part II, p 8, June 25, 1988.

Mills M: Classrooms in Compton cited as "horrible" by NEA chief, Los Angeles Times, part CC, p 1, May 28, 1987.

National Professional School Health Education Organizations: Comprehensive school health education: a definition, J Sch Health 54(8):312-315, 1984.

Newman I: Integrating health services and health education: seeking a balance, J Sch Health 52(8):490-501, 1982.

Noak M: State policy support for health education, Denver, 1982, Education Commission of the States.

Rabich T and others: The need for dental health screening and referral programs, J Sch Health 52(1):50-52, 1982.

Sauls C and Fuller A: School phobia: a paralyzing fear in a child's life, Early Years 17(1):88-90, 1986.

Scheiber B: Parents campaign for handicapped children and youth, Closer Look, Washington, DC, 1981.

Smardo F: Dental health of young children: how can we help them cope? Health Values 9:3, May-June 1985.

Sorenson E: Plan to prevent accidents, A Sch Board J 72:6, June 1985.

Tower C: Child abuse and neglect, Washington, DC 1984, NEA.

SUGGESTED READINGS

American Academy of Pediatrics, Committee on School Health: School health: A guide for health professionals, Elk Grove Village, Ill, 1987, AAP. Designed as reference for physicians, school nurses, teachers, and school administrators to help them understand how their roles interact. Purpose is to enable them to work together more effectively to help children remain healthy and benefit from their schooling. Covers functions and responsibilities of all personnel in school health program. Discusses characteristics and problems of school children, K through 12, appraisals, communicable disease control, and administration of total program including physical education and sports.

Andersen R and others: Infections in children: a source book for educators and child care providers. Rockville, Md 1986, Aspen Publishers, Inc. An easy-to-read, practical guide relative to many of the infectious diseases of childhood. Gives information on factors involved in disease development and spread; recommends immunizations and other control measures; describes usual treatment and patient care measures. Appendices include parent information handouts, glossary of terms, suggested additional readings, and lists of resources and agencies that may be contacted for assistance or further information.

Benenson, AS, editor: Control of communicable diseases in man, ed 14, Washington, DC 1985, American Public Health Association. Provides concise information on clinical nature, means of transmission, communicability, recommended care and preventive measures relative to 200 communicable diseases, including 12 separate reference pages dealing with AIDS.

Kolbe L and others: School health in America, ed 4, Kent, Ohio, 1987, ASHA. An assessment of state policies to protect and improve the health of students in kindergarten through twelfth grade. Provides data expressed as numbers and percentages of states including the District of Columbia. Reports the requirements and provisions for health instruction, health services, and a healthful school environment. Appendices present the survey instruments employed.

Lewis K and Thomson H: Manual of school health, Reading, Mass, 1986, Addison-Wesley. Prepared for use by nurses in school and community settings, but useful for anyone working in school health program. Summarizes practical information about children's and adolescents' health as affected by and affecting the school setting. Includes chapters on growth and development, vision and hearing, acute conditions, chronic conditions, drug and alcohol abuse, special education, and first aid.

McKenzie JF: Twelve steps in developing a school site health education promotion program for faculty and staff, J Sch Health, 58(4):149-153, 1988. It is asserted that a truly comprehensive school health program is concerned not solely with maintaining and promoting the health of students alone, but with that of faculty and staff as well. A framework of procedural steps for the guidance of school districts wishing to develop health promotion programs for faculty and staff is proposed for school site implementation. Although it can be argued that those steps might be better and more logically sequenced, they *do* nicely and succinctly cover those that must be included. Valuable cross references to the literature of workplace health education/promotion are listed.

Redican, K and others: Organization of school health programs, New York, 1986, Macmillan. Provides a vastly expanded discussion of the comprehensive school health program just outlined here. Organized into four sections: foundations, environment, services, and instruction. Each of these sections is carefully and thoroughly explored. Provides a current and balanced treatment and description of the total program.

Tower C: Child abuse and neglect, Washington, DC, 1984, National Education Association. An excellent and practical handbook for teacher use in detecting, reporting, and teaching children their rights and how to cope with abuse should it be a problem. Appendices provide further information by means of succinctly developed listings of resources, forms, immunity reporting laws, and more.

CHAPTER 3

Planning and Organizing the Health Curriculum

When you finish this chapter you should be able to:

- **Define the meanings of *planning* and *organizing* as they refer to curriculum development.**

- **Interpret the role of a school's philosophy of health education in determining scope.**

- **Compare advantages and disadvantages of using any particular curriculum design.**

- **Explain the teacher's special role in planning and organizing a curriculum for teaching.**

- **Describe ways to investigate each of the primary sources of the curriculum.**

- **Predict changes in children's health needs and interests as they grow and develop during elementary school years.**

- **Differentiate between horizontal and vertical organization of the scope of a discipline.**

- **Develop a feasible cycle plan for a selected level of elementary school health instruction.**

Planning and organizing are so closely related in their purposes that it is difficult to define where one leaves off and the other begins. Both are involved when decisions affecting the curriculum must be made. Generally, **planning** is concerned with determining the long-range goals and instructional objectives of teaching, and with designing effective means of attaining them. **Organizing** involves decisions defining the scope and sequence of the plans for teaching and learning.

Effective planning for health teaching depends on the worth and feasibility of proposed goals. Worthwhile goals must be synthesized from data gathered through careful investigation of three principal sources (Tyler, 1949). These are (1) the needs, interests, abilities, and concerns of the learners; (2) the culture and the community in which they must learn to live and to contribute effectively as citizens; and (3) the body of knowledge believed to be essential to the development of a person who is health educated. These are the sources fundamental to curriculum decision making in any discipline, yet in no field are the data generated through study of these sources more crucial than in health education. This is because we are basing teaching plans on the needs and concerns of real people, on human behaviors, and often on solvable or preventable community problems. The more current the curriculum, the more meaningful and the more transferable the learning.

By definition, goals are long-range plans. No one lesson or single course can assure their attainment. As a result, goals provide stability to a program so that instructional objectives there expressed at course- or lesson-planning levels can be responsive to what is relevant to a particular group of students yet, at the same time, can contribute to achievement of the broader aims. If thoughtfully derived goals are lacking, regardless of how unique or entertaining the lessons might be, it is like taking a trip without any destination in mind. It should not be surprising, in that case, if the teaching ends up nowhere and the students cannot tell you what they have learned or even what the purpose of the activity must have been.

The Aims of Health Instruction

In planning for effective teaching and learning a clear definition of aims is essential. The principal aim of school health instruction is to promote favorable health behavior. Broadly, the aim is to help children learn how to choose actions that enhance and protect health rather than the reverse. The acquisition of knowledge and the development of positive attitudes and beliefs about health and health behavior are also important goals. To impart information is easy, but whether that information will have much influence on a student's life style choices depends in part on the way it was acquired and also upon a variety of other factors over which no teacher has much control. For example, knowledge of the four food groups will have to vie with peer group pressures, cultural and family preferences, budgetary constraints, eating habits, and other forces affecting a youngster's dietary choices.

Attitudes and beliefs about health and the effects of unhealthful behaviors also determine what a person does in a given situation. Children come to school with a great many attitudes already firmly established. Still, these can be modified by learning new information. Knowledge that seems vital to a child because it has to do with his or her own concerns and interests is more apt to promote changes in behavior or attitudes than information having no apparent significance in real life.

The aims of health education might be expressed as follows:

1. To promote health behavior (choices, actions, habits) that is favorable to the development of a positive lifestyle.
2. To foster development of a well-balanced personality, based on a realistic acceptance of one's limitations as well as one's capacities.
3. To clarify misconceptions, remove superstitions, and provide accurate information about personal and public health matters.
4. To contribute to the health of the community through the development of health-educated citizens who will support future health measures intended to protect and promote the common good.
5. To develop ability in students to see causes and effects on health, to take preventive or remedial steps when possible, and thus to lengthen and improve the quality of life.

THE SOURCES OF THE HEALTH CURRICULUM

Planning a curriculum that is likely to help individuals achieve personally satisfying goals is difficult, as is devising learning opportunities relevant to present needs and issues. Added to these problems is the teacher's perennial dilemma—that is, how to create an educational program that has meaning for one's students and that can help them prepare to live effectively in a society that changes so rapidly. The kind of education that can facilitate the development of human capabilities must be directly related to the world outside of the school. The questions that need to be asked are: Who is to be educated? What does that person *need* and *want* to know about health? What are the important ideas that health education authorities believe are representative of its body of knowledge? How can these ideas become a functional part

of the learner's personal framework of knowledge? What skills are needed by and what behaviors are expected of members of our society?

Needs of the Learners

The primary source of data from which educational goals can be inferred is the learner—the needs, interests, concerns, the stage of maturation, skills, and abilities of the student.

Needs can be looked at in several ways. Some view a **need** as the degree to which the present condition of the individual differs from some acceptable norm. An educational objective based on this notion of a need would focus on a plan to provide learning opportunities designed to fill this gap—that is, to teach them what they need to know. Measurement of knowledge or its lack is probably the easiest aspect of needs assessment (see Chapters 6 and 7 for a detailed discussion of measurement techniques).

Another kind of need is reflected in the natural urge to maintain a balance between internal human drives and external conditions. These are the physiological needs such as those for food, water, and warmth; psychological needs such as those for affection, status, and belongingness; and integrative needs such as those for feelings of identity, self-fulfillment, and self-respect.

A third kind of need is revealed by the learner's interests and concerns. Felt needs are more readily identified, and it is easier to plan lessons that meet them. Planning lessons focused on needs that are not felt at all is more challenging. Children may need to know which people help keep them healthy and what they do to help, but recent studies show that this is a topic of little or no interest to children at all grade levels (Trucano, 1984).

Ways to identify needs. Considerable research has shown that similar needs are likely to be shared by children of the same age, developmental level, or sex living in the United States. A classic study carried out in Denver from 1948 to 1954 surveyed children, parents, and teachers on the health interests of 3,600 schoolchildren representative of a total school population of about 50,000. Analysis of the responses obtained showed that there was a consistent pattern of shifting interests that paralleled expected and actual physical and social development in these children (Denver Public Schools, 1954).

In 1969 a landmark Connecticut survey of student health interests was conducted that asked some 5,000 schoolchildren what they wanted to know about health (Byler, Lewis, and Totman, 1969). The findings were categorized by topics and in relation to age groups. Three main groups of age levels at the elementary level and another at the middle school level will be of interest to the elementary teacher.

As expected, interests of the very young child (kindergarten through grade 2) were found to be concrete and concerned with the here and now. Their questions tended to focus on "how" and "what." Many were directly related to their own health, growth, and development (e.g., "How does my heart beat?" "What makes the bones?" "How do you get colds?"). By grades 3 and 4 interest in the details of the entire body rises steadily. These youngsters want to know "how many" and "why" (e.g., "How many gallons of blood are there in my body?" "Why do we lose baby teeth?"). They want to know how the body works. Children in grades 5 and 6 continue to have great interest in the body, especially the organs, asking questions such as "How does the mind work?" and "What is inside the body?" Questions about puberty begin during grade 5 as boys and girls are maturing physically. These included "Why does a girl menstruate?" and "Why was I born male instead of female?" Their questions also reveal rising curiosity about drug abuse and its effects.

Many ask, "Why do people use drugs?" "What do they do to you?" or "Why do people want to smoke?" Children in both grades express a growing need to understand themselves, their peers, and their families.

It was discovered that the major health interest areas were common to all children of every age level, whether they lived in the inner city or in rural, suburban, or high-economic areas studied. However, the survey team urged that their findings not be regarded as universal, stating that "Teachers or curriculum workers will still need to answer questions such as 'What are the priorities in *my* class?' "

More recently, a sample of over 5,000 school children, representative of a population of 750,000 in grades K through 12, were surveyed in Washington State (Trucano, 1984). This study was a replication of the Connecticut study; however, the intention was not to make comparisons but to ascertain health interests and concerns in the eighties.

Data were gathered by (1) means of questionnaires written for and applied at four levels (grades K through 3, 4 through 5, 6 through 8, and 9 through 12), (2) classroom observations noted by teachers and aides, (3) open classroom discussions with students in grades K through 5, and (4) voluntary responses made by individual students during the procedures. All of the data were tabulated and reported by grades. Many of the health topics evoked questions and responses not dissimilar from those reported in the 1969 study. However, certain health topics were selected for additional discussion either because they were mentioned often, mentioned at every grade level, or seemed to be of special concern in the 1980s. These included: handicapping conditions/birth defects; genetics; child and sexual abuse; fears and worries (about divorce of parents, death, not being loved or losing love, suicide, and stress); self-concept enhancement; understanding human behavior;

effects of drugs and drug abuse; nutrition (including weight control from grade 4 on); aging; first aid/accident prevention; and sexuality/family/babies/pregnancy.

It was noted that although some health topics or areas appeared to be of high interest at all grade levels, different aspects of these topics became priorities at different age levels. It was speculated that part of this continued similarity of interests could be traced to the fact that students had not received enough health education along the way to answer their questions; hence, they continued to have them. Moreover, these findings shed light not only on health interests of students but on the growth and development patterns of students at these ages as well.

It is not fully possible to convey the richness of the data reported in *Students Speak* (Trucano, 1984). It would be well worth your while to obtain a copy and use it as a reference when planning for teaching and learning at any level of school.[1]

How can you determine the special concerns and interests of the students in your own class? There are several ways to do this. The most informed person about student interests is the student, and one way to learn about students' interests is to let them tell you what these are.

Student questions. Given the chance, children will ask questions in abundance, and for the most part these are reliable indicators of need. There are several ways in which such questions can be gathered and organized so they can be used in lesson planning.

1. Ask your students to hand in written lists of questions that they would like answers to. With *sixth-grade or older* students this is better done anonymously so they do not feel constrained and so they can ask questions that otherwise might embarrass them. Younger children's questions may need to be recorded for them by the teacher or an aide for later analysis.

2. Take note of significant questions asked during class, and file them for future reference under a classification system corresponding to the health topics or content areas specified in your district's curriculum plan. This will serve to identify those asked most frequently, thus reflecting common needs or interests of children of that age in your school.

3. Solicit the cooperation of other teachers, the school nurse, or other school personnel in recording on index cards any significant health-related questions asked them by the children. Such questions provide a different perspective on health interests, since they were motivated by situations outside the health class.

4. Develop a word list of perhaps 50 common words related to health actions or concepts. Ask the students to react to each word if it in any way suggests a question to them. Each child has had unique life experiences in connection with one or more of those words so the potential for new and unusual questions is great.

5. Prepare a health problem or interest checklist. This can be put together easily by using particularly interesting questions asked by earlier students. *Yarber (1977)* described such an instrument to be used with students in grades 3, 5, and 6 to ascertain their desire for much more, a little more, or no more information about specified health content areas. With younger children, such surveys can be read aloud by the teacher or an older child and their responses recorded by

---

[1]Comprehensive Health Education Foundation 20832 Pacific Highway South, Seattle, WA 98188

checking whichever answer best reflects their wish. Older children can read and check their own list and even participate in tabulating the results.

6. Arrange conferences, interviews, or informal discussions with individuals or groups of students to focus on their health concerns. When these shared concerns result in related learning opportunities, both interest and motivation to participate will be high.

Evaluation of school life. Consider what health problems may have had their origins in the school itself. Going to school is not always a totally healthful experience. Some children, as a direct consequence of being in school, become nervous and emotionally disturbed or develop such a strong sense of failure that they quit trying. Some suffer a series of communicable diseases contracted from other children and fall so far behind in their school work that they never quite catch up.

The emotional climate of the classroom needs careful analysis as a source of health problems. A child who frequently complains of being sick in the stomach may actually have severe stomach cramps or nausea, but the symptoms may be an emotional reaction to an unhappy teacher-student relationship or to peer group rejection. School experiences leave many marks. Most of these experiences enhance a child's well-being and growth, but others leave very real scars. The teacher who hopes to make health instruction vital and effective should arrange a social and emotional environment that helps a child cope with stress and learn at his or her own pace.

Analysis of health records. Since knowledge of health problems of individual students provides valuable data useful not only for lesson planning but also in preparing for any needed health care arrangements, you should be familiar with the information recorded in each student's cumulative health folder. Health needs and problems may also be identified through children's self-reports about personal health problems. Patterns of illness or disorders that frequently interrupt school attendance or hinder performance indicate needs for specific health instruction or conference with the school nurse or parent.

Growth and developmental characteristics. Knowledge of expected physical, social, mental, and emotional development makes it possible to predict what a child should be able to do at a particular age, and just as importantly, what a child should *not* be expected to do. This means that growth and development have more to do with readiness (i.e., *when* children can handle learning opportunities competently) than with *what* they should be taught at any age.

Consideration of the several dimensions of growth and development—physical, social, emotional, and intellectual—is not limited to decisions affecting cognitive development but needs to be involved in making classroom arrangements that facilitate affective and social growth (Moyer, 1986). However, readiness to learn will be the focus here.

It is a necessary assumption that prospective elementary teachers will have recently completed courses on growth and development of children and will be familiar with related learning and developmental theories, including those of Piaget (cognitive development), Erikson (psychosocial development), and Kohlberg (moral reasoning development). All of these have obvious applications for health teaching and learning. However, for the purposes of this section, discussion of growth and development characteristics will be limited to a brief application of Piaget's theories as they relate to planning curriculum sequence.

Children enter school during Piaget's preoperational period and progress to the period of concrete operations during elementary school grades. The preoperational child cannot consider the whole and the part simultaneously. Health and health behavior are viewed as a series of unrelated practices and ideas. Somewhere around age 7 or 8 a child begins to conserve ideas and to reverse thinking processes (the concrete operational stage); yet cause and effect are not well understood and the future is too abstract to contemplate. Health education that focuses on a child's immediate goals and desires will be more effective than education that promises future health benefits. The more health teaching is related to everyday actions, the more effective it will be.

Research shows that at age 8 or 9 children can begin to be active health consumers and make many of their own health decisions. It is recommended that health education be started before this age, but it should remain present-oriented despite the change in cognitive ability. Future-oriented teaching, stressing the value of health as a lifetime quality, is feasible only when children begin to understand abstractions and can formulate hypotheses based on reality testing (the formal operational stage) (Natapoff, 1982).

Kolbe and others (1981) concur in this view. They maintain that children do not possess the cognitive skills needed to make sound health-related decisions during the concrete operational stage of development. Instead, it is argued that either *training* or *indoctrinating* must be the process employed. They say:

When children are young, we need to train them to *do* so and so . . . and to teach them that so and so is the case (i.e., to believe something) . . . Thus as children mature developmentally we need to move away from training and indoctrinating them . . . and toward educating them (Kolbe and others, 1981).

Studies of the moral development of children have shown that they tend to reason egocentrically, being concerned mainly with consequences to themselves; yet when they are allowed to answer "why" questions and are then encouraged to examine consequences of an act on themselves and others—to develop reasons for behavior on their own—they are capable of higher reasoning with regard to concern for others (Dapice et al., 1988, p. 109).

Health concerns or problems of children, wherever they are found, should be identified, analyzed for their relevance and cruciality, and used in developing teaching-learning plans as much as possible. These may reflect persistent situations faced by all children in their daily life, as related to nutritional needs, safety rules, dental care, or worries about peer group acceptance and family disruptions. They may also involve health behavior standards such as personal health-care habits, certain social behaviors and manners, and acceptance of one's gender role. Of course, none of the aforementioned aspects of the learner are mutually exclusive. An interest exists because it is a concern. A concern or problem may be traced to a growth and developmental characteristic that occurs too early, too rapidly, or too late compared to the individual's peers, and so on.

Everything that can be learned about the children for whom a curriculum is to be planned should be considered when making decisions about what they need to know, what they want to know, and when it should be presented to them. This information cannot be used as the only basis for planning curricula, but it provides important clues that cannot be ignored if health teaching is to be meaningful to its audience.

Needs of the Community

The second source of data essential to sound curriculum development is the society in which we live. What does the student need to know about wise use of community health-care systems, and what concepts, skills, and abilities are needed to be an effective health consumer and a responsible neighbor, family member, and citizen? Some answers to these questions can be inferred by studying the social, economic, and political communities in which we work and live. National health concerns must be considered, as well as more immediate and local health issues and problems. If you are going to teach about health, it is necessary to look beyond school walls for clues to a curriculum that deals with life.

National health and education goals. There is an abundance of data on national health and education goals. The surgeon general's report on health promotion and disease prevention, *Healthy People* (U.S. Department of Health, Education and Welfare, 1979), emphasized four major factors that affect the nation's health. These are (1) unhealthy life styles; (2) inadequacies in the existing health-care system; (3) environmental hazards; and (4) human biological factors. Fifteen priority areas among preventable threats to health were named: high–blood pressure control; family planning; pregnancy and infant health; immunization; sexually transmitted diseases; toxic agent control; occupational health and safety; accident prevention and injury control; fluoridation and dental health; surveillance and control of infectious diseases; smoking and health; misuse of alcohol and drugs; nutrition; physical fitness and exercise; and control of stress and violent behavior.

Among the report's many recommendations, one specifically linked national health goals with school health education:

The schools may be the richest source of potential behavior change. Comprehensive school health education should include promoting health knowledge, the causes of disease, and the influence on health by personal decisions related to smoking, alcohol, and drug abuse, exercise, and sexual activity.

During the following year, *Objectives for the Nation* (U.S. Department of Health and Human Services, 1980) were proposed for each of the priority areas, including related health implications, specific objectives to be attained by 1990 or earlier, and other data.

Later, a two-day conference on *Prospects for a Healthier America: Achieving the Nation's Health Promotion Objectives* (U.S. Department of Health and Human Services, 1984) was held in Washington, D.C. The purpose was to study and discuss the objectives and make recommendations. Members of more than 50 national organizations representing health-care settings, health professions, business and industry, voluntary organizations, and schools were involved. The schools' work-group was made up of 10 members of major professional educational associations representing school administrators, teachers, and others.

The group quickly agreed that schools could best contribute to the achievement of the 1990 *Objectives for the Nation* by offering quality comprehensive health programs. Certain sub-recommendations are of special note:

#9 Categorical school health interventions (e.g., drug abuse, smoking, or cardiovascular diseases) developed through Federal agencies should be designed to be integrated with the broader comprehensive school health curriculum and school health services.

#13 Relevant Federal agencies should sponsor a meeting for prominent city and State school superintendents to provide the opportunity for them to experience an exemplary school health program, to participate in creative health education and health service activities, to practice healthful behaviors, and to appreciate a healthful school environment . . . At such a meeting, prominent superintendents could be informed about the role of the school in attaining the Objectives for the Nation (*Prospects for a Healthier America,* 1984).

All of this information is relevant in developing a curriculum for tomorrow's health classes.

Local community health needs and concerns. Green and others (1980) believe that local community needs assessment too often is overlooked entirely in school health curriculum planning. Certainly to base the goals and objectives for health education solely on national needs and objectives would be foolish and philosophically unsound. Knowledge of local health needs, especially those specific to a given school, neighborhood, or community is essential when planning a health education curriculum (Kunstel, 1978). Such needs are not difficult to identify. Look in any journal or newspaper, and you will find a wealth of social issues, problems, and trends with implications for health teaching. Various ethnic or socioeconomic factors may be unique in justifying curriculum emphases that are not as imperative in other communities. For example, poor nutrition may be a problem in a high-socioeconomic area, but it may exist for different reasons and be of a different nature than the same problem in an inner-city area. Health-related choices often are dictated by necessity or by ethnic or cultural forces rather than by willful neglect or ignorance. The kinds of teaching strategies that succeed with children in one school may be totally ineffective in another for a number of reasons.

Community influences on curriculum planning. Although the community is a source of the kinds of data previously listed, the curriculum is in many ways the *product* of the community as well. For example, local morbidity statistics may show that the incidence of sexually transmitted diseases has increased alarmingly among school-aged children; nevertheless, parent groups may be so opposed to education planned to counter this problem that they act to prevent any related instruction.

Legislative and political factors have a powerful impact on curriculum decisions. State legislatures decide what the requirements for teacher credentials will be. Whether elementary school teachers receive specific preparation for their health teaching responsibilities depends to a great extent on state laws. A current investigation of teacher certification requirements reveals that 26 states (51%) do not require prospective elementary school teachers to take course work in health education, even though some of those states mandate some health instruction at elementary levels (ASHA, 1987). Furthermore, lawmakers, not educators, decide whether health education will be provided and if so how comprehensive it will be. Local and state boards of education are usually elected bodies, and no public school can carry out a program contrary to board policy, regardless of how urgent a community need may be judged to be by school personnel.

Other external influences on decisions about the health curriculum are the values or philosophy of the community regarding the need for or the worth of health education. It is not likely that a teacher would propose an educational goal that was inconsistent with her or his own value system. However, an educator's values may conflict with those of some other members of the community. This kind of conflict is exemplified by the flaps about health topics such as human sexuality or family planning. Somehow such issues must be resolved with the needs of the learner as the primary consideration.

The health curriculum for the 1990s probably will continue to reflect the increasing national concern with drug abuse among children and youth and with the crucial problems of AIDS prevention, environmental pollution, teenage pregnancies, and stress and violence control. These priorities will change if other health problems are later perceived as having greater urgency. That urgency will come from the community in most cases.

Crisis-generated community pressures are more often the cause of curriculum priority-setting, changes in health education than in most subjects commonly taught in the public schools. Unfortunately, such a bandwagon approach is categorical and reactive, whereas health education, to be effective, should be comprehensive and proactive. If health education is to be effective, it must consider the whole person, not merely the diseases and disorders to which humans are prey. Children need and want to know more about wellness than how to cope with next year's diseases. A set of lessons designed to keep one jump ahead of specified health problems, year after year, would be dreary. Another problem is that, as we have already suggested, young children, at least, don't really relate to future problems or benefits. They want to know about what is happening now. Health education for the 1990s and beyond seeks to emphasize promotion far more than prevention or control, as has been the case. The goal is a healthful life style and abundant wellness—now and tomorrow too.

The Body of Knowledge

The body of knowledge, the third source of information affecting curriculum planning, is defined by consensus of its subject matter specialists. Every subject area lays claim to some broad but definite range of principles, concepts, and generalizations. But information, however well it may be structured and organized, is not by itself the content of a discipline. There is also process, the constellation of intellectual skills employed in acquiring and using that knowledge. Neither content nor process can exist or be taught or learned in the absence of the other. Parker and Rubin (1966) argue that process is in fact the life blood of content. In classrooms where transmission of information is primary, learners play a passive role. Where the emphasis is instead placed on process (e.g., analyzing, decision making, problem solving), the learners are actively involved. Transmission or assimilation of information is not less important, but subject matter becomes the vehicle for learning rather than merely a destination selected for the learners by the teacher. This outcome has been aptly described as representing the difference between knowing something, and knowing what it is good for (Parker & Rubin, 1966, p. 2).

Students need to learn how to search out what is known about a problem and how to analyze, compare, and sensibly choose the best among alternative solutions. Use of problem-solving and decision-making skills is stimulating in elementary school years and it may be more important to begin using them then than at later levels of education. Thinking should not be a process deferred until secondary school levels, or its happening left to assumption. Bruner (1963) says that "intellectual activity anywhere is the same, whether at the frontier of knowledge or in a third grade classroom . . . the difference is in degree, not in kind." The subject matter used in investigating health topics arises from the problem being worked on and should never be viewed as the primary goal of instruction. The teacher becomes a facilitator of learning, not a communicator of information.

Health information doesn't long stay the same, and even if it did, no system for presenting that information could equip children with enough of it to deal sensibly with every manner of health-related problem or decision over a lifetime. Learning *how* to learn is imperative in education today, because it has lifelong utility and application. Information can become obsolete or irrelevant, but the ability to discover fresh facts when they are needed increases each time it is used. The person who has mastered problem solving and informed decision making has the versatility needed to cope with new challenges, technologies, and health problems if they occur.

However, there must be a system for selecting the principal topics to be used to structure the subject matter of concern, so it follows that content and values will be inseparable. The questions that must be addressed to the subject specialists in a field are these: What knowledge is of most worth in today's world? What knowledge does an educated person need to function effectively as an individual and as a worthwhile member of our society? The answers will always be somewhat different over time because the essential knowledge about health and health behavior is changing more rapidly than it can be communicated to the public. So much is being learned about life and health and at so fast a pace that teachers are hard pressed to keep up to date. However, unless they do and adjust their teaching plans accordingly, their students may have to cope with tomorrow's problems using yesterday's information.

The trend in every discipline has been to abandon any attempt to describe its total body of knowledge, since this is impossible. Faced with this reality, scholars have sought to identify the most powerful concepts and generalizations in their fields to structure and define the scope of their discipline. This is the most logical and economical way to organize a field's content matter. As Bruner (1963) has said, "To focus on structure is to learn how things are related." Once a student has grasped the fundamentals of healthful living, each new idea fits in neatly and is quickly understood because it belongs. Even young children can learn how things affect and are connected to each other.

A Philosophy Statement: Curriculum Guidelines

Curriculum planning waits upon data gathering, needs assessments and synthesis of the resulting data. An important first step must now be taken. The beginning point in planning an instructional program is the development of an effective statement of the set of basic beliefs upon which subsequent curriculum decisions will be based. In effect, this is the function of the United States Constitution. Without the guidance and justification of such a document, planning curricula is like starting a difficult journey in the absence of a dependable map. Given the existence of an effective statement of philosophy, schools can resist pressures to add or delete studies according to every passing fad. Teachers are able to plan instruction consonant with the purposes spelled out in the statement. In short, every curriculum decision is provided with focused direction if the document is a good one.

Perrin (1986) argues that many statements purporting to be "philosophies" are instead descriptions of methods of operation, personal thoughts about educational methods and programs, or prescriptive lists of "shoulds" relative to administration, organization or curriculum.

Instead, Tyler (1963) says that such a statement seeks to define the nature of a good life and a good society. Perrin (1986) concurs, saying: "A philosophy should describe the ideal 'educated' person whom the public schools seek to produce and the conditions of society which demand an individual with that kind of education." He believes that the 1961 Educational Policies Commission produced one of the best examples of philosophy stated properly. A section relevant to health education follows:

The traditionally accepted obligation of the school to teach the *fundamental processes*—an obligation stressed in the 1918 and 1938 statements of educational purposes—is obviously directed toward the development of the ability to think. Each of the schools' other traditional objectives can be better achieved as pupils develop this ability and learn to apply it to all the problems that face them.

Health, for example, depends upon a reasoned awareness of the value of mental and physical fitness and of the means by which it may be developed and maintained. Fitness is not merely a function of living and acting; it requires that the individual understand the connection among health, nutrition, activity, and environment, and that he take action to improve his mental and physical condition.

The document abounds with statements no less applicable and satisfying as acceptable goals and objectives. Whatever curriculum design selected for a program, there should be a statement justifying its selection as an effective means of developing the kind of health-educated person needed today.

DEFINING THE SCOPE OF HEALTH EDUCATION

The term **scope** in health education refers to the total range of subject areas or health topics selected to represent the body of knowledge of the discipline. It is usually categorized and ordered by means of a series of units, referred to as its "organizing elements." To use a simple analogy, if we were to speak of an ordinary ruler as a scope having 12 units, then we might say that its organizing elements were inches, and the plan was the "Inches system." The way any scope is described depends on the point of view of those given responsibility for determining how it is to be organized. Although in essence it is always the same material, the form in which it is presented differs somewhat. Whatever the plan chosen, the subject matter considered by all of its organizing elements together is its scope.

The organizing elements most commonly employed are the major body systems, current health problems, traditional content areas, health topics, or health concepts. For example, those viewing the appropriate focus of health instruction as being physiological-anatomical

would probably use body systems as their organizing elements. Each plan has certain strengths and weaknesses. Whichever structure is chosen for a school curriculum, there will unavoidably be some effect on the way the body of knowledge titled "Health Education" will be perceived and taught.

Which of the following plans fits your own beliefs concerning the best possible presentation of health instruction? In your opinion, which one seems most oriented to wellness promotion?

Body Systems Design

Obviously the body systems design focuses on an anatomical and physiological study of the body and its functions. The strength of this plan, particularly at the elementary level is that young children do have great interest in learning about their bodies and how they work. The weakness in using body systems as a curriculum framework is that the focus tends to be more on physiology than on health education. Also, there is no logical reason for including health content, other than that implicit in the area of optimum physical growth and development. Consumer health, prevention and control of diseases, community health, and environmental health must be tacked on, if they are to be considered at all. Teachers who lack preparation in health teaching cannot be blamed if they mistake the systems for the total body of knowledge. Moreover, since some communities object to any mention of the reproductive system, especially at the elementary level, the teacher is in the awkward position of having to avoid discussion of the system about which student interest is greatest.

The body systems design was used in the Primary Grades Health Curriculum Project (PGHCP) and the School Health Curriculum Project (SHCP). Each grade's study focused on a body system, part, or sense. However, attention

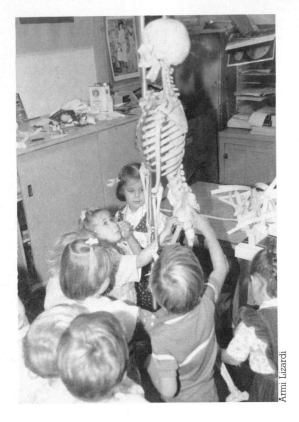

Armi Lizardi

focuses on the crucial health problems of the day. An early example of this rationale was the development of a guide to instruction by a Commission of the American Association for Health, Physical Education, and Recreation (AAHPER, 1967). Their first step was to identify the most crucial health problems for the 1960s and 1970s. This judgment was determined by a process of consensus among the members. By inference, those not specified did not meet the criterion of cruciality. The problem areas selected were accident prevention; aging; alcohol; disaster preparedness; disease and disease control; economics of health care; environmental conditions; ionizing radiation; evaluation of health information; family health; international health; mental health; nutrition; and smoking. The list was not intended to be representative of the total scope of health education, but the exclusion of drug abuse and misuse as a problem area is surprising.

A more recent example is the 15 priority areas identified in the surgeon general's report *Healthy People* (U.S. Department of Health, Education and Welfare, 1979). In fact, these are also *problems,* so the title could as aptly have been *Unhealthy People*).

The advantage of using health problems to structure health teaching and curricula is that the greatest emphasis can be given to the prevention or control of threats to health that are most likely to be encountered by the learner. As such, the material is both current and meaningful. The disadvantage is that related health instruction is limited to the selected problems, which may or may not be crucial by the time the instruction occurs. Moreover, what seems crucial to adults may be far less threatening to healthy youngsters.

There are other disadvantages. For example, a problem-focused curriculum is based on the assumption that students need know nothing more about healthful behaviors than how to

was later given to the need for comprehensiveness during the revision of the original units between 1979 and 1982. At that time the organization plan was changed from the body system design and expanded to encompass ten more or less traditional content areas into which the earlier objectives and activities were interwoven as appropriate. Retitled, "Growing Healthy," the curriculum today reportedly reaches more than 600,000 students in grades K through 7 nationwide (National Center, 1984).

Health Problems Design

The scope in the health problems design reflects the conviction that effective use of the limited time and resources available for health instruction is possible only if the curriculum

cope with those problems. Learning how to prevent or solve common health problems is not the same as learning how to make wise everyday choices that affect wellness in important ways. The approach also ignores the pressures that motivate unhealthful actions. As Neubauer and Pratt (1981) point out:

In very concrete ways the health of individuals is a reflection of the social, economic, and political patterns of the community, and is in fact simply a symptom of those patterns. To talk about "health" as if it were disconnected from dominant institutions and community life is to fall into the trap that tells us that isolating events gives us control over them.

To focus on disease as though knowledge about symptoms, causes, and prevention or risk reduction were the primary or only requisite factor in health promotion is the very opposite of what health education should be.

Health Content Area Design

The use of content areas as the organizing elements for curriculum development is the traditional and most familiar form by which the scope of health instruction is defined. There are many strengths associated with this plan, one of which is that when fully developed and implemented it provides a comprehensive survey of the body of knowledge. The format is so well accepted that a wealth of resource materials (e.g., books, textbooks, pamphlets, articles, films, filmstrips, and tapes) keyed to those areas is easily obtainable and frequently updated. For the same reasons, school health educators anywhere in the country will interpret and teach the subject matter in much the same way. The content area titles are consistent with the actual subject matter and serve to define the boundaries of the information contained in each.

Content areas are often used as the organizing elements in official curriculum documents such as those formulated by state boards of education, state departments of education, and national health organizations, both voluntary and professional. Two such lists of recommended content areas illustrate how nearly universal their titles are:

California State Board of Education (1978)

1. Personal health
2. Family health
3. Nutrition
4. Mental-emotional health
5. Use and misuse of substances
6. Diseases and disorders
7. Consumer health
8. Accident prevention and emergency care
9. Community health
10. Environmental health

National Comprehensive School Health Guidelines Committee (1984)

1. Community health
2. Consumer health
3. Environmental health
4. Family life
5. Growth and development
6. Nutritional health
7. Personal health
8. Prevention and control of diseases and disorders
9. Safety and accident prevention
10. Substance use and abuse

The latter list was endorsed and accepted by all of the school health-interested national professional groups (ASHA, AAHE, SHES/APHA, and the Society for State Directors of HPER). The seeming omission of mental-emotional health as an area is based upon the belief that these dimensions of health are always a part of all ten content areas.

A weakness associated with use of content areas is that the very compactness and neatness of those titles leads to division and compartmentalization of instruction. Unless care is taken to plan meaningful and logical transitions between the areas, the result can be a series of short courses with little to link them other than their concern with health or its absence. Also, because the cue for instruction is taken from the content area titles, what is taught or learned tends to be subject matter, not processes, with the focus on *knowing* rather than *doing* or thinking. Finally, when there is not enough time allocated for full study of all the areas, those left until last are given little attention or are omitted entirely. This diminishes the effectiveness and comprehensiveness of the program as it was intended to be taught.

Topic Design

A topic differs from a content area in that it is usually a subordinate area or a theme. A subordinate area might be oral health, stress reduction, or rest, sleep, and relaxation. Stated as a theme, it might be ''eating for energy and health,'' ''living safely at school and at home,'' or ''protecting the world we live in.'' An advantage of using a topic design is its flexibility in planning health instruction according to student interests and curriculum time constraints. Topics meaningful to a given grade level can be studied in ways that contribute to learning in other basic studies.

Topics tend to be built around life styles or day-to-day health decisions so that they relate well to specific needs and concerns of the learner. A weakness is that they seldom encompass the total scope of health instruction, even added together after the entire elementary school experience. Another weakness is that it takes a very skilled teacher, who knows the difference between health education and physiology or hygiene, to plan and integrate health topics into a day's teaching so that it has real impact. A busy elementary school teacher, already burdened with teaching so many subjects, may not have time to do the special planning this requires. The topic design works best when it is

promoted vigorously by the school administrator and coordinated by someone who is qualified and given the free time needed to do so.

Conceptual Approach

A conceptual approach to curriculum planning might be described as one that (1) employs powerful generalizations or concepts as a means of structuring a given area of subject matter, (2) derives its scope from those concepts, (3) stresses teaching strategies that provide practice in applying cognitive skills, and (4) uses factual data to facilitate conceptualization rather than as bits of information to be memorized.

Conceptual teaching takes advantage of the fact that conceptual learning is the way people learn naturally. It is centered on the learner, not the teacher. The classroom is not a scene typified by rows of passive students listening or filling out worksheets. Instead it is characterized by the vital sounds and sights of active participation in the investigation of real problems and interests. The goal of conceptual teaching is the discovery of answers to questions that lead to meaningful conclusions. Conceptual learning goes on all the time, in and out of school. In the conceptual approach the teacher provides an accepting environment, arranges experiences facilitative of that kind of learning, and then simply allows it to happen.

Probably the best-known example of a conceptual framework defining the body of knowledge in health education is the SHES curriculum (1967). Based upon the results of a carefully designed and implemented research project, its ten concepts have had a lasting impact on health education curricula. For example, when the study was begun more than 35 different subject areas were commonly listed in curricula across the country. Somehow, few curricula offered since those ten concepts were devised to categorize the subject matter have either

SHES CONCEPTS FOR DEFINING BODY OF KNOWLEDGE IMPORTANT IN HEALTH EDUCATION

1. Growth and development influences and is influenced by the structure and functioning of the individual.
2. Growing and developing follows a predictable sequence, yet is unique for each individual.
3. Protection and promotion of health is an individual, community, and international responsibility.
4. The potential for hazards and accidents exists whatever the environment.
5. There are reciprocal relationships involving man, disease, and the environment.
6. The family serves to perpetuate man and to fulfill certain health needs.
7. Personal health practices are affected by a complexity of forces, often conflicting.
8. Utilization of health information, products, and services is guided by values and perceptions.
9. Use of substances that modify mood and behavior arises from a variety of motivations.
10. Food selection and eating patterns are determined by physical, social, economic, and cultural patterns.

changed the number of organizing elements or departed very much from its basic categorization scheme. In fact, the project was very possibly too far ahead of the profession when it was introduced to be understood or well accepted. In a very real sense, the SHES curriculum was fated to succeed by osmosis rather than by acclamation although a great many school districts adopted the full curriculum during the 1970s.

Since the concepts are stated as complete ideas, they provide far more guidance as to their meaning than do other kinds of organizing elements. For example, the concept "Use of substances that modify mood and behavior arises from a variety of motivations" is a complete idea and probably has been understood as long as humans have known of substances that can do that. When one reduces the concept to a couple of words like "substance abuse," as in a

content area designation, the real meaning of the concept is lost along with much of its power as an idea. In the first place, there are lots of substances that we eat or drink or ingest somehow. Which of them is intended by the word "substance," even when linked with "abuse," is uncertain. Ice cream modifies one's mood, but if you eat too much of it too often you tend to add unwanted pounds. The real point of the concept is that whatever the substance may be, the motives for taking it can differ widely.

When the physical, social, mental, and emotional dimensions of these concepts (big ideas) are explored, the outcome is a holistic view of health and health behavior, not one limited to the physical alone. In addition, the conceptual approach provides a rationale for study at every grade level. Although specific enabling objectives must be designed for every level of teaching, the concept keeps them on target. Krueter

(1980) observed, ''The SHES approach remains the most conceptually and philosophically sound guide to the development of school health education curriculum.''

The weakness of the conceptual approach probably lies in the fact that it takes more skill and planning to teach concepts instead of facts. Green and others (1980) opined that ''Paradoxically, the philosophical and conceptual strength of the SHES curriculum may have been its major weakness. Many health educators apparently found it hard to understand and apply in the classroom situation.'' The problem is not in arranging for children to conceptualize. The challenge lies in arranging the kinds of perceptual experiences (lessons) that will lead to the formulation of the concept wanted. Elementary teachers do not always possess the background in health sciences needed to plan meaningful and valid learning opportunities. It is often desirable and necessary to arrange inservice training in health teaching, whatever the curriculum plan chosen for a school. The provision of at least a part-time consultant to advise and suggest ways to enrich the program would be a valuable addition.

DETERMINING THE SEQUENCE OF HEALTH INSTRUCTION

Sequence, the ordering of the organizing elements, is a problem that must be dealt with once the scope is defined. Vertical sequence is the ordering of organizing elements from year to year, kindergarten through grade 12, and is usually established at the administrative or district level. Horizontal sequence involves a plan for ordering the elements within the time allotted for direct teaching, whether as a semester course or as a single grade's curriculum plan. Specific decisions concerning horizontal sequence are best made by school curriculum committees and teachers (Hartoonian & Laughlin, 1986).

Determining when study of any particular organizing element (concept, topic, content area, health problem, or body system) should be scheduled is a complex problem. There must be a reason for the position assigned in every case. There is no one right sequence, but there must be logic connecting one element to the next. The sequence represented by the chapters in the textbook you are using provides a sequence but it is somebody else's sequence. Ask yourself, ''Since this is what I know about children of this age (their concerns, what they need to know, their cognitive abilities etc.), what would get their interest on the very first day of school, and what would they feel most confident and comfortable about discussing in a new situation like that?'' When that has been decided, look at the other elements of the scope that you are asked to teach and choose the one that seems appropriate as a next step. For example, suppose you decide that, since second-grade students typically are very interested in having friends and being a friend, you will plan a way that helps them to get to know each other during the health lesson. That has to do with social health and with growing and developing, and so it easily leads into discussions of a number of ways in which children grow and develop. Once growth and development has been studied in all its dimensions, what might reasonably be considered next? Whatever the sequence you adopt, whether your own or as recommended, the important thing is that there *is* a plan and that the children can see what it is. A little time spent during the first day or even the first week of school might profitably be spent asking them to tell you what they would like to know and what they would like to learn first. The more you can involve them in making these kinds of decisions the more likely it is that the health lesson will be their favorite time of the day.

It is not always possible to schedule the total scope of health instruction during any one grade or course of study. This means that the task of planning horizontal sequence involves a sort of vertical aspect. In general, two scheduling schemes are employed in order to accommodate all of the subject matter within a period of time encompassing two or more school grades. These are a cycle plan and a spiral plan. A cycle plan is illustrated in Table 3-1.

Placement of each of the content areas in the grades as indicated has been based on known needs, interests, and the physical, social, mental, and emotional growth and development characteristic of each age or grade level. Notice that all of the content areas are emphasized three times during the K through 8 school years, although more of them are covered in some years than in others. Such a plan does not preclude natural overlaps into unscheduled content areas as a consequence of the planned study. The advantage of the cycle plan is that every teacher knows the minimum that each student in his or her class is expected to learn in that year. The disadvantage is that it rests upon the interest and competence of each teacher to accomplish the goals of the total curriculum if later grades are to progress as intended. Unless there is careful coordination of these units and commitment to the goals of the total health curriculum, the minimum is apt also to be the maximum.

A spiral horizontal scheme is implicit in the SHES scope and sequence chart (see Table 3-2). The school years are divided into four levels, K through 3, 4 through 6, 7 through 9, and 10 through 12. The spiral plan is built into the sets of measurable objectives proposed for each concept at every grade. The lower the grade, the

TABLE 3-1. Proposed organization of cycle plan health curriculum

	Level								
	I				II			III	
Content areas	K	1	2	3	4	5	6	7	8
Community health				X			X		X
Consumer health			X			X		X	
Disease prevention and control			X			X			X
Use and abuse of drugs				X		X		X	
Environmental health				X			X		X
Family life education				X			X		X
Mental and emotional health			X			X			X
Nutrition	X	X			X			X	
Personal health	X	X			X			X	
Accident prevention and safety education	X	X			X			X	

simpler the cognitive skill elicited and the more concrete and simple the subject matter involved. As the students progress through the level, the teacher is free to select the objectives students must achieve if they are to be successful at the next level. The notion of "spiral" comes from the gradual broadening of subject matter and greater complexity of the cognitive processes represented in the objectives.

The advantage of the spiral plan is its greater flexibility and adaptability to the learners involved. Actually, the SHES curriculum objectives as proposed could be used to plan instruction for any age group assuming only that those being taught had the necessary background information and skills to cope with the objectives selected for them. The disadvantage is that teachers must be able to design learning opportunities that match the objectives as proposed or must be able to devise enabling objectives of the same nature that would lead toward achievement of the general objectives. During the lower two levels, a supplementary cycle plan might need to be worked out if time allocations were too few or too short. Some ways that the objectives developed as the framework can be sequenced to fit both the subject matter and the students' existing abilities are explained in Chapter 4.

CHOOSING CURRICULUM PATTERNS FOR HEALTH TEACHING

If those responsible for the administration of a school or school system believe that comprehensive school health education should be provided, or if it is mandated and supported by state funding, then health education will be included in the school's curriculum plan. How it will be implemented depends again on decisions made at the administrative level. Patterns of organization at the elementary level may be integration or direct teaching. The latter pattern

is most typical of upper elementary and middle school organization.

Integration

To integrate is to relate the parts of something within the whole. To employ integration in planning for teaching and learning is to focus on relationships, generalizations, or concepts that tie experiences or facts together. As a curriculum plan, **integration** refers to the means by which a subject area is introduced and treated in a given educational situation. In traditional educational patterns, from elementary school onward, learning is often compartmentalized and specialized. Each subject area is dealt with in turn as a separate entity. The relevance of what is learned in one subject area to that learned in others may be less than clear if students are not helped to see significant relationships between them.

As a process, integration functions as a part of *any* effective teaching and learning program, however it may be organized. For example, teaching in the conceptual approach engages the learners in activities that require the use of a whole array of cognitive skills and affective experiences as they progress through the elementary school years. Students actively participate in investigations dealing with their own needs and those of the community. They learn about living, and at the same time they learn ways of processing the flood of data that pours in daily. These are the kinds of lessons that children must have if they are to live in the twenty-first century as effective family members and citizens.

Health instruction in elementary schools is often integrated with social studies and science. Goodlad (1984) concluded that development of truly integrated programs of study (those that involve a wide number of disciplines in a program focused on larger themes) is something that no level of school does well. His investigation revealed that many first-grade and second-grade classes put together the theme of understanding self and others, with discussion of the family and community as part of social studies. By the third grade, children were frequently studying community needs such as those for health care. As a part of science studies, grades 1 through 3 were focusing on personal orientation to the natural world, and fourth graders were learning about nutrition and drugs/alcohol problems. In general, he noted that the science curriculum at the elementary level appeared to link with health.

A weakness of the integration model is that its success depends so heavily on the individual teacher's understanding of comprehensive health education. Elementary teachers are prepared to be generalists, and they do a remarkable job of teaching the many basic subjects for which they are responsible. Some become interested enough as undergraduates to take electives that help them fulfill this important aspect of the curriculum. Many states employ health teaching specialists as coordinators or instructors in junior high or middle schools. These are individuals whose preparation has been in health education and who are credentialed as health teachers.

Direct Teaching

The most successful pattern is **direct teaching,** with a regular class period allotted to health instruction. How much time is scheduled is ordinarily an administrative decision. What is covered in direct teaching, its scope, often depends on the content of the textbook or the curriculum plan adopted by the school. Therefore, the scope and sequence of health education in the elementary schools are essentially determined less by schools than by authors and publishers.

When direct teaching will be provided is an administrative decision and varies with the phi-

losophy of the school or its principal. There is no standard practice in elementary schools regarding the content or grades in which health instruction is provided. Some health instruction usually is given each year, based on recognized health problems and the growth and developmental characteristics of the age group of concern. The quality and quantity of that instruction depends to a great extent on the interest of individual teachers.

Many organizations, professional groups, and experts in health education recommend that elementary school children should be given a minimum of 20 minutes of health instruction each day. Students in grades 7 and 8 should have *at least* a full class period once a week for a year, and preferably a full semester of daily health instruction. Specified health topics usually are emphasized in some years and not in others according to a determined plan. (See Table 3-2.) For example, accident prevention and safety may be stressed every year from kindergarten through grade 6. Another topic often included in the primary grades is dental health. Topics such as drug misuse and abuse and boy-girl relationships often are not approached until grade 7 or 8. What do you already know about the health needs and interests and the growth and development of children that justifies these decisions regarding the sequence of this study?

When the administrative commitment is to direct teaching, the program must be of high quality and coordinated by qualified health education specialists. The subject must be given time, space, and material support equal to those provided other basic subjects. Unfortunately, there is not enough time, even with daily health lessons, to teach children all they want and need to know.

There are many advantages to direct teaching. It is the traditional pattern, so teachers are most familiar and comfortable with it. Health

TABLE 3-2. Health education: a conceptual approach to curriculum design

CONCEPT 1 Growth and development influences and is influenced by the structure and functioning of the individual.	CONCEPT 2 Growing and developing follows a predictable sequence, yet is unique for each individual.	CONCEPT 3 Protection and promotion of health is an individual, community, and international responsibility.	CONCEPT 4 The potential for hazards and accidents exists, whatever the environment.	CONCEPT 5 There are reciprocal relationships involving man, disease, and environment.
Level I: Approximate grade levels K-3				
A. Relates good nutrition, adequate sleep, and physical activity to optimal growth and development. **B.** Names major body parts and organs and their related functions. **C.** Explains how body types and other factors determine differences in height and weight. **D.** Defines the meanings of heredity and environment. **E.** Identifies ways in which plants, animals, and children resemble their parents.	**A.** Cites examples showing how people of the same age differ and yet are similar while growing and developing. **B.** Explains why differences in the rate and stage of growth and development among children of the same age are to be expected. **C.** Identifies ways in which one grows over a given period of time. **D.** Describes how each person becomes unique.	**A.** Defines the meanings of health and of community. **B.** Describes the relationships of health and community. **C.** Identifies familiar health problems which are the joint responsibility of individuals and groups. **D.** Recognizes local community efforts designed to meet common health needs. **E.** Is aware of the variety of health personnel involved in solution of community problems.	**A.** Describes what accidents are and the need for their prevention and control. **B.** Detects environmental factors which affect health and safety. **C.** Indicates hazards existing in the home, school, and community. **D.** Identifies procedures which help protect personal health and safety and that of others. **E.** Is aware that groups exist to help prevent accidents and eliminate or control hazards.	**A.** Distinguishes between being ill and being well. **B.** Identifies factors which affect wellness. **C.** Discusses ways in which disease-causing organisms can be transmitted from person to person. **D.** Identifies ways in which a person can protect himself and others from disease.
Level II: Approximate grade levels 4-6				
A. Describes the basic structure and function of the human organism as it relates to growing and developing. **B.** Concludes that although each organ and system has a special task, each is dependent on the other in meeting body needs. **C.** Identifies ways in which girls are both physiologically ahead of boys and different in behavior and interests at some stages of growth. **D.** Explains the importance of certain personal health practices as they relate to the process of growing and developing. **E.** Illustrates the effects of heredity and environment on growth and development.	**A.** Describes how growing and developing occurs unevenly for body parts, systems, and functions. **B.** Identifies different ways children grow physically, mentally, and socially. **C.** Discusses the variety of influences which affect growing and developing. **D.** Compares individual growth status with information contained in growth charts. **E.** Predicts the kind of growth and development changes that may occur during adolescence.	**A.** Explains why some health-related efforts are common to all communities while others are unique to certain communities. **B.** Identifies factors that influence the nature of community health activities. **C.** Compares health programs, facilities, and services provided by organized segments of society. **D.** Describes skills and techniques required to meet existing and emerging community health needs. **E.** Explores functions of and the range of career opportunities in health-service professions and allied fields.	**A.** Cites authoritative data related to the occurrence of accidents. **B.** Illustrates relationships between accidents and human behavior. **C.** Reports the effects of environmental factors on the health and safety of individuals and groups. **D.** Relates precautions to the reductions of hazards and accidents.	**A.** Names various methods by which disease can be prevented, controlled, or cured. **B.** Identifies various sources of disease. **C.** Concludes that immunization prevents and controls some diseases. **D.** Cites examples of the effects of disease upon individuals, families, communities, countries. **E.** Recognizes that a concern for wellness motivates individuals and organizations.

Modified from the School Health Education Study: Scope and sequence chart for a unified and comprehensive program for health education, K-12

Published in 1971

CONCEPT 6	CONCEPT 7	CONCEPT 8	CONCEPT 9	CONCEPT 10
The family serves to perpetuate man and to fulfill certain health needs.	**Personal health practices are affected by a complexity of forces, often conflicting.**	**Utilization of health information products, and services is guided by values and perceptions.**	**Use of substances that modify mood and behavior arises from a variety of motivations.**	**Food selection and eating patterns are determined by physical, social, mental, economic, and cultural factors.**
A. Describes the role and responsibilities of individuals within the family. **B.** Describes how family members contribute to the health of each other. **C.** Lists similarities and differences between boys and girls in appearance, interests, and activities. **D.** Discovers that all living things come from other living things.	**A.** Tells why personal health practices affect participation in life activities. **B.** Identifies practices which affect oral health. **C.** Is aware of the influence of growing and developing on personal health practices. **D.** Discovers that decision making is involved in personal health practices.	**A.** Names familiar people who promote, protect, and maintain health. **B.** Is aware that there are differences among health products and among health services. **C.** Identifies various sources of health information. **D.** Recognizes that laws and regulations exist to protect the consumer.	**A.** Identifies substances commonly used by many individuals in society that modify mood and behavior. **B.** Names ways common mood and behavior modifying substances are used in homes and community. **C.** Is aware that there are differences between alcoholic beverages and other beverages. **D.** Realizes there are differences in family practices and feelings about use of tobacco and of alcoholic beverages.	**A.** Distinguishes among a wide range of foods. **B.** States reasons for eating a variety of foods. **C.** Is aware of factors that detract from or enhance eating certain foods. **D.** Identifies types of foods and patterns of eating that are related to different cultures.
A. Illustrates relationships within a family that influence the degree of health and happiness of all members. **B.** Is aware of families in present day society display a wide range of characteristics. **C.** Describes personal qualities which affect peer group relationships. **D.** Explains body changes which occur during puberty. **E.** Is aware of the reproductive process and how life begins. **F.** Defines heredity and is aware of inherited and acquired characteristics.	**A.** Discusses why guidance is necessary in determining a balance of sleep, rest and activity. **B.** Distinguishes between practices that promote and those that hinder development of the oral structures. **C.** Illustrates ways in which personal choices affect health practices. **D.** Identifies conflicting forces affecting personal health practices. **E.** Illustrates relationships between personal health practices and well-being.	**A.** Is aware that emotions, family patterns, and values influence selection and use of health information, products, and services. **B.** Compares and contrasts health information, products, and services. **C.** Identifies different kinds of medical, dental, and health related specialists and their role in health services. **D.** Cites examples of agencies, groups, laws, and standards that protect the health consumer. **E.** Applies the knowledge that harm can result from self-diagnosis, self-medication, and the unwise use of drugs, medicines, devices, cosmetics, and dietary supplements.	**A.** Describes the range of substances used by man to modify mood and behavior. **B.** Differentiates among controls on purchase, possession, and use of substances that modify mood and behavior. **C.** Illustrates how, when, and where certain mood and behavior modifying substances are used for dietary, ceremonial, social, pain relieving, and other reasons. **D.** Discusses why certain mood and behavior modifying substances are used rather commonly and others only under special circumstances.	**A.** Describes functions of food as they relate to health. **B.** Develops acceptable criteria for food selection and patterns for eating. **C.** Cites examples of social and emotional influences on attitudes and eating habits. **D.** Relates different eating patterns to circumstances of living.

textbooks are written with direct teaching in mind. The teachers' editions or supplements include suggestions for lessons designed to be used in separate courses. The packaged curriculum guides widely used in schools are similarly designed to be implemented by direct teaching. And with the set amount of regularly scheduled class time typical of direct teaching patterns, a teacher can be more responsive to current needs and concerns. Interest and motivation are naturally sustained when a daily program is possible. Health can be considered in all of its dimensions.

A disadvantage of direct teaching is that, where it exists, there is a tendency to view health education as having been given complete coverage. Potential enrichment by means of integrating experiences in other subject areas is forgotten. When health instruction is assigned to unqualified or uninterested teachers, instruction may be limited to reading the book. Although "health is more than hygiene," the student in such a class may be lucky to learn even that much. As a result of dependence on the textbook, the sequence may be a lockstep march through the chapters with no attempt to give priority or emphasis to those topics most relevant to a given group of learners. Finally, where teaching is confused with "telling," lecture becomes the sole technique used. Health instruction becomes a series of "no-no's," health rules, and warnings instead of stimulating learning opportunities that offer ideas and strategies for self-care and maintenance of wellness.

Nevertheless, direct teaching has been shown to be the most effective single pattern for organizing the health curriculum. School health education at its best develops a student who has learned to generalize and has formulated a set of useful concepts and skills that will remain long after specific facts have been forgotten. Direct teaching provided by a competent instructor is, potentially at least, health education at its best.

THE TEACHER'S ROLE IN CURRICULUM DECISIONS

Because of its complexities, curriculum development has emerged as a major field in education. Curriculum specialists have to be knowledgeable about current and past research findings related to curriculum problems. They must be skilled in conducting and interpreting research. They must have the ability to design and carry out valid program evaluation procedures. They must be thoroughly grounded in curriculum theory and methodology. Extraordinary skill in writing and creating curriculum materials is a must. Fortunately, although teachers need to be able to speak the language of curriculum developers, it is not necessary that they be curriculum specialists. Teachers should not be expected to add curriculum designing to all the responsibilities already given them.

Sliepcevich (1969) differentiates between two levels of curriculum planning, one no more essential than the other, and each essential to the effectiveness of the other. The broader, more general view of curriculum development entails careful research leading to a product applicable in any community because it is based upon universal needs and concerns. She terms this level the *macroscopic* view of curriculum organization. The more specific curriculum problems encountered at the classroom level are termed the *microscopic* view of curriculum organization. This is the teacher's special area of decision making and curriculum planning.

A teacher brings unique competencies, skills, insights, and practical experience to the tasks of adapting, modifying, and implementing programs proposed by the specialists. Where this division of labor exists, the teacher and cur-

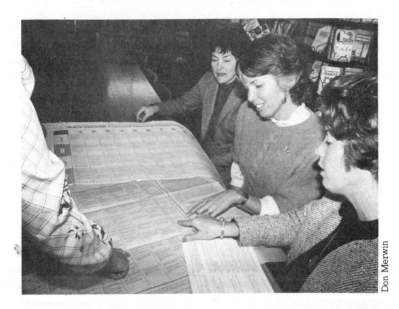

Don Merwin

riculum specialist complement each other's skills. The result of such a dynamic partnership is increased efficiency, economy of effort, and effectiveness of the total school health program. Sliepcevich concludes that teachers are not *less* involved as a consequence, but *more* involved, and at a more sophisticated and meaningful level.

Developing packaged curriculum materials for schools requires the macroscopic view of the problems and goals of health education. A set of broadly described objectives forms the framework of such documents. Each of these general objectives specifies a measurable skill as well as some significant subject matter with which it is to be employed. However, instead of listing a series of lesson ideas, **learning opportunities** are described that could be used in achieving that objective. The principal difference between a learning opportunity and a lesson is that the first focuses on a curriculum-level objective, is described in general terms, and requires several lessons for its accomplishment. A lesson plan focuses on enabling objectives subordinate to a general objective and describes an activity that

can be accomplished within the limits of a day's class, yet contributes to the achievement of the learning opportunities.

The words "packaged curriculum guide" may suggest a mechanistic approach to health instruction, reducing the teacher's role to that of the tool used to activate the plan. Nothing could be further from the truth; in fact, it is quite the other way around. In the absence of skilled teachers who can interpret and adapt such materials to fit their students' needs and abilities, the finest and most innovative curriculum package is just a lot of words and paper. When you think of it, a textbook is a packaged learning system, especially the teacher's edition, and it is how the teacher uses that textbook that makes it as effective as it is intended to be. If nobody reads it, a book is just a lot of paper and words, too. And if teachers do nothing more with a textbook than use it for quiet work, those words cannot make much of an impact on the reader. In the case of packaged curriculum guides, the emphasis is on *how,* not just *what.* It cannot be handed to the students; it is a teacher's aid.

The testing and adaptation of a curriculum guide must take place in the classroom, and the responsibility will be yours. You have to know what it ought to include and how to judge the quality and validity of its goals and objectives. Remember that the use you make of it must be appropriate to the needs and interests of *your* students, and not students in general. Base your plans on the information you have gathered about your own students and the communities of which they and your school are a part.

SUMMARY

There are but three basic sources of information to be analyzed in curriculum development. These are the learners, their needs, interests, problems, maturity, and abilities; the demands and problems of the society in which they live; and the valued subject matter. There was a time when the only consideration when planning for instruction was the named subject matter. That might have worked even 75 years ago, but it is no longer possible for anyone to know everything there is to know about anything. So the problem is to decide what knowledge is of most worth today, and that depends on many other things (e.g., the nature of the students, where they live, and what they need to know how to do in that environment and society).

In recent years, the study of curriculum has become a discipline in its own right, having a special vocabulary and distinctive modes of procedure. Teachers need not be experts in curriculum design, but they do need to be comfortable in their grasp of its language and relevant data sources, first, because they are responsible for the interpretation and application of curriculum plans where it counts most, at the classroom level; second, because they are so often asked to participate in the development or updating of school or district level curricula; and

third, because the processes employed and the information needed are no less applicable and essential to the development of resource units, learning opportunities, and lessons.

Any vocabulary that might seem strange or new is just a matter of using another word or words to mean what is already familiar language for teachers. What curriculum specialists call **organizing elements,** teachers often refer to as "units." In health education, units are ordinarily titled according to the design selected for a particular curriculum, i.e., as health content areas, topics, health problems, body systems, or concepts. A *scope* lists the number and kind of organizing elements chosen for a curriculum plan. **Sequence** is the word used to describe the plan for ordering the organizing elements, from kindergarten through twelfth grade so that one learning experience builds on another by intention. **Horizontal sequence** is the planned arrangement of elements side by side so that they buttress each other in effect and logic. When curriculum specialists refer to **organizing centers,** what they are talking about are the suggested learning opportunities as proposed in a curriculum guide.

However thorough the investigation of the sources of a curriculum may be, an essential preliminary statement must be prepared. This is the philosophy or set of basic beliefs about health education held by those who will plan the curriculum. Such a document specifies the nature and skills of the health educated person the schools seek to develop, and justifies this goal on the basis of demonstrated needs. Subsequent decisions setting goals, objectives, content focus, learning activities, and the rest are based upon and guided by that philosophy. The result is a plan that is consistent with the avowed purpose of the program, whatever the level of instruction.

How the scope of the curriculum is taught

requires another set of decisions, similarly based upon what we learn about the learners, the community and the body of knowledge. Health teaching at the elementary and middle school levels may be integrated with other subjects such as social studies, science, or physical education. Or it may be accorded equal treatment with other basic subjects, and allotted single subject status including adequate amounts of time, resources, and facilities. Ideally, a combination of both patterns is provided, which requires careful coordination of activities and objectives, and inservice training for all of the teachers who will be doing the teaching.

QUESTIONS AND EXERCISES

Discussion questions

1. What would be the advantages and disadvantages of basing curriculum decisions solely on interests of the learner?

2. Differentiate between needs and interests and the developmental characteristics of children. Which set of data do you see as having the greater influence on *what* is taught and which one on *how* it is taught?

3. What is the relationship between general education and health education?

4. Which plan for organizing the scope of health instruction seems best suited to a focus on wellness? Which plan might present the greatest problem if health promotion were to be the goal of instruction? Why would it be difficult?

5. If health is viewed as a concept with interacting physical, social, mental, and emotional dimensions, can mental health be dealt with as a distinct and separate area? If so, explain your rationale for such a separation. If not, explain why not.

6. In what ways do community values influence health curriculum planning? Give examples of some ways you perceive to be significant.

7. What do you see as the major differences between integrated and direct teaching of health science? What would be the best way to correct the weaknesses of each?

Exercises and problems

1a. For an elementary school grade of your choice, find out as much as you can about the needs and interests of the students as reported in the literature; the levels of physical, social, mental and emotional development to be expected of these children; the scope of health instruction recommended or mandated in your state or school district; and a listing of the local health needs and problems relevant to a health curriculum for children of that age.

1b. Based on careful consideration of all these data, (1) define the scope of health instruction by means of the organizing elements that you believe to be most suitable, and (2) order these elements according to a stated logic for a horizontal sequence for one year. Present your plan to the class and be prepared to support your decisions by reference to the data from which they were inferred.

2. Make a scrapbook of current news clippings collected from local, state, or national publications that have implications for health curriculum planning. Organize them according to their relevance to the organizing elements you have chosen, whether these are content areas, topics, or others. Note which elements are most often a community concern and which are mentioned least. How could this information affect your plans concerning sequence?

3. Interview at least five children of either primary, upper elementary or middle school age, and ask them to tell you what they want to know about health or health problems. Encourage them to think about health as a means of enjoying life and growing up to be what they would like to be. Record every question that they ask. Share your list with others in your group and draw some conclusions, based on the accumulation of questions, about the interests and the needs revealed, as well as about the frequency with which each of these is expressed. Which kinds of questions were asked most frequently? Were there questions you expected but did not get? Speculate about the reasons that this might have been the case.

4. Obtain a copy of a local school health curriculum guide (or one prepared by a community health agency or professional health organization) and analyze its components. What are the organizing elements used to structure the subject matter? What is the scope of the curriculum? Is there a plan for horizontal sequence? If so, what is suggested for first consideration? Is there a plan for vertical sequence? Does the scope reflect a comprehensive view of health education, or is it limited in any way? If it is limited, what is missing? What would you add if it were in your power to amend the plan? Write a report of your analysis.

REFERENCES

American Alliances For Health, Physical Educational Recreation: Health concepts: guides for instruction, Washington, DC, 1967, AAHPER.

American School Health Association: School health in America, ed 4, Kent, Ohio, 1987, ASHA.

Bruner: The process of education, Cambridge, Mass, 1963, Harvard University Press.

Byler, Lewis, G, and Totman, R: Teach us what we want to know, Connecticut State Board of Educ., New York 1969. Mental health materials center, Inc.

Dapice, Ann, et al.: Teaching and learning values, Educ Horizons **66**:3, Spring 1988, pp. 107-109.

Denver Public Schools: The health interests of children, Denver, 1954.

Educational Policies Commission: The central purpose of education, Washington, DC, 1961, National Education Association.

Goodlad J: A place called school, New York, 1984, McGraw-Hill.

Green, LW and others: Health education planning: a diagnostic approach, Palo Alto, Calif, 1980 Mayfield.

Hartoonian H and Laughlin M: Designing a scope and sequence, Social Educ 50:7, Nov/Dec 1986.

Kolbe L and others: Propositions for an alternate and complementary health education paradigm, Health Educ 12:3, May-June 1981.

Kreuter MW: Considering realistic outcomes for school health education. Unpublished paper presented at Promoting Health through Schools Conference, Denver, 1980.

Kunstel F: Assessing community needs: implications for school and staff development in health education, J Sch Health, 48:220, April 1978.

Moyer J: Child development as a base for decision making, Child Educ 62 (5): 325-329, 1986.

Natapoff J: A developmental analysis of children's ideas of health, Health Educ Q, 9:2, 3, Summer/Fall 1982.

National Center for Health Education: Growing healthy, vol 3, New York, p 41, 1984.

National Center for Health Education: Primary Grades Health Curriculum Project and School Health Curriculum Project, San Bruno, CA, 1981.

National Comprehensive School Health Education Guidelines Committee: Comprehensive school health education, J Sch Health, 54 (8): 312-315, 1984.

Newbauer D and Pratt R: The second public health revolution: a critical appraisal, J Health Politics, Policy Law, 6:205, Summer 1981.

Parker J and Rubin L: Process as content, Chicago, 1966, Rand McNally.

Perrin K: Instructional leadership: a statement of philosophy is the first step, NASSP Bulletin, 70 (494): 65-73, 1986.

School Health Education Study: Scope and Sequence Chart, 1971.

Sliepcevich E: Curriculum development: a macroscopic or microscopic view. National Elem Principal, 48:2, 1969.

Trucano L: Students speak, Seattle, Wash, 1984, Comprehensive Health Education Foundation.

Tyler R: Basic principles of curriculum and instruction, Chicago, 1963, University of Chicago Press. (Originally published in 1949.)

US Department of Health and Human Services: Public Health Services, Prospects for a healthier America, Washington, DC, 1984.

US Department of Health and Human Services: Public Health Services, Objectives for the Nation, Washington, DC, 1980.

US Department of Health, Education, and Welfare. Healthy people, Washington, DC, 1979.

Yarber W: Accounting for health instruction, Health Educ, 8:4, July/Aug 1977.

SUGGESTED READINGS

Anspaugh D and Ezell G: Teaching the developmental process to elementary children, Health Educ, 15:2, March/April 1984. Describes ''Body Timetable'' activity providing needed information about pubertal developmental changes for fourth-grade to sixth-grade children.

Harris J and Liebert R: The child, Englewood Cliffs, NJ, 1984, Prentice Hall. A textbook written for those who want or need to learn about the growth and development of children. Begins at conception and considers every aspect of development in chronological fashion through adolescence. Discusses cognitive, motor, intellectual, social, moral, and every other aspect of growth and development. Thoroughly researched and documented, yet easy to read, it provides a wealth of valuable information.

Jones H and others: Planning for health instruction in the schools, Eta Sigma Gamma Monograph Series, 2:1 Feb 1984. Outlines and describes ten essential steps to be taken in planning local and school district comprehensive school health education. Includes listings of health-concerned federal agencies as well as reprints of relevant articles discussing expectancies for school health program contributions to promotion of health among students and in the community.

Schaller W: The school health program, ed 5, Philadelphia, 1981, WB Saunders, Chapter 8. Gives tabulated descriptions of physical, emotional, social, and intellectual characteristics of school-aged children, including preschool (ages 3 to 5); primary grades (ages 5 to 8); upper elementary (ages 8 to 11); and middle school, (ages 11 to 14). Discusses factors that affect growth and development.

CHAPTER 4

Defining Goals and Objectives for Health Teaching

When you finish this chapter you should be able to:

■ Differentiate between the structure and functions of educational goals and instructional objectives.

■ Analyze the advantages of using measurable objectives as the framework for planning health teaching.

■ Evaluate the worth and functionality of goals and objectives proposed for health teaching in elementary schools.

■ Apply the criteria for preparing clearly stated objectives to the development of a set of classroom-level objectives.

Since it is your intention to become an elementary school teacher, you may already have had some experience in writing goals and objectives. Is there anything about doing the same thing for health teaching that is different? We think so. The other basics of the elementary school curriculum focus on communication and computation skills (i.e., reading, writing, and arithmetic). What is to be learned is clearly defined, and what is taught is much the same anywhere in the country. Health teaching has to do with helping children learn and apply problem-solving skills in making everyday choices that will build and maintain a healthful life style. Its subject matter is far more complex and dynamic in scope and its objectives must elicit activities involving active participation rather than passive listening or desk work. The goals of health teaching do not propose ends without real-life utility, nor can its instructional objectives be effective in attaining those ends in the absence of relevance to the learners.

Can you write an objective that describes an educational outcome with potential use in solving an actual health problem? Can you differentiate between a goal statement and an operational objective? The following eight statements labeled *objectives* are taken from as many current elementary school curriculum guides published by major health-concerned organizations:

1. To understand some of the reciprocal relationships involving man, disease, and environment.
2. Be able to state that the heart is a muscle that never stops working.
3. Explains why certain foods have limited nutritional value.
4. The student will be able to discuss three major differences between active and passive immunity.
5. Students will have opportunities to identify the characteristics of human blood.
6. Children will recognize what they can do to maintain and protect the environment.
7. After listening to, completing, and discussing several riddles and poems, the pupil will be able to identify the function several body parts can perform by completing the given worksheet with 80% accuracy.
8. Recalls why individual, community, and international health problems prevail on the local, state, national, and international scenes.

Do you see any differences among these eight statements? How many of them would you accept as being meaningful and achievable objectives for health teaching in elementary schools? If they all look good to you now, we hope that you will read on before you make up your mind definitely.

FUNCTION OF GOAL STATEMENTS IN CURRICULUM DESIGN

Goal statements describe the *ends* or purposes of a curriculum plan. Whatever their level of specificity, **objectives** always describe ways and means of attaining those ends. Differences between goals and objectives also depend on their intended function in curriculum development and on their distance from the students themselves. Krathwohl (1965) divides these distances into three levels. At the most remote level—farthest from the classroom and the student—are the broad, abstract, and most general statements describing the educational goals for a total program, for grades K through 12. At the next level are the general objectives used to structure plans for a semester course or curriculum unit. Such an objective is broad enough in content to require many learning opportunities for its achievement. The third level—that closest in impact to the learner—is composed of the most specific objectives, used to structure a single lesson or part of a lesson.

The broadest statements are those referred to as goals or aims. The subordinate and more specific general objectives and instructional objectives allow teachers flexibility in choosing among them and in selecting the strategies and techniques to be used in carrying them out.

Goodlad (1963) has said that the term *objectives* should be used only when referring to purposes stated in terms of learner activities, and that for purposes to be carried out by schools or teachers, the terms *goals* or *aims* are appropriate. He, too, defines three educational decision-making levels of remoteness from the classroom, but they differ from those of Krathwohl. Most remote, says Goodlad, is the *societal* level, which includes the educational goals set by school boards, legislators, and federal agencies.

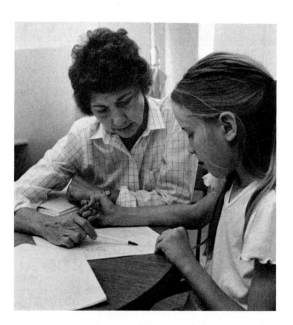

Closer are the institutional goals—those set by school administrators and teachers when making curriculum plans intended for an entire school or school district. Closest to the students, is the instructional level, and only these, he says, should be termed behavioral or educational objectives.

FORMULATING LONG-RANGE GOALS

Every statement of educational purposes, whatever its level of generality, includes the same two dimensions: (1) behavior and (2) some amount of subject matter. The differences between goals and objectives are most apparent in the behaviors used in each case and the relative abstractness of the content prescribed. The behavior or verb used to state long-range goals is often ambiguous, such as *knows, understands,* or *believes.* This is acceptable for goal statements because, in effect, the meaning of the ambiguous behavior will be defined by the objectives proposed as means of achieving that goal.

In health teaching, long-range goals represent target outcomes and remain the same throughout the entire curriculum plan. Thus, they provide stability and give direction at every level of teaching responsible for their achievement. Typically, goals are stated in terms of what is hoped the students will know, believe, and do about health-related practices and problems. Accordingly, they are categorized as belonging to the cognitive, affective, or action domains of behaviors. The cognitive domain includes those objectives that deal with recalling or recognizing knowledge, and those requiring higher intellectual skills and abilities such as comprehension, application, analysis, synthesis, and evaluation. The affective domain includes those that describe desired changes in

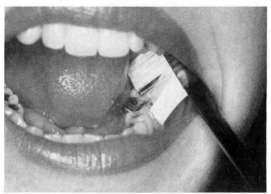

Copyright by the American Dental Association. Reprinted by permission.

interests, attitudes, and values. There is a third domain, the psychomotor, which has to do with manipulation or motor skills and which has greater application in physical education (Harrow, 1972).

There *are* health education objectives with psychomotor components. These are the kinds of objectives that can be practiced and evaluated observably such as the ability to carry out cardiopulmonary resuscitation (CPR), use dental floss or a toothbrush correctly, apply certain first-aid procedures, or perform recommended personal health care practices such as those involving care of the skin, hair, and nails.

Rather than using the psychomotor domain as its third category of long-range goals, the writing team of the School Health Education Study (1967) devised a new term, *action,* as more descriptive of desired adult health actions. The action domain was defined as those aspects of health behaviors in which one applies health knowledge, attitudes, and problem-solving skills to an actual life situation. Since its introduction, the term *action* has been used by many health educators to categorize the third group of health education goals.

Exemplary goals categorized according to the three domains are

Cognitive: Knows that body parts, systems, and functions grow and develop at varying rates both among and within individuals.

Affective: Believes that the potential for growth and development can be fostered or hindered by an individual's own choices and actions.

Action: Exhibits health behaviors that promote or maintain optimum growth and development.

COMPETENCIES AS GOALS

In many states and school districts, instead of long-range goals, competency statements have been proposed as descriptors of desired learning outcomes. The notion of competency as a goal has gained wide acceptance and competencies have been recommended for every level of instruction from kindergarten through graduate school.

Competencies written in regard to health education are usually stated at two levels of abstraction. The high-level competencies are virtually indistinguishable from statements otherwise termed goals, and the specific competency statements, inferred from the broader statements, are in no way different from behavioral objectives.

The principal difference between the two levels appears to depend on whether the behavior is ambiguous (e.g., *knows, appreciates, behaves*) or specific (e.g., *identifies, names, lists*), and whether the total statement describes an outcome that corresponds to one of the previously mentioned domains of learning.

A general competency and its supporting objectives, adapted from those specified for a high school in California, is as follows:

Competency: Students will understand the effects of nutrition on their immediate and long-term personal well-being.

Objectives: Names the essential nutrients and their functions.

Identifies beneficial effects of common food.

Explains long-term effects of poor nutrition.

The following long-range goal with a similar purpose is almost identical to the preceding competency statement. ''The student comprehends that the choice of foods determines the nutrient balance vital to effective functioning of the body.'' The form has not been altered; only the label is different. Nevertheless, the use of competencies as desired outcomes of instruction has brought much greater attention to the quality of the instructional objectives designed to attain them. Goal statements are apt to be forgotten by those who write instructional objectives. Competency statements seem to be more provocative targets; hence, the objectives that are subsumed tend to be more relevant and interesting than they otherwise might be. In fact, the greatest contribution of the competency movement may have been this emphasis on measurement of student learning in terms of predetermined abilities and the consequent sharpening of the objectives designed with that in mind.

RELATIONSHIP OF GENERAL TO SPECIFIC OBJECTIVES

Curriculum-level, or general, objectives are inferred from the long-range goals. Instructional objectives, in turn, are inferred from the general objectives. At every level, these statements attempt to answer the question, ''What are the skills and knowledge an educated person needs to know in order to build a positive life style and to solve health-related problems effectively when they arise?''

The objectives designed to implement goals should be stated at the classroom level. Whether they are broadly or narrowly defined depends on their intended function. A few broadly stated general objectives can be used to structure a unit or course of study with considerable economy of detail and no loss of clarity. The most specific objectives subordinate to these general statements are best left for the classroom teacher to prepare, since different groups of students have different interests, past experiences, and abilities. Only the teacher should tailor the specific objectives designed to fulfill the purposes expressed in a general objective. As long as the specific objectives collectively result in the achievement of the general objectives, small differences in the enabling (specific) objectives have little, if any, importance. For example, if a

FIG. 4-1

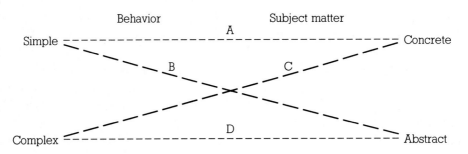

proposed general objective were, "Develops criteria for choosing among commonly used personal health products," some enabling objectives that a teacher might use as a means to that end are the following:

1. Defines the meaning of the term "health product."
2. Names health products commonly used at home.
3. Identifies reasons that certain health products were chosen.
4. Lists criteria used by parents and friends when choosing health products.
5. Describes the key factors involved in determining each criterion.

Although general objectives do not differ in form from the specific objectives, they *are* different in the breadth of the subject matter they encompass, or in the complexity of the behavior they elicit. The more complex the behavior, the more maturity and skill the learner needs to carry it out. The broader the content, the more elaborate the learner's system of previously learned concepts must be. These two major components, behavior and content, can be manipulated to suit a given level of student readiness. The accompanying diagram illustrates four possible patterns for combining the two dimensions to adjust for the needs and abilities of individual groups of students.

Examples of each of the four possible combinations, from the simplest to the most complex objectives, are these:

A. Lists ways to avoid exposure to germs.
B. Names characteristics common to all living things.
C. Classifies foods according to the four food groups.
D. Evaluates social, cultural, and economic influences on health behavior.

It is important to remember that the objectives you devise must be attainable by your students. Within a set of general *or* instructional objectives, each objective must be consistent with the others at that level of generality, that is, in a given set, all objectives must have the same combination of the two dimensions which you decide is best suited to the abilities and needs of your students (the A, B, C, or D combination). For students at a given level, a mixture of two or more of these patterns confuses both the purposes and the results.

MEASURABLE VERSUS BEHAVIORAL OBJECTIVES

Most educators are willing to admit that anyone planning to teach needs to decide what the objectives are to be. The principal issue seems to center on the degree of measurability such statements should possess. This point has been debated for some time without much resolution, probably because the two sides are not all that far apart in their approaches. The curious thing is that despite all this debate, few instructors find it easy to write objectives and fewer still bother to write them at all. Nevertheless, whether or not you believe that precision and measurability are essential elements of an instructional objective, you should know how to write one and how to use them to facilitate lesson planning. Objectives that are measurable should describe *what the learner will be able to do following instruction that she or he could not have done before.*

Perhaps the problem is not that educators believe that there is no need to write objectives that describe actions or behaviors that can be seen and measured, but that the word *behavioral* is not clear in meaning. Often behavioral objectives are descriptive of lesson-specific activities, for instance, "Given a diagram of a

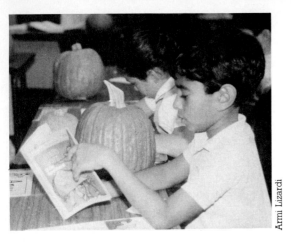

Armi Lizardi

Stating Measurable Objectives

Authorities differ somewhat in their recommendations regarding the form of a well-stated objective. Most agree that it should propose a behavior that can be practiced and observed in the classroom (as opposed to the ambiguous long-range behaviors used in stating goals). Major differences in opinion, as we have said, center around the relative precision with which those behaviors should be stated, and whether the criterion of achievement must be included in the objective. In general, three patterns of handling objectives seem to have evolved. One is the *programmed instruction model,* another has been influenced by the Bloom taxonomy of educational objectives (1956), and the third will be termed the *operational model* in this discussion.

Programmed instruction model. Those who have adopted a programmed instruction pattern would write an objective of this kind: "Given a list of ten common foodstuffs, the student will be able to identify each according to its food group with at least 80% accuracy." Use of this very specific, criterion-associated objective had its origin in Mager's little book, *Preparing Objectives for Programmed Instruction* (1961). The book gained such immediate and popular acceptance that at the second printing it was given a broader title, *Preparing Instructional Objectives* (1962). Although no change was made in the content, the new title led to the belief that what had been intended as an aid in developing programmed instructional materials was equally appropriate for all kinds of education. However, the Mager kind of objective focuses on the very specific learning outcome essential for programmed instruction. In an attempt to apply this model at all levels—lesson, course, school, and district,—curriculum workers found themselves drowning in a sea of ob-

particular part of the body (e.g., the eye) the student will be able to correctly label that diagram." *(Feuerstein and Galli, 1983).* Some see "behavioral" as referring only to cognitive skills which have been sharpened and increased as a result of the activity called for in the objective, for example, "Describes the structure and function of the eye and ear" (SHEP, 1981). Others reject the word in this sense because the resulting objectives seem to them trivial, mechanistic, and therefore dehumanizing, or part of a plan to mold or control the minds and behaviors of children. Still others see "behavioral" as referring to changes effected in actual health practices, for example, the learner no longer exhibits a harmful behavior or adopts a healthful behavior as a result of the learning experience provided.

For the purposes of this book, when the word *measurable* is used, it will simply mean that the objective describes an activity, mastery of which can be assessed in the classroom. Whatever you call it, an instructional objective for health education specifies a measurable cognitive or affective behavior associated with some amount of meaningful health content.

jectives. Critics looked at the mass of minutiae and decided that *any* objectives that attempted to specify learning outcomes were useless.

Popham (1972), an early advocate of behavioral objectives, commented:

Certainly there are abuses of instructional objectives. These are usually perpetrated by administrators, who having read Mager's little volume on objectives feel themselves blessed with instant expertise and thus institute a free-wheeling circus in their schools.

A related problem is the fact that objectives so narrowly conceived and rigidly prescriptive tend to stifle teaching creativity and flexibility. Moreover, individualization of instruction in such a situation becomes difficult, if not impossible.

Taxonomy model. If care were taken to give equal emphasis to all of the six categories of cognition identified in the Bloom taxonomy (Bloom et al., 1956), this model would be a useful framework for the design of health education objectives. However, studies show that the overwhelming majority of objectives based on this approach focus on the lowest level of the hierarchy, *knowing.* At that level it is the *content* dimension on which the specificity depends, particularly in the case of objectives designed for the elementary school years. An example of such a fact-oriented statement is: "Knows that a food which is derived from the flesh of animals belongs to the meat group." Use of the single behavior "knows" for so many objectives gives the teacher no guidance in selecting an activity but only in deciding *what* to teach, yet the goal of health education is to develop the ability to think and use the information learned in making decisions, not the acquisition of a lot of facts about health.

A set of consumer health objectives, devised according to the Bloom taxonomy (Bloom et al., 1956), illustrates the hierarchy of cognitive skills that were identified. Each level of cognition presupposes achievement of that preceding it.

Knowledge: Names people whose job it is to keep us well.

Comprehension: Explains ways advertising influences choices of foods and other health products.

Application: Interprets the meaning of information on food labels.

Analysis: Distinguishes between health quackery and reliable health advice.

Synthesis: Formulates a set of criteria for the selection of health products.

Evaluation: Evaluates the reliability of claims promoting the sale and use of health products.

Operational model. Instructional objectives intended to structure health teaching are most efficiently stated in operational terms. *Operational* means that the statement clearly describes what the student will be able to do after instruction and what she or he will be practicing during instruction. Furthermore, the criterion or test of its achievement can be inferred from the objective itself, exactly as stated. Objectives can be broadly stated as to the content, yet measurable so long as the associated skill can be demonstrated by the student. An example of an operational objective is: "Explains the influence of peer pressure on one's health behavior."

Both teaching and evaluation can be based on such an objective by *any* means a teacher chooses as long as the students are (1) helped to learn how to accomplish the objective, and (2) ultimately asked to demonstrate their new ability. Operational objectives provide direction but do not restrict teachers in choosing how they will be implemented. They allow teachers freedom to vary techniques to suit their own style and the special needs of their own students.

Another problem that can be avoided by use of operational objectives is ambiguity. For example, consider this objective: "Identifies foods that are essential for a balanced diet." There is no single list of foods which are essential for a balanced and nutritious diet. In other words, health is not like mathematics. There is not always one right answer. The goals of health teaching are not to develop singular abilities. What might be a good list in this country for a person of a certain age and sex could be totally inapplicable in another situation. What needs to be learned is the ability to choose, from the total range of available foodstuffs, a diet that fulfills one's current nutritional needs.

CRITERIA FOR THE DEVELOPMENT OF INSTRUCTIONAL OBJECTIVES

Before the functions of an objective or sequence of objectives are discussed, some guidelines for the development of objectives that work well must be considered. As Mager has said, "If you don't know where you are going, you might wind up somewhere else" (Mager, 1962). However specific or general it may be, a well-stated objective satisfies at least these criteria:

1. It is stated in terms of a learner behavior, not in terms of a teacher's intentions.
2. It specifies both the behavior and the content matter of interest.
3. It describes just one behavior and one content component.
4. It is operational, meaning that the learner can practice the skill and work with the subject matter in the classroom setting.
5. It specifies a behavior that is explicit, not ambiguous.
6. It describes a cognitive or affective outcome rather than an activity that is an end in itself.

7. It describes an outcome with apparent life-long application and worth.
8. It is feasible for the students for whom it is designed.

Criterion 1

An operational objective is stated in terms of a proposed learner activity, not as descriptive of something the teacher plans to do, for example, "To teach reasons why so many people continue to smoke despite official warnings of possible ill effects." Learning happens in the learner. The stated objective could be carried out by the teacher in an empty room, speaking for the benefit of an admiring tape recorder. A better objective is, "The student explains why people begin and continue to smoke cigarettes." This statement says exactly what the student is expected to be doing during the learning opportunity, yet the teacher has considerable latitude in planning since there are many ways that practice in explaining the reasons involved could be provided.

Criterion 2

An objective must have two basic components: a measurable behavior and some clearly defined subject matter. "The effects of drug abuse" is a topic and not an objective since it merely states generally *what* will be covered. On the other hand, "To analyze critically" is a behavior without any subject matter. A complete objective would be: "The student describes hazards associated with abuse of any drug." Both components, the behavior and the subject matter, are included, and achievement of purpose of the objective can be demonstrated several ways.

Criterion 3

An objective must specify just one behavior and one element of content. The statement, "Names methods of disease control and explains how each method is most appropriately applied," combines two objectives. Separately stated, they are easier to carry out, and, in sum, the outcome is at least the same and probably better.

"Identifies and describes methods of disease control" is an objective with two behaviors but only one element of subject matter. These behaviors will have to be practiced one at a time. A better statement might simply ask the student to "describe," since "identify" would be a necessary first step in doing any describing of those methods.

"Describes methods of disease control and how each control is applied" has two content elements. The student will have to deal with these one at a time, so there is no avoiding the fact that there are two objectives to be reached. In fact, a better behavior might have been suggested for the second content element if two objectives had been proposed; for example, "Describes methods of disease control," and "Explains how different methods of disease control are applied."

Criterion 4

An operational objective elicits a teaching strategy that allows the student appropriate practice and permits its achievement to be immediately demonstrated in the classroom.

"Refrains from using substances that are harmful to health" is a goal, not an objective. The teacher would have to monitor the student's behavior for the rest of his or her life in order to evaluate its success. A better objective is, "Differentiates between uses of mind-altering substances that may be helpful and those that are harmful." A number of hypothetical problems or simulated situations could be devised to evaluate achievement of that objective. The student either can or cannot do it. Whether the ability to differentiate between these kinds of uses leads to wise decisions in later life is not something that the teacher can or should attempt to test.

Criterion 5

An operational objective specifies a behavior that is measurable rather than ambiguous. Certain action words or verbs are more descriptive of skills and therefore communicate their meaning more universally than others. Cognitive behaviors commonly used in objectives and accepted as being measurable include *identify, describe, compare, analyze, explain,* and *evaluate.* Although individual teachers may interpret these behaviors somewhat differently, most would generally agree about what was happening when a student is describing, or listing, or comparing things.

Verbs that are too ambiguous (open to many equally plausible interpretations) to dependably communicate the intended behavior include *know, understand, comprehend, appreciate, learn, recognize,* and *realize.* What would you ask a student to do to show that she or he appreciates, or knows, or comprehends? The teacher who bases learning opportunities on these kinds of fuzzy behaviors may not decide what the student will be asked to do until the examinations are being written. However, whatever the examination asks the student to do, the task will not be ambiguous but specific. If the teacher does not know what will be asked while the lesson is going on, who can blame the hapless students who have no way of knowing what they will be asked about the lesson later? For example, "Appreciates the value of good health" is nice but also ambiguous. Everybody appreciates good health (although those who appreciate it most are those who have it least).

But how would you measure how much a person's appreciation had increased as a result of your instruction? And how would that objective help you plan a lesson that would contribute to your students' appreciation? "Explains the relationship between good health and the enjoyment of work and play" might get at the same thing. Even small children could carry out a lesson giving them appropriate practice in doing that, and could later explain the relationship to others.

Criterion 6

An operational objective specifies a cognitive or affective skill or behavior that transfers to other times and other problems, rather than a word that simply describes a *means* of exhibiting or expressing such a skill. Words such as *discuss, write, state* and *tell* verbally express what is happening cognitively or emotionally. But is it possible to discuss something without explaining, describing, or comparing, for example? *Discuss,* which is the most overworked word in the lexicon of curriculum developers, actually describes a means of verbalizing cognitive skills. Other words such as *observe, participate,* or *demonstrate* usually describe an activity, or assignment. The real objective, which should tell us why this would be done, is unstated. *Do not confuse a description of an assignment with a statement of an instructional objective.*

An objective such as "Discuss the correct use of dental floss" poses several questions. Who is to discuss it? Is it to be the teacher? What does "discussing" mean in that event—lecturing or telling? If it is to be the students who are doing the discussing, won't they actually be describing the way to use dental floss? If so, why not say so? And how would you devise a means of evaluating a discussion?

"Demonstrates ability to take a pulse rate" is another activity. It is not an objective, but rather the outcome of the unspecified objective. What happens once the student can demonstrate the skill? How does that relate to health behavior? Do the children learn the relevance of this activity to their own health or later learnings? Or, as is more likely, is it simply an end in itself?

Criterion 7

An educational objective should describe an outcome with potential life-long utility and value. Thus, a worthwhile objective requires problem solving and deals with content that can be generalized to similar problems at other times and places. Only rarely are decisions made that do not in some way affect health, both our own and that of others. Not only should an objective be measurable in the classroom, but what has been learned should also be useful in the future. At the very least, an objective ought to contribute to the ultimate achievement of another objective that does have that potential. For instance, study of the physiology of the heart might be justified as a part of health education if it were integrated with learning how diet choices are a factor in preventing coronary heart disease.

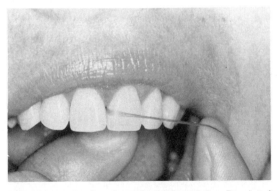

Copyright by the American Dental Association. Reprinted by permission.

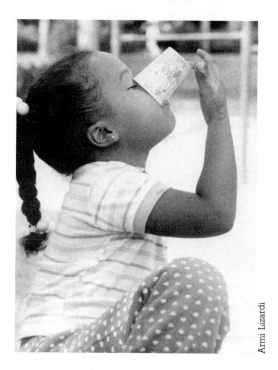

Armi Lizardi

"Names the principal bones of the human skeleton" is not an objective clearly relevant to health behavior. How does ability to name bones help the student of health education? Can it help a person to walk better, run faster, or stand straighter? Unless it is deemed an asset to be able to pass a test on the names of bones, achievement of such an objective is simply an end in itself.

On the other hand, "Explains how adequate fluoride levels in drinking water can affect the development of teeth and bones" has both physical and social uses beyond the immediate learning situation. The learner discovers the implications of fluoride use for the growth of children and in the maintenance of healthy bone tissue in the elderly. As a potential voter, the learner is better prepared to make a reasoned decision about the addition of fluorides to public water supplies.

Criterion 8

An instructional objective must be feasible. An objective might satisfy all the foregoing criteria and yet fail this test. The abilities and comprehension of the subject matter specified in the objective must be within the range of possibility for the students for whom it is intended.

For example, "Analyzes the impact of environmental pollution on the quality of urban living" might be feasible for high school students but not for those in the third grade. The appropriateness of an objective must be justified on the basis of studies of the learners, as recommended previously, so that the objective reasonably matches expected skill development and builds on past content learnings. Grade-3 students probably will not be able to demonstrate ability to analyze or to deal with the concept of quality as it relates to urban living.

"Identifies physical characteristics that are inherited" is a relatively simple behavior, and the content element is factual rather than abstract. The Trucano Study (Students Speak, 1984) revealed that interest in genetics was high at all grade levels. Such an objective should be interesting and feasible for elementary students, given appropriate enabling objectives developed for each grade.

Another aspect of feasibility has to do with the available time, money, and facilities. It is pointless to develop objectives that cannot possibly be achieved. Questions of cost, time requirements, and the availability of qualified staff and supplies that can have a significant influence on implementation must also be considered when defining teaching objectives. Thus the objective "Develops a videotaped survey of sources of water, air, and noise pollution" could result in a dramatic production and give great satisfaction to both students and their parents. However, it probably involves more sophisticated and expensive equipment, technical expertise, and more time than schools are able to devote to health education at any level of schooling. A substitute objective needs to be devised that describes something that *can* be done and is just as satisfying, but is also feasible.

COGNITIVE BEHAVIORS

Certain behaviors descriptive of cognitive processes are more useful in stating measurable objectives than others. Some verbs have wide acceptance because their meaning is specific enough to be interpreted in much the same way by most educators. However, even slight differences in interpretation can alter both the approach selected and the outcome of the instruction. It is wise to specify the meaning of the behaviors to be used, rather than to assume that each will be perceived by everyone else exactly as intended by its developer. Whenever you set out to design a series of instructional objectives, define the terms you are going to use before you begin. It simplifies the task of choosing behaviors that are feasible for your students, promotes consistency in form, and facilitates the development of lessons that provide appropriate practice. The following are examples of definitions that might help establish what the learners should be doing as they carry out the objective. Each of these has been tentatively categorized according to the hierarchy proposed by the Bloom Taxonomy of Educational Objectives (Bloom et al., 1956). Remember that these are not *the* definitions—only possible examples.

1. *Knowledge*
   a. Naming: using the correct word to designate a given person, object, or idea.
   b. Defining: stating the exact meaning of a word or sense of a word.
   c. Listing: making an ordered record of persons or objects, usually of the same nature.
   d. Identifying: ascertaining the nature or definitive characteristics of a thing or person.
2. *Comprehension*
   a. Explaining: verbally making the nature or meaning of something clear; offering reasons.
   b. Describing: telling about something in detail; picturing with words.
   c. Interpreting: translating complex ideas or concepts into simpler terms.
3. *Application*
   a. Illustrating: clarifying by using examples and comparisons with words, pictures, or actions.
   b. Predicting: stating what might happen in a given situation on the basis of prior or newly obtained information.
   c. Discriminating: distinguishing relationships or differences among elements of a communication or problem.
   d. Applying: transferring learned concepts and skills, as needed, to solve new problems.
4. *Analysis*
   a. Analyzing: separating a communication, problem, or concept into its component parts as a means of clarifying the meaning of the whole.
   b. Categorizing: determining the placement of an idea or object in a specific division of a classification system.
   c. Classifying: arranging or sorting items according to a set of shared characteristics.
   d. Differentiating: noting or showing specific variations in or between objects.
5. *Synthesis*
   a. Concluding: making a reasoned judg-

ment or inference based on all the data available.

   b. Proposing: suggesting a novel plan or solution to a problem for consideration and adoption.

   c. Synthesizing: combining separate substances, elements or ideas to form a wholly new product.

  6. *Evaluation*

   a. Contrasting (with): showing or emphasizing differences between or among objects, persons, or ideas.

   b. Comparing (with): examining objects, persons, or ideas to note similarities between or among them.

   c. Evaluating: appraising the quality of a product or plan according to a set of predetermined standards.

AFFECTIVE OBJECTIVES

Although all the objectives discussed so far have been drawn from the cognitive domain, this does not mean that affective objectives cannot be defined in a form that is measurable to some degree. Affective objectives are primarily concerned with the development of positive attitudes, values, and interests. Krathwohl, Bloom and Masia (1964), who devised a taxonomy of affective educational objectives, believe that the term *internalization,* used to describe these kinds of learnings, refers to the inner growth that occurs as one becomes aware of and then adopts attitudes, codes of behavior, and values that make up the personal system of beliefs that influences health-related decisions. The five categories of objectives in the affective domain range from the lowest and nearly cognitive level of learning, termed *awareness,* followed by *responding, valuing,* and *organization,* to the highest level of the taxonomy, *characterization by a value or value concept.*

Achievement of an affective objective may be as difficult to measure as it is to define. For this reason, some educators neither try to write them nor consider an objective that seeks to modify an attitude as feasible or necessary; yet the goals of health education are inextricably linked to the promotion and maintenance of attitudes favorable to their attainment.

Learning activities can be planned to help students analyze their existing beliefs and make a reasoned interpretation of the impact of those beliefs on their daily choices among behaviors. Objectives for this purpose can be stated nearly as operationally as those for cognitive purposes (AERA, 1975). Affective objectives have been specified by health educators, such as the following: "Volunteers to participate in a campaign to promote a neighborhood cleanup program"; "Seeks to persuade family members to improve poor health practices when these are noted"; or "Evidences willingness to comply with school safety procedures."

Admittedly, these are more exactly descriptions of desired outcomes of instruction based upon meaningful cognitive objectives, whether stated or not.

Meaningful cognitive objectives have much to contribute to affective outcomes. For example, in one classroom two students, whose existing negative attitude toward fluoridation of drinking water made them reject any information that supported its worth, were permitted to argue their point of view as a class project. It was agreed that they would first study both sides of the issue as carefully and thoroughly as they could. To their own surprise they found themselves persuaded that fluoridation of drinking water supplies does in fact have a positive effect on the development of strong teeth and bones. Their prior convictions and attitudes had been entirely reversed as a result of what could have been perceived as a cognitive objective such as, "Describes the effect of fluoridated water on growth and development of teeth and bones." Had a measurable affective objective also been defined, it might have been, ''Believes that fluoridation of water supplies promotes optimum bone and teeth development.''

ADVANTAGES OF USING MEASURABLE OBJECTIVES

Although it cannot be argued that good teaching is impossible in the absence of guidelines in the form of measurable objectives, neither can it be denied that their use makes good teaching more likely. There is no one set of health instructional objectives whose mastery is essential to the achievement of the goals of every elementary school. Even if there were, it would be necessary to evaluate and revise it continually in order to adjust for changes in needs, conditions, health problems, and health information. Nevertheless, there are some very concrete advantages to using objectives as tools for planning and implementing effective health instruction.

First, specifying educational objectives in terms of the cognitive processes to be practiced is the most meaningful and powerful way to begin the task of planning learning activities which are relevant to curriculum goals whatever the discipline involved. The teacher must decide on the purpose of a lesson before deciding how to teach it. Process-focused objectives make teaching a professional, decision-making function instead of an accumulation of fuzzy plans such as to ''discuss how body parts grow,'' ''talk about the chapter that was assigned,'' ''draw a picture that describes one's family,'' ''show a film about drug abuse,'' or ''invite a dentist to talk to the class about dental hygiene.'' Such plans are formulated day by day as coping strategies based not on skill development, but on subject matter alone. With specific objectives, skill and subject matter are not two things, but one. Guided by these kinds of statements, teaching is a reasoned process rather

than a haphazard mixture of activities and textbook reading.

A teacher who knows exactly what a student needs to be able to do and know when the lesson has been completed is more effective in planning matching learning opportunities. That is what an operational objective describes. On the other hand, a teacher who is guided by ambiguous objectives such as, ''To help the students understand and appreciate the role of the family,'' understandably confuses teaching with telling.

Second, an operational objective facilitates teaching because it contains within itself clues to the four basic teaching tasks. (1) The cognitive skill to be practiced in a lesson or lessons is explicit in the specified behavior. (2) The technique or strategy appropriate to that behavior is implicit in the statement as well. Certain techniques are suited to practicing a given behavior, whereas others are not. Panel discussions, debates, or preparation and presentation of a report would allow the student practice in synthesizing. But if the behavior were ''describe'' or ''explain,'' a lecture or film could not be the sole technique employed because only watching or listening are required. (Whether the students actually see and hear what is being presented is another problem). So the operational objective suggests which techniques you can use as well as which ones are unsuitable. (3) The objective sets the boundaries of the subject matter to be studied. If the content specified is ''effects of drug abuse,'' any other information, such as their chemical components, slang names, laws concerning their use, or historical highlights of usage is completely irrelevant. If any of that seems essential to the goals of the unit being studied, then you need to develop additional enabling objectives that deal with that information. A measurable objective tells you what subject needs to be included as well as what ought not to be covered. (4) A measur-

Rating scale for instructional objectives

	Objective	Acceptable	Unacceptable	Criterion or criteria not met
1	The pupil can indicate the number of primary teeth.			
2	Learns to say no.			
3	The student will demonstrate an increase in cognitive knowledge by taking a test.			
4	The pupil can name the three basic functions of teeth and tell why teeth are important.			
5	Keep the fingernails clean.			
6	Students will list their five favorite foods and their five least-liked foods.			
7	Understands the major factors that influence healthful living.			
8	Describes the structure of the eye and ear and explains the functions of each.			
9	The principal causes of premature death and disability.			
10	Cooperates with others to promote a healthful environment at school, in the home, and in the community.			
11	To teach the techniques of CPR.			
12	To use problem-solving skills correctly.			
13	Discusses the benefits of wellness versus illness.			
14	Analyzes the cost effectiveness of preventive medical treatment as a means of controlling health care expenditures.			
15	Recognizes qualities of a good friend.			
16	Knows the relationship between food choices and dental health.			

able objective is the best guide to its own evaluation. Evaluation is not just facilitated, but its validity is assured when it is based on a measurable objective since it matches what the student presumably has been helped to learn.

Often classroom tests bear little relationship to what actually has been taught and learned; this is especially the case when the objectives of the teaching have never been clearly defined and employed as guidelines to the teaching.

When the expressed intention is unclear, as in, "The student will really appreciate the potential harmfulness of misusing or abusing drugs," how would you arrange for practice or evaluation of that behavior? What is a student doing when appreciation is being practiced or really exhibited? The ability to recall facts about the subject matter is usually what is assessed, the assumption apparently being that the more facts students know, the greater their appreciation.

Third, evaluation of the teacher's success and of the feasibility of the objective itself is facilitated when a measurable objective is used. If students cannot yet demonstrate mastery of the specified subject matter and skill, new or different learning opportunities can be devised to give added practice or broadened study of the subject matter. If it seems likely that failure to achieve the objective is not an indication of inadequate teaching, but instead due to the fact that the objective simply was not feasible for these students, the statement can be discarded or rewritten, as the teacher decides.

Fourth, use of measurable objectives as a framework for curriculum development at any level of implementation minimizes the risk of irrelevance to student needs or educational goals, with a waste of time and materials as a consequence. The clarity of such statements, as derived from careful analysis of the sources described in Chapter 3, makes it easier to assess both the worth and potential contribution of each to the overall plan.

Fifth, supervision and inservice education are facilitated when what the teacher expects to accomplish has been clearly specified in advance of instruction. The degree of success or failure can be assessed and the strengths and weaknesses can be diagnosed based on the criteria implicit in the objectives.

Sixth, communication is facilitated, especially between teacher and student, but also between teacher and supervisor, and between one teacher and another who are teaching the same material. Carefully planned and clearly defined objectives, developed at levels of increasing complexity and comprehension from kindergarten through middle school and beyond, allow successive teachers to build on and reinforce desired competencies. Each teacher can see what the student needs to have learned at any particular level in order to participate effectively in the objective proposed for the next. When objectives are stated clearly and unambiguously enough to convey a similar meaning to any teacher, then the final outcome should be much the same whatever the means chosen to carry them out.

Finally, and perhaps most importantly, students who are involved actively in the learning process (and measurable objectives are far more apt to motivate choices for these kinds of teaching strategies than are the "knows" and "appreciates" kinds of statements) are more likely to adopt and value the behaviors basic to positive health attitudes than students who are merely passive recipients of health information or health rules (Black and Newton, 1981).

SUMMARY

Education holds no patent on the terms "goals" and "objectives," nor on the manner in which they are stated and employed. The National Health Goals and subsequent supportive Objectives for the Nation illustrate this point quite well (Hew, 1979). This is to say that the models and criteria we have recommended for use in planning and organizing health teaching should be perceived as tailored to the purposes of teachers and curriculum developers. Even in education you will find "goals" that are not really goals, and "objectives" that do not satisfy some of the criteria proposed in these pages. Some statements labelled objectives may not satisfy any of them, in fact.

Goodlad's (1984) study of the nation's schools found that, while state education guides were a "conceptual swamp," district guides were usually more directly oriented to the classroom, proposing more and better goal statements; yet even district guides listed a combination of behaviors desired in students, purposes for teachers, and admonitions to schools under the title of goals. He concludes that those working at all levels of the educational system must be accountable for the quality of the education planned for and offered children in our schools.

Elementary teachers may not think of themselves as sharing in the responsibility for establishing or fulfilling the long-range goals for health education. In reality, they have a key role to play in fulfilling the hopes and plans implicit in those goals. At the bottom line, it is the classroom teacher who brings them to life. Elementary teachers need to know what the goals and general objectives proposed for district schools at all levels are, and how to infer from them a set of instructional objectives capable of contributing to their achievement.

Whatever grade level at which you teach, you also need to know what objectives your students will have already completed, and what they will need to know and be able to do at the level that follows your own teaching. Only when successive elementary teachers know how to define meaningful and measurable objectives with full knowledge of what has preceded them and what is to follow, will children be afforded the firm foundation of health-related information basic to effective problem solving and decision making essential in promoting a healthful life style.

QUESTIONS AND EXERCISES

Discussion questions

1. What difficulties do you see in planning a health education curriculum in the absence of stated long-range goals?

2. Explain the advantages of basing health instruction plans on clearly stated operational objectives.

3. Which of the criteria for the development of well-stated objectives would not apply to goal statements?

4. What would be the disadvantage of specifying performance standards as part of an instructional objective?

5. Why is it nearly impossible to write an instructional objective that is totally cognitive or affective in its intent and outcome?

6. Which element of an instructional objective would you identify as the most apt to be the cause of complaints that "behavioral" objectives focus on trivialities? What could you do to avoid that problem?

7. Based on examples provided in the literature, how would you explain the difference between a competency statement and a measurable objective?

8. Why is it important that an instructional objective be demonstrable in the classroom setting?

9. Explain the criterion of feasibility as it applies to objectives of health teaching in particular.

Exercises and problems

1. Using the categories described by Krathwohl, Bloom, and Masia (1964), (see page 4-24) develop for each a set of affective behaviors. Formulate a definition for each behavior to serve as a guide for planning a lesson so the students can practice that skill.

2. Develop a general objective that would require a number of enabling, or subordinate, objectives for its achievement. Then define a list of such

enabling objectives to allow for as many different levels of ability and knowledge as might be expected among children of a given age. Which of those you propose would be essential for all children, and which ones would probably be needed by only a few?

3. The chart on p. 111 contains a list of "objectives" taken from many kinds of publications for health education in elementary schools. Read each one, and decide whether it meets all the criteria for a measurable objective. If it does not, enter the number of the criterion or criteria it fails to meet in the appropriate space.

4. Rewrite each of the objectives you judged unacceptable in the previous question to make it acceptable. Which criterion or criteria were most often the problem? What is your conclusion about objectives and the problems involved in writing operational statements?

5. Select a health content area or concept that interests you and develop long-range goals for the cognitive, affective, and action domains. Next define a curriculum (general) objective for each of the first two goals. Finally, prepare an instructional, or enabling, objective for each of these two curriculum objectives. Study the progression that you have established. Do the statements at each level meet the criteria? Does each logically depend on those below it for its achievement? Does the behavior become more explicit and the subject matter more narrow as the concern of the statements moves closer to the classroom?

REFERENCES

Black JL and Newton J: Should health behavior change be an objective of school health personnel? J Sch Health 51(3):189-190, 1981.

Bloom BS and others: Taxonomy of educational objectives, Handbook I, Cognitive domain, New York, 1956, David McKay Co, Inc.

Feuerstein, P and Galli, N: Linking Health Screening to Health Education Learning Modules For Elementary School Student: A Feasibility Study, J Sch Health 53(1): 10-13, Jan 1983.

Goodlad JI: Planning and organizing for teaching, Project on the instructional program of the public schools, Washington DC, 1963, Rand McNally & Co.

Goodlad, JI: A place called school: prospects for the future, New York, 1984, McGraw-Hill.

Harrow, AJ: A taxonomy of the psychomotor domain, New York, 1972, David McKay Co, Inc.

Krathwohl, DR: Stating objectives appropriately for programs, for curriculums, and for instructional materials development, J Teach Educ, March 1965, p. 83.

Krathwohl DR, Bloom BS, and Masia BB: Taxonomy of educational objectives, Handbook II, Affective domain, New York, 1964, David McKay Co, Inc.

Mager RF: Preparing instructional objectives, Palo Alto, Calif, 1962, Fearon Publishers.

Pollock MB: Speaking of competencies, Health Edu 12:9, Jan/Feb 1981.

Popham WJ: Objectives '72, Phi Delta Kappan 53:433, 1972.

Popham WJ: Two-plus decades of educational objectives. In Wolf, editor: Educational objectives in educational evaluation: the state of the field, International J of Educ Res 11:1, London, 1988.

School Health Education Study (SHES): Health education: a conceptual approach to curriculum design, St Paul, 1967, 3M Education Press.

School Health Education Project (SHEP): Health education curricular progression chart, 1981, National Center for Health Education.

Thayer L and Beeler K: Activities and exercises for affective education, Washington, DC, 1975, American Educational Research Association.

Trucano L: Students speak, Seattle, 1984, Comprehensive Health Education Foundation.

US Department of Health and Human Services, Promoting health/preventing disease: objectives for the nation, Fall 1980, DHHS, PHS.

US Department of Health, Education and Welfare (HEW): Healthy people: The Surgeon General's report on health promotion and disease prevention, Washington, DC, 1979, DHEW, PHS.

SUGGESTED READINGS

Ebel, Robert L., and Frisbie, David A.: The role of instructional objectives. In $\frac{6}{M}$: Essentials of educational measurement (4th edition), Englewood Cliffs, N.J., 1986, Prentice-Hall, pp. 36-40. Explains the connection between broad educational goals and the derivation of instructional objectives. Categorizes the purposes of objectives as instructional planning, learner information, and evaluation planning.

Flanders, R: When goals and objectives multiplied, we learned to divide and conquer, The American School Board J. 173: 8, August 1986. Describes the steps taken by members of a school board, working with school administrators and community leaders, to streamline what had become an impossibly long list of goals and objectives.

Kibler Robert and others: Objectives for instruction and evaluation, ed 2, Boston, 1981, Allyn & Bacon. Major focus of the book is on the nature and uses of instructional objectives, defined as statements describing what students will be able to do after completing a prescribed unit of instruction. It describes procedures for matching objectives and evaluation strategies, and discusses the relationship between instructional objectives, criterion-referenced learning, and mastery learning. Instructional procedures for implementing cognitive and affective objectives are included.

McGreevy P: Performance and learning: key elements in continuous assessment, The Pointer 30(2): 19-21, Winter 1986. Argues that there is no relationship between a handicapped child's initial performance on an objective and subsequent learning related to the same objective. Ideally, an objective should initially be "hard to do" from the child's point of view, and made "easy to learn" by instructional and reward strategies based on continuous assessment of progress. At the conclusion of instruction the competence expressed in the objective should be performed accurately and well.

Popham WJ: Two-plus decades of educational objectives (Chapter 3 in Educational evaluation: the state of the field.), Int J Educ Res 11(1): 31-41, 1987. Traces the behavioral objective movement from its beginnings in the mid-sixties to the present. Proposes five guidelines regarding objectives for use by educational evaluators. Concludes that clearly stated objectives, skillfully employed, can contribute to more defensible evaluations.

White R and Tisher R: Research on natural sciences. In Wittrock, M (ed.): Handbook of research on teaching. Chicago, 1986, American Educational Research Association, p. 876. A section on research regarding the effect of behavioral objectives on learning in science cites specific studies and general support findings on the basis of clustered studies on the use of such objectives as promoting learning and retention.

CHAPTER 5

Developing
Effective Teaching
and Learning Plans

When you finish this chapter you should be able to:

- **Analyze the interdependence of process and content in the promotion of problem solving and thinking abilities.**

- **Synthesize cognitive and social learning theories in the design of lessons.**

- **Describe the procedures and purposes of commonly employed active teaching techniques.**

- **Explain the problem-solving method.**

- **Design experiential health teaching strategies appropriate to the needs and abilities of specified students.**

- **Interpret the influence of values on an individual's health-related actions.**

- **Develop adequately detailed lesson plans based upon instructional objectives attainable by selected students.**

However laudable and carefully crafted the stated goals and objectives of a curriculum for health teaching, without the enthusiasm and skillful planning of a classroom teacher, they are just a lot of words. Typically, the broadest statements of purpose have been agreed upon by consensus of state or district curriculum committees composed of school administrators, curriculum specialists and content consultants (who may be teachers). *Sometimes,* as frequently occurs today, they may have been supplied as components of commercially developed curriculum packages complete with objectives, lesson plans, and coordinated resource materials.

This chapter will consider the basic questions that teachers must continually ask themselves as they infer enabling objectives from the general objectives they are expected to implement. It is the content and behaviors specified in their own objectives that should guide the choices among techniques that are appropriate for their lessons. Remember that achievement of the objectives you prepare must be (1) feasible for your students in terms of their readiness, experience, and the time and resources you have; (2) a legitimate concern of the schools; and (3) consistent with school and district curriculum goals and policies.

Given that goals represent overall target competencies to be sought, remember that every class is different in some ways. These differences must be kept in mind when lessons are being planned because they must influence the choice of teaching techniques and the choice of content.

Madeline Hunter (1971), probably the best-known and most influential authority on elementary school teaching today, says: Regardless of any particular method or program, the planning of the teacher is probably the most critical element in generating the transfer which yields student productivity and cre-

ativity. This planning makes the difference between "hoping that it will happen" and "seeing that it does."

When to teach the content and skills explicit in your objectives is a problem of horizontal sequence. The chapters in the textbook provided for your students may or may not present a logical sequence of subject matter that matches class needs. If you like the way the textbook is organized, it can be used as it is. If you like the book, but not the sequence, you can change the order in which the chapters are to be studied to fit your own plan.

What content would you choose as the focus of your first lesson in health education for a group of second grade children? Why would you choose to introduce that subject matter over any other for the introductory lesson? Are there any health content areas that you would *not* schedule first? Why? How could knowledge of the needs and interests of 7-year-old children help you to make sensible choices among content areas and teaching strategies for their health lessons? It is generally agreed that decisions affecting curriculum need to be based on knowledge of all aspects of child growth and development—physical, social, emotional, and intellectual (Moyer, 1986). Think about what you have learned about Piaget's stages of cognitive development. What implicaions for sequence for either subject matter or skills do you find in that information?

To plan a sequence of instruction that fits every aspect of student readiness is not easy, nor is it easy to distinguish between unnecessary repetition and desirable reinforcement. It depends, to a great degree, on your students; you will have to be sensitive to their special needs as you make your plans. Some revisiting of subject matter is needed every year for most students. What they need to know about nutrition, for example, cannot be mastered in a few

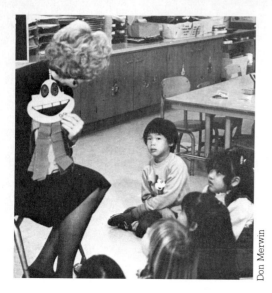

Don Merwin

lessons even if a few were provided every year. As students grow older they have more control over food choices. Lessons have to shift from learning about basic facts, such as the nutrients categorized within the four food groups, to understanding some of the many forces that motivate diet choices.

Health problems keep recurring, but in different forms and with different degrees of severity. The social and emotional needs of children in grade 6 are very different from those typical of children in first grade or eighth grade. Although Bruner (1960) proposed that any subject can be taught effectively in some intellectually honest form at any stage of development, cognitive and moral developmental abilities are of a higher order among children in upper elementary grades. This means that during early school years more emphasis has to be given to *training* children to practice desirable health behaviors. Only as abilities increase can health teaching activities begin to focus on decision-making skills (Kolbe, et al. 1981).

These are some of the kinds of things we have talked about in Chapter 3 that must be considered before you can decide how to teach and what techniques are best suited to the implementation of any particular objective.

PROCESS-FOCUSED INSTRUCTION

Health education is not limited to the communication of health-related information. It is as concerned with the development of cognitive skills as with providing the learner with information. As Combs (1981) has said:

The information explosion has made the concept of the teacher as the fountain-head of knowledge ridiculous. Science has provided us with marvelous techniques for the dissemination of information; radio, television, movies, computers, recordings and many more. These devices are capable of placing vast amounts of information in the hands of anyone quickly and efficiently. They have also made the role of the teacher as information provider obsolete.

Because we have spoken of the two dimensions of an instructional objective as being content and a measurable cognitive skill, it might seem that the two are separate elements of a teaching-learning plan. What do we mean by *process* in this context? The term is used in education to describe all the operations of which the human mind is capable. It encompasses theorizing, conceptualizing, analyzing, decision-making, thinking, and generalizing, to name just a few of the cognitive skills employed in active learning. Content, as we use the word in health teaching, refers to the fund of accurate information with which the discipline is concerned. That information consists of the set of concepts, principles, and generalizations that, by agreement of its scholars, represents its body of knowledge. These are categorized under general headings such as content areas, subject matter, topics, or problems.

Content is static. It becomes dynamic only as we use it in employing the processes with which humans carry on their work and do their thinking (Parker and Rubin, 1966). Paradoxically, cognitive skills, once mastered, have life-long utility and transferability, whereas content can only be considered tentative. Content needs to be tested frequently for its dependability because its application is crucial in solving a problem.

Health behavior is the result of decision making, which must be based on a reasoned examination of possible alternatives. The belief that the purpose of education is to develop intellectual skills is not new, but sometimes it has been assumed that stuffing students' minds with facts is the most effective way to do this; yet encyclopedias and computers are filled with facts, none of which are of any use without the ability of a human being to retrieve and apply those facts productively.

Like any others, intellectual skills must be practiced to be mastered. Learning opportunities must be planned as much for their potential contribution to the development of mental processes as for the accumulation of health information. Whether the health problems or behaviors of interest to children are real or hypothetical, the processes employed in investigating them are the same. Problem solving is perhaps *the* method of health education, and the way humans decide on any particular health behavior.

Emphasis on reasoning rather than information is essential for health teaching. Combs (1981) supports this view when he describes problem solving as a creative process that is useful whatever the subject or whenever the need. Use of this method as appropriate during elementary school years seems implicit in these remarks:

The student's own personal problems seem like a logical place to begin. In problem solving, process takes precedence over subject matter. Moreover, personal problems have the distinct advantage of built-in

motivation. A review of research on motivation suggests that students are most likely to be motivated when problems are real and personally relevant, when students feel solutions are reasonably within their capabilities, and when results are immediately discernible.

The use of cognitive skills or of productive thinking goes on all the time, whenever people need something or want to do something they don't know how to do—in short, whenever a problem occurs. This is true at every age. It is the schools' responsibility to help students from kindergarten upward to learn and use those skills effectively so that they can live better both now and in the future. Other disciplines besides health education recognize their obligation to teach thinking and decision making. For example, here is a statement taken from social science literature:

The emphasis of elementary social studies should be on process, not content, specifically the process of gathering, categorizing, and analyzing information, and then making generalizations based on this analysis. (Resnik, 1985).

Measurable objectives provide direction in selecting teaching strategies that require learners to practice cognitive skills.

LEARNING AS CONCEPTUALIZING

Conceptual learning is the way people learn naturally, without (and sometimes in spite of) formal teaching, yet it depends entirely on the senses as receivers of information. Interpretation of that information is heavily influenced by the individual's past perceptions. Communication between the teacher and the learner is bounded by two realities: (1) the five senses are the only avenues of communication, and (2) what is perceived will always be affected by related past experiences.

In order to plan how to teach, you have to

understand how a person learns. Learning is a very personal thing, first because no two people have had exactly the same experience in life, and second because every one of us has different abilities, interests, learning styles, and motivations.

An infant begins to sense almost at once that certain things or experiences belong to a family of like things or experiences. One of the first generalizations a human being formulates is from a myriad of perceptions about food. At first the infant reacts with pleasure when hunger has been satisfied and begins to associate that contented state with the touch of familiar food on the lips and in the mouth. Then more senses—taste, smell, and sight—are stimulated, and the infant adds those perceptions to the first ones. As time goes by, colors, sounds, odors, even textures of food begin to be added to the "things that bring relief of hunger" pleasure. All the while, the senses are also yielding information about things that can be put in the mouth but are *not* food. Very soon, long before he or she has learned a word for it, the concept of food is well established in the baby's mind. Anyone who has tried to persuade an infant to eat something new or disliked knows this quite well. In short, generalizing is a natural process, and generalizations based on our perceptions are the milestones of learning.

A teacher who depends on nothing but *telling* could be successfully replaced by a tape recorder. Lecturing limits the number of senses that are stimulated and thus the range of kinds of perceptual experiences afforded the audience. The more senses involved in a learning experience, the more effective the lesson will be. Think about your own experiences as a student. What kinds of learning activities have you found to be the most rewarding and interesting? What kinds have seemed least absorbing and memorable? How many senses have been involved in each category of those *teaching strategies?*

LEARNING AS BEHAVIORAL CHANGE

Health education in schools isn't hygiene any more, nor is it limited to ways to avoid illness or chronic diseases. In the case of AIDS, a problem that at this writing appears to have no medical solution, behavioral change effected through health education currently offers the only hope for any sort of control.

It is a long held assumption of health educators that health-informed people are more likely to behave in ways that are beneficial to their physical and emotional health. Alas, it isn't that simple. Behavior is the result of decisions, whether conscious or subconscious in origin, and may be either negative or positive in effect. Decisions affecting health behavior are not always good ones nor are they always rational. They may be based on too little information or on misinformation, and they often reflect some miscalculation of the consequences of the chosen behavior. And even when they know what can happen, people don't always do what they know is best. Risky behavior is more fun— that's what makes roller coasters so popular. Because something is risky, it is a lot more exciting, whether the actual activity is fun or not. Clearly, cognitive learning is a necessary— but not sufficient—outcome of health education if the learner is to adopt a pattern of behaviors that adds up to a healthful life style.

Owing to its significance in understanding the complexity of human behavior choices, many health educators and behavioral scientists view social learning theory (SLT) as paramount among the learning theories with application to health teaching. Briefly, social learning theory posits that every person exhibits a variety of behaviors, some of which are reinforced and will recur when the stimulus is the same. Those that are reinforced often enough eventually become the behavior of choice or habit. Bandura (1977) says

It is largely through their actions that people produce the environmental conditions that affect their behavior in a reciprocal manner. The experiences generated by behavior also partly determine what a person becomes, or can do, which in turn affects subsequent behavior.

Behaviors can be learned, or changed, according to social learning theory *directly,* by directly providing the reinforcement as in an experiential lesson; *vicariously,* by arranging for the learner to observe someone else being reinforced for a behavior (social modeling); or by *self-management,* having learners monitor their own behaviors and provide their own rewards (by encouraging them to carry out a healthful behavior for a specified period of time, at the end of which they grant themselves a predetermined prize). All of this has great potential for the development of lessons that stimulate thinking, foster creativity, and generate positive behaviors among children and youth. Moreover it dramatically changes an erroneous concept of health education as simply being concerned with teaching good grooming, physiology, or the symptoms and avoidance of diseases or disorders.

Educational techniques based on social learning theory include modeling, skill training, contracting, and self-control (Parcel and Baranowski, 1981). In the case of elementary school children, these concepts seem promising as sources of lesson plans designed to motivate development of decision-making skills and favorable health behaviors.

Modeling affords children an opportunity to observe others performing a desired behavior, which is an effective way of promoting that behavior's adoption. Content is communicated as they watch the action and listen to the dialogue. Concrete examples of how it is done are provided simultaneously as in real life. Vicarious modeling can be provided through films (in which the focus is on behaviors rather than information), video tapes, role playing, puppetry, and dramatizations. For example, children can be shown models for how to resist peer pressure to try drugs, how to be a friend, how to select healthful snack foods, how to behave in social situations with poise, and so on.

Health behaviors are actions, and nobody learns to demonstrate an action solely through observation; there must also be *skill training.* An essential element in teaching desirable health behaviors is the provision of opportunities to practice the behavior, first in small steps separated out and practiced as means of learning its component skills, and finally as a whole when these have been mastered. For example, in order to teach youngsters how to use dental floss and a toothbrush correctly, the following steps might be practiced: as a preliminary motivating experience, self-application of disclosing tablets to reveal any existing plaque; then learning how to measure off the amount of floss to be used, and the manner in which it is held between the fingers; then learning the technique to be employed in cleaning between the

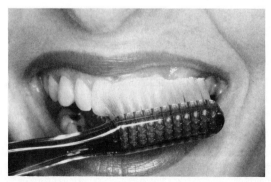

Copyright by the American Dental Association. Reprinted by permission.

teeth and under the gum line; then learning the manner in which the brush is positioned depending on the shape and function of the teeth; and finally, learning the brushing motion most effective in removing plaque. At each of these steps, there should be immediate feedback to the student reinforcing correct practice and correcting any as needed. These practices could be combined with the technique of *self-monitoring* and *self-rewarding,* where students would agree to follow these procedures as carefully and completely as possible for a specified period of time, at the end of which a test by application of disclosing dyes would provide an indisputable measure of the results. The reward would be a mouthful of very clean teeth, and whatever recognition the students might have stipulated as worthy of their efforts.

SPECIAL CHARACTERISTICS OF LEARNERS

Spend some time during the first weeks of school finding out as much as you can about the students in your class. Instruction has to begin "where they are" if it is to interest them. Do any or all of them have the necessary educational background for what you plan to teach? What are their cultural and socioeconomic characteristics? Assumptions about prior experience, whether in or out of school, must be avoided; for example, so called "middle class values" will not be held by all children and, in some areas, not by any of them. Some youngsters learn less from what they hear than from what they can see or touch (indeed, this is probably true of all children). More attention may have to be given to teaching listening skills to the child from an inner city environment, where the ability to shut out unwanted sound is an effective way of coping with it. Children who are living in poverty may be less interested in learning activities

that promise something as nebulous as "good health," or that have little to do with their real problems. For these children, teaching strategies that deal with the immediate and concrete may be more effective.

Many children have feelings of low self-esteem or shyness that make them distrust their own judgment and conclusions. During the first weeks, task setting should be planned so that success is inevitable. Success is essential to self-esteem, and self-esteem breeds the confidence that allows its possessor to risk failure, suggest theories, propose tentative solutions to problems, and try new ways of doing things. Confidence flourishes in a classroom environment where failure is viewed as a learning experience and that kind of risk taking is viewed as fun.

The time needed to learn certain skills varies among people. Children learn and develop intellectually, as in all ways, at their own pace and in their own style. Teaching and learning methods should not be tied to a "one style fits all" criterion of selection. Bloom's concept of mastery teaching (1981) is based on the conviction that, given enough time, all students can attain mastery of a learning task. He says:

Each student should be allowed the time he needs to learn a subject. And the time he needs is likely to be affected by his aptitudes and verbal ability, the quality of instruction he receives in class, and the quality of help he receives out of class. The task of a strategy for mastery learning is to find ways of altering the time individual students need for learning as well as finding ways of providing whatever time is needed by each (Bloom et al., 1981, p. 51).

The same teaching goals can be attained for most children. The differences between children do not change the goals as much as the teaching strategies selected to achieve them. The teacher's task is to provide an experience that will make a child's active participation both likely and productive. Assimilation of useful information is a logical outcome of that kind of activity.

Skill in diagnosing a student's special needs is basic to the selection of appropriate learning opportunities. It is not enough to know how to carry out teaching techniques or follow specific procedures. That's like confusing the cookbook with cooking. Choosing a technique must be based on analysis of needs rather than on whim or habit. The question to ask yourself is, ''What has this plan to do with the needs of these students?'' The answer to that question should be as clear to them as it is to you.

RECITING VERSUS THINKING

The Bloom taxonomy of objectives (Bloom et al., 1956) identifies six categories of cognitive skills—knowing, comprehending, applying, analyzing, synthesizing, and evaluating. The first category is the simplest since the only process required is remembering. Knowledge is basic to all of the categories and essential in the practice of complex cognitive skills such as categorizing, interpreting, judging, organizing, and thinking.

The tendency to focus on simple recall as the desired outcome of learning persists at every level of education, up to and beyond the doctoral; yet information is useless without the cognitive skills needed to apply it appropriately. Cognitive processes are not fostered by means of lessons and curricula that emphasize memorization. Nevertheless, this is the pattern of instruction predominantly found in schools. In his 1984 study, Goodlad says, with regard to science teaching (which is typically the host area for health teaching in elementary grades), ''The tests used emphasized heavily the recall of specific information rather than exercise of higher intellectual functions'' (p.216).

Children will learn to think if lessons are planned to elicit thinking rather than reciting. Feldman (1986) says that although we are doing a good job of teaching the ''basics,'' too many kids are not learning to think. She adds,

We know for a fact that thinking can be taught and that it flourishes in a school environment that encourages initiative, independence, and originality, rather than obedience and docility. Encourage them to think of themselves as thinkers. Be a good role model. State the reasons for your actions, admit errors or lack of knowledge, and show them how you get back on track.

Wales et al. (1986) suggest a new paradigm for education to replace the long-standing focus on transmission of factual information. The new paradigm is ''schooling based on decision making, the thinking skills that serve it, and the knowledge that supports it.'' Before that can happen, those thinking skills will have to be learned.

Focusing on higher cognitive skills does not change the subject matter used in teaching, only the way the learner handles it. The activity called for in a lesson changes, and in most cases learning becomes a lot more fun, without losing one iota of its worth and transferability.

The following tasks illustrate how thinking about and using subject matter can involve increasingly complex cognitive behaviors. They represent different levels of cognition, arranged as nearly as possible according to Bloom's taxonomy. The subject matter remains the same (sources and functions of protein in human nutrition) and all tasks require the student to apply the basic knowledge. Only the first is limited to remembering; the others require thinking. Most importantly, the thinking tasks bring the facts to life:

Knowing: Name the group of nutrients to which meat, poultry, fish, nuts, and peas belong.

Comprehending: Explain why protein is essential to good nutrition and human growth.

Applying: Predict what the outcome would be if an infant were given enough food but a diet nearly lacking in protein.

Analyzing: A 4-year-old child is given the following daily diet:

Breakfast: 1 cup of dry cereal, a half cup of skim milk, a slice of toast with jelly, and 1 pat of butter.

Lunch: 1 peanut butter sandwich, a cup of skim milk, 4 vanilla cookies.

Dinner: 1 small hamburger patty, 1 cup of french fries with catsup, 1 ear of corn, 1 glass of cola, 1 piece of apple pie.

What changes would you make in order to ensure adequate amounts of protein for a child of this age?

Synthesizing: Make up a day's diet that contains only one serving of meat yet supplies adequate amounts of protein for a student of your own age, sex, body build, and level of activity.

Evaluating: Protein can be obtained from a wide variety of foods derived from animal flesh, animal products (eggs, milk, and cheese), and vegetables. Which of these two sources, animal or vegetable, is the better source of protein? State the reasons why you think one is better than the other.

Measurable instructional objectives in which higher level behaviors are specified facilitate creative teaching. Ambiguous behaviors such as *knows, understands,* and *appreciates* lead to teacher-centered activities with memorizing and reciting as outcomes.

Even the most clearly stated objective is useless unless a teacher develops a lesson that matches its expressed intention. If the behavior is not elicited in the lesson, or if the objective serves only as a decoration, then it might as well have been ambiguous. Suppose that an objec-tive called for a psychomotor skill rather than a cognitive skill, for example, "The student demonstrates ability to perform CPR techniques." The teacher *tells* the students how CPR is done, gives them a pamphlet to read that describes the separate steps involved, shows them a film illustrating the procedures, and then arranges for an actual demonstration of CPR techniques. Satisfied that they should now know how to carry out CPR, the instructor asks each student to demonstrate what has been learned. How well do you think the students would do? Can you suggest anything that would have increased the quality of the performance of learners who had had all of these experiences? Right you are. They needed to have had a chance to practice the techniques.

Failure to implement the objective as stated is more obvious when it concerns a physical skill that can be evaluated on the basis of "can do" versus "can't do." Practicing the specified behavior is just as imperative when it is a cognitive skill and you can't see it happening.

Blackwood (1967) proposed the following criteria to appraise the worth of an elementary school science learning activity. They are equally applicable to health teaching plans and are as appropriate twenty years later as when written. Ask yourself these questions as you review a lesson plan you have prepared or carried out.

1. Did the activity involve the children in describing or explaining the phenomenon?
2. Did the children collect original data from which to draw conclusions?
3. Did the children organize and communicate about the data in useful ways?
4. Did the children have opportunities to speculate and predict?
5. Did the experience relate clearly to the development of a major science (health) concept?

6. Did some of the questions provide stimulation for further study?

If the answer to all of those questions is "No," then the chances are that you are teaching the facts as ends in themselves, not as vehicles for thinking.

METHODS AND TECHNIQUES OF TEACHING

Methods courses provided for prospective teachers usually stress specific ways of imparting information, rather than strategies for practicing creative thinking and decision making. We think that these specific ways are techniques and the primary method of health education is problem solving. Activities such as field trips, lectures, debates, role-playing, panel discussions, and buzz-group discussions are techniques, and they, along with written materials, audiovisual equipment, and other teaching aids, constitute the set of tools from which a teacher can choose in designing teaching strategies.

Problem Solving: the Primary Method in Health Teaching

At the very heart of thinking processes is a problem of some sort. It may be something as ordinary as deciding whether to sleep another fifteen minutes and give up breakfast or deciding what to wear to a party, but the process is the same whenever a decision has to be made. Problems devised by teachers, for which there are neat, predetermined solutions, are no substitute for realistic, open-ended problems, for which there may be no pat answers or "correct" solutions. Children should be encouraged to formulate and solve their own problems—problems they care about.

A person's ability to do anything improves with practice. There is no better way to learn problem-solving processes than by solving problems. The method is always the same, consisting of a series of steps that move the thinker from the point where no solution exists, to the discovery of some new information that leads to a verifiable solution. These steps are generally described as follows.

Defining the problem. Health problems often are perceived by the individual as primarily physical (e.g., diabetes, obesity, or dental caries), social (e.g., shyness, overaggressiveness, or rejection), or emotional (e.g., feelings of loneliness, depression, or unworthiness). It is essential that activities focused on this step help the learner perceive the interacting influence of all three dimensions, since all three are involved in every health problem. When the problem is clearly identified and is perceived as real, and when a solution seems desirable and possible, the student is far more motivated to try to find a solution.

Theorizing about solutions. Some thought must be given first to a reasonable theory as a means of limiting the search for relevant information. Even small children are capable of

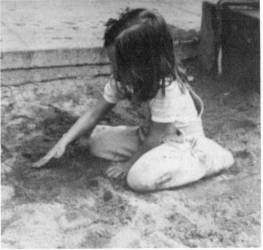

Armi Lizardi

theorizing if they are encouraged to do so. Let them brainstorm in this step. Instruction may be necessary at this point to give them guidelines for identifying a theory as a logical starting point for their investigations, thereby avoiding blind-alley searches as much as possible.

Data gathering. Depending on the problem and the individual, the basic information may already be available through past experience. Some information may have to be discovered, increased, or broadened. The teacher may act as adviser to help the students channel their search efficiently, but should not serve as a source of ready-made answers. Whatever sources of information are used, they must be demonstrably sound and authoritative.

The process of collecting these data will be limited by the individual student's experience and ability. Children in grades 5 or 6 are capable of searching for information in popular and professional magazines and journals, as well as many other kinds of references. Younger children will have to be supplied with the needed data through carefully selected audiovisual materials or appropriate readings. Reading for problem solving must always be purposeful, so that students read to find answers that they realize are necessary to fill in the gaps between what they know and what they need to know. In any case, the process of collecting data should be thorough and orderly, rather than incomplete and haphazard. Whatever sources are used, they must be objective and not slanted or biased.

Proposing solutions. During this step, the student categorizes and analyzes the data she or he has gathered and tries to arrive at a good solution. A teacher may have to provide some guidance here to avoid wasting time on implausible solutions.

Verifying the solution. This may be the final step if the student finds success on repeated testing of the tentative solution. If the first proposed solution does not solve the problem, then another promising approach is tried and another, if necessary, until the problem is solved.

Although these steps have been presented in a logical order the process doesn't have to be developed exactly so. Instead of beginning by identifying a problem, the problem may suggest itself as an outcome of data gathering for an entirely different purpose. Some agile minds leap from the definition of a problem to a valid solution almost by intuition. Creative thinking is often unstructured, rather than methodical, yet both approaches can produce solutions.

Theories are actually tentative solutions for which data gathering may be more of a verifying process than an investigation. Many cognitive skills are being developed in the total process of problem solving; analyzing, identifying, ordering, categorizing, evaluating, interpreting, concluding, and more—all of which are employed in thinking.

Solving problems builds competence in decision-making skills, and decision making determines health behavior. Good problem solvers are confident and persistent. They can live with uncertainty and do not jump to conclusions, but they make decisions when they must. They can risk being wrong or looking foolish. They act on hunches and change direction if it seems necessary, and they don't give up easily or look to others for their answers (Feldman, 1986, p. 39). Problem solving is a skill with total transferability.

A teacher can choose from a wide array of teaching techniques and instructional aids when planning lessons that help the student discover reliable information on which to base decisions affecting any aspect of human behavior.

Criteria for Selecting Teaching Techniques

The first step in selecting a technique to use with a particular instructional objective is to look at the proposed cognitive skill to be practiced. An objective, in effect, says "This is where the student should be." The lesson should answer the implicit question, "How can we best help him or her to get there?" Whatever technique is chosen, it must give the learners an opportunity to practice the specified behavior. For example, suppose the objective calls for *evaluating.* You cannot simply tell the students or show them a film that tells them about the subject and be satisfied that you have provided practice in anything other than listening or observing. A student *may* be evaluating what was heard or seen, but that is an assumption at best, and not an outcome on which you can depend or for which you can take any credit.

Thus the first two criteria in a plan for teaching are that the learner is given a chance to practice the behavior and to deal with the content described by the objective. In addition, the lesson should be appropriate to the present abilities of the students for which it is intended. Lessons that promote the development of cognitive skills can be tailored to the needs of individual students according to their abilities, or employed with the entire class, depending on grade level in general and individual abilities in particular. Some children may not be ready for the more advanced ways of thinking about a specific subject because they have not learned the facts needed; others who have learned the facts would be bored if they were forced to go over them again. Tasks can be varied to conform to individual readiness. The child who has learned enough to handle tasks at the level of knowing can succeed because what is required matches exactly what has been taught. At the same time, that child benefits from hearing how others have dealt with the same information in other ways.

There are other kinds of skills to be considered. For example, it is deceptively easy to plan a lesson that depends on the technique of discussion, but disconcerting to discover that your students don't know how to discuss. Discussion skills have to be learned, and discussion leading is a skill, too. "Discussion" often turns out to be teacher answers to student questions, or vice versa. It may be more satisfying to the students when they are asking the questions (although these often stray from the intended topic), but the outcome is not discussion; it is telling or reciting.

A fourth test of an effective lesson is its worth as perceived by the students, based not on its entertainment value but on its relevance to their present needs and interests. The *worth* of a lesson is measured by the sense of satisfaction generated by having achieved the objective.

Since any number of different teaching techniques might be equally effective in satisfying the preceding four criteria, it is best to pick the one that can provide the greatest number of concurrent desirable outcomes. For example, while preparing for a group presentation on a health-related topic, the student improves library skills, learns to read with better comprehension and purpose, to organize data logically, to generalize, to make oral presentations, to work and plan cooperatively with others, and more.

However, not all concomitant learnings are positive in effect; the outcome of teaching can be negative, too. Even small children tire of "health" lessons that focus on the four food groups or the mechanics of toothbrushing year after year, or that use scare tactics to prevent unwanted health behaviors. Health instruction for some luckless youngsters comes to mean,

''Don't do anything that grown-ups seem to like to do; it's bad for your health.'' Unwanted negative outcomes are far more common when instruction focuses solely on facts, with no attention given to problem-solving processes. If the learner has helped to define a health problem, interest is nearly ensured, and discovering a solution to that problem can be very satisfying. Growth in knowledge is a desirable outcome, but the ability to obtain and apply needed information in similar situations is a primary goal of comprehensive health education.

ACTIVE TEACHING TECHNIQUES

The specific teaching strategies or techniques used in health teaching are the same as those in any other subject area. Those commonly used for health instruction may be categorized as either **direct** (the learner is directly involved intellectually, physically, and emotionally) or **vicarious** (the learner views activities recorded at another time and place). Both of these types can be carried out as group activities or as individual procedures. Group activities include buzz sessions, brainstorming, committee projects, panel discussions, forums, lecture-discussions, role playing, and field trips. Individual procedures, in which each student works independently, include textbook study, computer-assisted work, and individual projects. Overlaps are inevitable; for example, role playing or a field trip assignment can be an individual or group activity.

Vicarious teaching techniques involve audiovisual and other material resources, including television, overhead projection transparencies, films, slides, filmstrips, radio, videotapes, audiotapes, models, and mock-ups (simplified and clarified parts or working models of a real device, e.g., a working portion of an automobile used for driver training).

Direct Teaching Techniques

Lecture. In the past, lecturing has been the most commonly practiced technique. The rule used to be: ''Tell them what you are going to tell them. Tell them. Then tell them what you told them.'' The notion of a lecture has strong negative overtones for many students because of past experiences. Admittedly there are dull lectures, but there are also absorbing lectures; the difference can be traced to the speaking skills of the lecturer.

A lecture has its own uses and several advantages over any other techniques. It facilitates the quick communication of a common fund of information so that every student can start with the same background data. It functions as a stage-setting and focusing activity for discussions and other group procedures. It can also offer a welcome change of pace when it is not overused (which is true of all techniques).

Use demonstrations or visual aids (e.g., transparencies, pictures, models, posters, or puppets) to enliven your talks. Never simply read a prepared lecture. If your students fail to understand what you are trying to explain, you will know at once from their expressions if you watch, and you can't do that if you are reading to them. Don't continue until you have cleared up any misunderstanding or confusion. Urge them to ask questions. That takes skill, too. Often students prefer not to appear slow at understanding, so they wait until the class is finished and then ask each other what the teacher said. Sometimes if you pause after making a point instead of plunging ahead after a second or two, someone will venture a question, and that will usually result in more questions. Maintain eye contact, move about the room, show enthusiasm about the topic you are explaining.

Don't be afraid to admit that you don't have all the answers. If a student's question is beyond your own expertise, if it is relevant and of common interest, use it as a departure point for a class research project, a visiting speaker, a field trip or any other means of investigation that is feasible and appropriate.

Once the lecture is completed, ask the students to summarize what they have learned, either verbally or in writing. What you learn about the effectiveness of the talk can be disappointing, but it is a very good way to find out how you need to modify your talk to make it a better communication technique.

Discussion. Judging by the frequency with which the word *discuss* appears in curriculum guides as a suggested activity, discussion must be the predominant technique used in health teaching. Since the suggestion is seldom accompanied by further advice it is difficult to predict how it is interpreted or carried out. Feldman (1986) asserts that

True discussion, in which we join students in trying to resolve questions with unknown or indefinite answers, is rare. Our questions too often call for factual, one-word responses. In fact, it's been noted that most of us answer two thirds of our own questions.

Discussion is *supposed* to be a dynamic interchange of ideas that build, one on the other, until an issue is resolved or a conclusion is reached. This is difficult to do. Some teachers cannot seem to resist the urge to do most of the talking. Goodlad et al. (1984) found that, on the average, about 75% of class time was spent on instruction, and that nearly 70% of this was talk, usually teacher to students. "Teachers outtalked the entire class of students by a ratio of about three to one."

Some teachers have difficulty tolerating the relatively unstructured classroom environment necessary for a pupil to pupil dialogue to build to vital discussion, so they limit discussion to teacher-pupil interactions. White (1986) says that teachers often act as if they "own" the knowledge, claiming the right to ask all the questions, as well as "owning" the right to decide if the answers supplied by students are correct or not.

Even where pupil-to-pupil dialogue is encouraged, it is difficult to prevent "class talkers" from dominating the action. Generally, the larger the group, the more difficult it is to motivate and direct discussions without losing the spontaneity and freedom required.

A good way to facilitate productive discussions is to first provide the group with a common background of information about the issue or problem of interest. Any technique that results in the quick communication of the information needed can be used. Often audiovisual materials are effective, but the students must be given cues to indicate the points for which they will be responsible in the discussion to follow. Once everyone has an established fund of information, the discussion can be initiated with a related, thought-provoking question, for which there is no one right answer but which has meaning for the children. For example, "How many teeth are there in the full primary set?" may be relevant, but it leads to a factual answer not likely to lead to further comment. A better question might be "What are some foods that you like that you couldn't eat if you had no teeth?" The question, "What are the safety rules to follow when playing on school grounds?" is certainly relevant but is not as likely to motivate thinking and application of information as "What can *you* do every day to make play time safer and more fun for everyone?"

Each person's ideas must be given consideration and everyone's participation is essential to at least some degree. This balance is not easy to achieve. Be careful to avoid dominating the discussion so that in the end it is always your conclusions or solutions that are adopted. Let

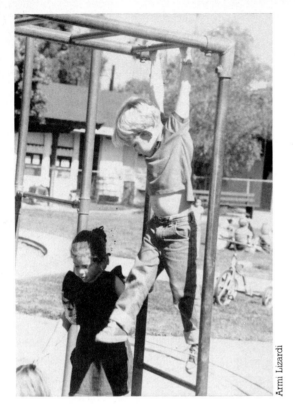

Armi Lizardi

the students summarize and decide what they have learned.

Discussion is probably a part of *every* teaching and learning activity. However, there are a number of recognized forms by which a discussion may be organized. Four of these are discussed here, the first three of which can be used with any age group. The fourth is probably more effective with middle school students. Before you plan any kind of discussion, find out whether your students know how to discuss. If they don't, spend some time introducing them to the joys of being free to offer ideas and to react to those of others just as they are accustomed to doing among their friends outside of school. Plan short sessions initially, setting some ground rules for speaking as the first step.

Lecture-discussion. Teachers often describe their mode of teaching as a lecture-discussion. This usually means that some new material is first introduced by the teacher in a direct lecture, after which the students are encouraged to ask questions, express any reactions, and talk about what has been offered. A lecture-discussion allows the teacher to set the stage for learning by providing a common base of information to the class in a short time, but there is typically more lecture than discussion. Its success depends primarily on the subject matter and the skill of the instructor in engaging the interest of the class during the lecture and in leading the subsequent discussion so that it is the students who are doing the thinking and talking.

Brainstorming. This activity can be led by the teacher for the whole class or employed in small groups as a quick means of obtaining a number of ideas for later analysis or evaluation. As an initiating procedure, the teacher or class identifies a problem or question such as, ''How many ways can one person's actions affect his or her own health as well as that of others?'' The teacher asks the children to think of as many physical, social, economic, environmental or other effects as they can. Every idea should be recorded without judging its worth until no more can be suggested. The tenor of the activity should be the free flow of ideas and complete acceptivity. When no more ideas can be elicited, each is then considered and classified as either positive or negative in its effect on personal or community health.

When the whole class is participating, the teacher acts as moderator and recorder. Use of the chalkboard or overhead transparency is an effective means of recording and summarizing any conclusions. Small groups can be led by an appointed or elected leader and notes taken by a group recorder. Each group brainstorms, considers their results, and categorizes its ideas as either positive or negative in effect.

As a culminating activity, the teacher *might* poll each group in turn for one effect that they identified as positive until all of them have been shared. Next, the negative effects *are* reported. Since the first group *might* have hit on most of the important effects, only one idea should be accepted from any one group at a time. Otherwise later groups are robbed of the satisfaction of contributing their work to the outcome.

Brainstorming is useful as a means of generating the ideas needed to define a problem of concern, to identify ways of locating needed data, and to theorize about possible solutions.

Buzz sessions. This activity must be carried out in small groups of not more than five or six persons, *who* are given a specified amount of time (usually 6 to 10 minutes) to talk over a problem or issue and to decide on a tentative solution. The buzz session gets its name from the sounds that result, since the format promotes active participation by everyone. Each group may work with the same topic or each may be assigned a different topic. In either case, the culminating activity involves communicating the groups' conclusions or recommendations to the total class. This can be done by means of individual reports given by the group leaders, or by forming an impromptu panel of representatives from each group which would then share the groups' viewpoints. The remainder of the class forms the audience and should be encouraged to question or offer suggestions. Buzz sessions are useful in fostering creative thinking, building confidence in expressing new ideas, and promoting communication skills. They can be used effectively as preliminary planning activities for role playing, group projects, dramatizations, or any other procedure for which creativity is essential.

Panel discussions. In the more formally organized panel discussions the panel members spend some time in advance preparation for the presentation. As a teaching and learning strategy, preparation for a panel discussion usually requires considerable time, spent both in and out of the classroom. This kind of discussion needs to be somewhat structured. Each group should be provided with a list of its responsibilities, along with suggestions for completing the assignment. Panel discussion projects may include more members than are required to participate in the final presentation. Time should be given in class for each group to elect a leader, prepare a tentative outline of their presentation, allocate the work to be done, and set a due date for each step involved. The leader should be given responsibility for submitting, before the presentation, an outline indicating what part each member will play in the total project.

Planning the presentation, its theme, how it will be presented, and what visual or audio material, if any, will be required should be done by the total group. The specific tasks involved in preparation, such as doing research, producing the posters or other visual aids, writing the individual reports, and making the actual presentations, can be assigned by volunteering or drawing lots. Individual differences between students are best accommodated by allowing each person to choose the task that interests him or her most, when possible.

When the panel makes its presentation, usually as a conversational interaction among the group members, the leader is the discussion moderator and summarizer. The presentation also could be a series of brief descriptions of key aspects of the issue, after which the rest of the class is encouraged to join in the discussion. It is better to limit such panel discussions to no more than one a day. When there are more, each successive group's work and conclusions are diminished in importance and effect. Too much of the same kind of activity can pall, even at the college level. Elementary school children need frequent changes of pace to keep their interest level high.

Panel discussions are particularly successful for considering issues or problems, such as boy-girl relationships, dress codes, environmental pollution, drug use or abuse, and any other topic that currently concerns the community or the school.

Whatever the form of discussion employed, help the class formulate summarizing conclusions or ideas for future action. These need not always be clear-cut but may be developed in the form of promising alternatives. Never let the outcome be lost because the bell rings and cuts off discussion. You know when the bell is going to ring and should anticipate it. If time is running out and there will not be enough time to reach any conclusions, propose a postponement of that part of the activity until another day. But the students should be left with some kind of summarizing thoughts and the clear expectation of further discussion on the topic. If the timing works out well, the class can make some decision or recommend a position to be taken. Most of all, it is essential that everyone sees the significance of what has been learned in relation to what is to come next.

Committee projects. The cooperative participation of a small group of students in exploring some designated topic is sometimes preliminary to other techniques. As already described, committee work is involved in preparations for panel discussions. It also precedes other forms of presentations, such as plays, skits, films, puppet shows, slide presentations accompanied by recorded narration, debates, or demonstrations. Committee work can help children learn how to discover answers to questions, work effectively as members of a team, and differentiate between fruitful and fruitless

searches for valid information. A careful structure is essential to the success of this technique, however. It is not enough to simply make the assignment, since the result may be a project to which only a few members contributed, or a committee whose reports are largely derived from encyclopedias and are as boring to hear as they were meaningless to prepare.

A good way to structure committee work is to prepare reporting forms that uniformly channel planning and reporting. The first form might ask the group to report the preliminary sources used to make plans, the second to specify what every committee member will do and when the work is due, and the last to indicate the title of the project, the format that will be employed (e.g., dramatization, debate, or media study), plans for involving the rest of the class in either the discussion or evaluation, and so on.

Committee projects can be a stimulating means to investigate health problems such as quackery, malnutrition, and local or school health needs. Whatever the issue, the important outcome is the development of valid conclusions by the students that tie the purpose of the project to those of the unit or course.

Role playing. This technique appeals to all ages. It is an ad-lib, 3- to 5-minute informal acting out of a social situation in which the participants assume fictitious identities and then dramatize their parts. Role playing can be used to illustrate a concept or problem. Two or more persons may take part, and ordinarily a short amount of time is allowed for planning the action. Although informality and fun are associated with role playing, it should never be used simply for entertainment but always as a means of implementing a clearly evident instructional objective.

Role playing can be used to introduce a new area of study or to give students practice in applying what they have learned in another lesson. It can demonstrate the impact of tradition,

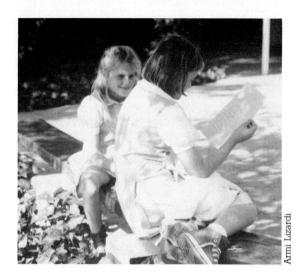

Armi Lizardi

values, attitudes, cultural beliefs, or social pressure on individual behaviors. Thus it can provide an outlet for feelings or convey ideas that, if approached more directly, might be awkward or uncomfortable for the students. For example, children may be too embarrassed to ask about some personal dilemma or health behavior, whereas role playing enables them to portray the unspoken query in the safe anonymity of the role being played. Understanding and empathy for the problems and responsibilities of others can be promoted by allowing a child to first play a role with one point of view and then switch to that of the other person in the situation. For example, a student might gain valuable insight into a parent's or teacher's problems by trying to play that role. When it is possible to present more than one dramatization without the players having seen the other version(s), the fact that differing perceptions can result in different behaviors can be demonstrated by giving the same problem to two or more groups.

In general, the teacher should first provide a well-structured explanation of the activity and its intent, either verbally or in writing, as on a transparency or prepared cards. Whatever the subject of the role playing, it should not have too personal a meaning for any one class member. The situation and resulting reactions should be those of people in general. It may be especially wise, when the students have not had experience in this kind of activity, to call for volunteers rather than require everyone to take part.

Any nonparticipating class members should be given a feeling of belonging by being assigned something to do while the role players are planning their act. One way to ensure active participation of the audience is to allow the role players to choose and illustrate some principle, problem, or other health-related concept that the class members are challenged to interpret from the action. For example, teams of two or three persons might be given generalizations drawn from previous lessons such as, "Stress can be helpful or harmful in its effect on health." Each team should be given at least 5 minutes to plan a way of presenting this idea through role playing. Those who are shy or not ready to attempt this activity might be allowed to develop the generalizations or create the plan for portraying them. Role playing is an effective summarizing device, with the other students asking questions or commenting on how it was done. Used in this manner, it is employed only after lessons that have provided the students with the information needed to play the role.

Field trips. A dynamic means of linking the course's purposes with individual concerns and responsibilities is a visit to a local community health agency or an on-the-spot exploration of a health hazard or problem. As with any teaching and learning strategy, this technique should be chosen for its potential contribution to a desired instructional objective and offer evidence of being the best way of doing so. Although there is no reason why a field trip cannot be either an individual or small group activity, the term usually describes a total class movement to some place other than the classroom. The area can be on the school grounds or at a considerable distance from the school.

Much preliminary planning is needed for a trip away from the school grounds. A class discussion might be used to identify the exact place to be visited, the information desired, and the relationship between this information and the health concepts being studied at the time. Depending on their age and ability, the class members may make some or all of the actual arrangements, such as arranging for the visit by telephone or interview, setting the date and time for the visit, providing the hosts with necessary information about the class and the purpose of the visit, and *always following up with a letter of appreciation signed by everyone.* In such a situation the teacher can act as a counselor but should stay in the background, allowing the students to practice the social skills and processes they need to develop.

The primary purpose of a field trip should not be to divert (although diversion it may be), but to provide the kinds of experiences that contribute to the acquisition of some powerful idea related to health protection or behavior. For example, on a field trip to a neighborhood health facility, rather than focusing on the services available simply by listing them, the students could find out what new services are being provided and what changing circumstances made them important (the idea being that community health programs must change as the community itself changes). The field trip should not be structured as a fact-finding endeavor but as a way to investigate and infer answers to questions such as, "Why are these services or facilities offered?" or, "Why aren't some provided here that are offered elsewhere?"

All safety precautions for the students making the trip must be planned in accordance with school or district policy and state liability laws. Transportation, teacher aids, parental permission or assistance, and other logistical problems should be identified and solved well in advance of the scheduled travel.

After the field trip, it is essential to discuss what was observed. Cause and effect inferences should be examined and recommendations for change or improvement developed where appropriate. Another profitable field trip activity is to encourage interested students to take photographs, which can later be organized and a commentary dictated, taped, or written.

Public-opinion surveys concerning health issues or needs, searching for traffic or fire hazards that need to be corrected, or investigating prices and ingredients of over-the-counter medications are just a few examples of individual or small group projects that could be conducted outside the classroom.

Experiential activities. There is more than one concept of experiential education. It is commonly described as the outcome of activities that take place off-campus, most particularly as provided for college and university students. For example, Conrad and Hedin (1981) define experiential programs as "educational programs offered as part of the general school curriculum, but taking place outside of the conventional classroom." James (1981) urges that students be provided opportunities for small group community-based experiences and services. He says, "Cognitive learning and experiential learning need not be viewed as adversaries," which suggests that they usually are. Kierstead (1985) agrees that the two are not mutually exclusive but complementary in the hands of teachers who know how to synthesize the two.

What seems to be the common denominator in any plan labeled *experiential* is not its setting but the use of techniques termed "hands-on." Hands-on learning activities are those that approximate reality as nearly as possible and provide the learner with an experience often having powerful physical, social, and emotional dimensions. For example, one health educator obtained the loan of a number of wheel chairs, and students had an opportunity to propel themselves around the school and carry out commonplace activities while chairbound. As a follow up, they shared the insights they had gained relative to the difficulties a paraplegic or other handicapped person has in satisfying what might have seemed to be simple personal needs otherwise. To learn how arthritis might make it difficult to use one's hands, children put on mittens and then tried to work the computer that they had learned to operate, or tried to open a milk carton or soft drink can. They tried to use the telephone or, accompanied by a guide, cross the street with their eyes covered or their ears stopped up in some way. They examined animal lungs and watched them expand when air was blown through a straw into the principal airway. They took each other's pulse before and after running in place for a specified length of time, and drew some conclusions about the effects of smoking on the efficiency of lungs in supplying the heart with oxygen during exercise.

The possibilities for experiential activities are limited only by the creativity and willingness of the teacher to spend the time and energy it takes to make these kinds of arrangements. A word of caution, however, must be given; be sure to check any plans for experiential activities with your school administrator in advance. There may be school policies or other problems of which you are not aware that would prevent your carrying them out. Should there be any complaint, you will be on safer ground if you have obtained approval beforehand.

The success of experiential teaching depends on the meaningfulness of the activity to the learners and the degree to which they are involved. Most simply, in experiential learning the students practice what the teacher used to preach. They learn by doing, and as many of the senses are involved as possible. Simulation games are experiential, as are many of the techniques commonly employed in health education . . . role playing, experimenting, demonstrations, dramatizations, and so on. In fact, effective health teaching is always experiential. Every lesson should have experiential elements.

Values-related activities. Inescapably, a person's values, or what seems important to her or him, shape the beliefs that underlie and give direction to every decision and resulting action that person takes. Like their first cousins, attitudes, values are essentially learned standards of behavior and products of the wide range of influences each person experiences from the moment of birth. What a person believes and does about his or her health perhaps is influenced more by values than by knowledge. The decision to begin smoking, stop smoking, eat sensibly, exercise appropriately, or do anything at all that affects health is inevitably based on values.

If you believe that health education needs to recognize this powerful influence, does consideration of values belong in the cognitive or the affective domain? Opinions on this issue are strong and they differ. According to those who favor the affective approach, values cannot be dealt with as though they were facts to be memorized in the way that people learn that two times two is four. Since values involve feelings and beliefs, they can be approached only through activities that stir reactions. This includes the use of role-playing situations, thought-provoking visual materials, and devil's advocate discussions.

Those who favor the cognitive approach believe that values and moral judgments should be based on reasoning rather than on opinions or feelings. According to this view, affective education is perceived as manipulative rather than educational and is more aptly labelled *excitement education*. The primary purpose of role playing, in their view, should be to promote understanding. An affective impact will inevitably occur as a desirable secondary outcome of a meaningful experiential activity.

Tyler suggests that "clarifying values is an essential part of being an intelligent person. It is simply a sensible way of helping children as they go through life to find a way to think about the things they do and ask questions about the thinking involved in their actions." However, he suggests that the term "values clarification" be discarded because it is too often misunderstood (Mickler, 1985).

Whatever strategies you choose as the means of promoting positive health attitudes, take care not to ask your students to discuss matters that could be interpreted as an invasion of personal or family privacy. Also, because some of the published values-clarifying activities are relatively unstructured and even fun, their purpose can get lost in the excitement. Be certain that you never lose sight of your objective, and that the strategy you have chosen is best suited to its achievement. Above all, be certain that the students know *why* they have participated in that activity. Help them to interpret the meaning of what has happened and to relate their conclusions to future health-related decisions and actions.

Vicarious Teaching Techniques

Televised instruction. Although the use of television in teaching is not universal, there is no question that it works as an educational tool. Students can learn from television as well as they can from teachers, textbooks, and other educational devices, as demonstrated by the success of *Sesame Street.* Where closed-circuit television equipment (a means of sending and receiving programs originated and received only within the school) is available, the potential for more effective use of demonstrations and experiments is obvious. Each student has a far

better view than when everybody must crowd around a small area in order to see, and many classes can have a close look at a single show. Increasing use of videotapes makes it possible to record presentations by specialists or students themselves for future use. Taped demonstrations and presentations may even be better than live sessions for observation and study.

Many teachers use scheduled educational television broadcasts as supplementary instructional material. Very large school districts, such as that in Los Angeles, have their own educational television channel with programs available for public, as well as school, viewing. The weekly program schedules of both commercial and educational channels provide a means of identifying current shows with relevance to health education. Documentaries on topics such as environmental pollution, consumer issues, substance abuse problems, AIDS and other health-related concerns are frequent. Such programs usually are given advance publicity and can be announced and used as a homework assignment or recommended as voluntary viewing for extra points and subsequent class discussion. Effective use can be made of audiotape recorders for preserving the sound portions of televised materials where this does not affect its comprehensibility. For example, a taped series of commercials can be used to demonstrate kinds of sales appeals or to evaluate the student's ability to identify those appeals when they are heard and seen.

Software Applications

Overhead projection materials. Professionally prepared transparencies are available for use in connection with most aspects of health instruction. Drawings used for transparencies differ from photographs in that they are simplified line drawings, which are the most effective in promoting understanding of structure and function. The transparencies enliven verbal descriptions and illustrate what is said. They can be used to introduce new topics, stimulate discussion, summarize, stress key points of a lesson, structure and explain assignments, or evaluate students. For example, instead of reproducing copies of tests, a transparency can be used to exhibit the questions and then stored for future use.

The development of original transparencies by students is a worthwhile and enjoyable project. Transparencies can be used to present the results of buzz sessions or to illustrate committee project or panel discussion points. A blank transparency is an effective substitute for the chalkboard, since the writing is easier to read (if care is taken to print or write in inch-high letters), and the writer can face the class and thus is more audible and effective.

Films, slides, and filmstrips. Through the use of film media, a vicarious field trip, experiment, or demonstration can be arranged that otherwise might be difficult or impossible to do. Often a 15-minute film can cover an experience more effectively than an hour-long field trip or lecture. All students see and hear the same material, and certain details can be emphasized so that every part and its function are better described and observed than during an actual field trip. This is not to say that a film is always preferable to a field trip, since there is undeniably greater impact and interest generated by seeing the real thing.

The effectiveness of filmed presentations depends as much on the way they are used as on the skill with which they were developed. Few films are of much value if they are shown without comment or discussion. The instructor must preview and note the key points that make up the message of the film. The entertainment quality of a film can be such that the educational purpose is overlooked. It is doubly important in such cases that the students be told in

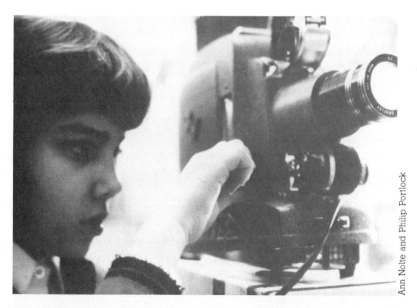

Ann Nolte and Philip Portlock

FIG. 5-1. The filmstrip is a common tool used in health teaching. To use it effectively, the filmstrip can be stopped at appropriate times in the presentation to discuss issues or content addressed.

advance which points to look for while they are enjoying the story. As a means of further ensuring the students' close attention, it can be rewarding to ask for and use their evaluation of the film's worth as a learning activity. It is essential to establish in advance what objective the film is expected to fulfill. Although it may require more time than is available, research shows that learning is greatly enhanced when a film is shown, discussed, and then shown a second time.

Slides and filmstrips do not have quite the dynamic realism of films, but they have the advantage of greater versatility. Individual frames can be viewed for as long as needed, (Fig. 5-1) and the sequence can be altered as desired. Slide presentations are the most flexible of all. New pictures can be added, old ones deleted, and the sequence changed at any time. Slides can be created easily and inexpensively even by young children. When combined with a taped commentary, a slide presentation rivals the dynamic quality of a motion picture. For example, a group of seventh-grade students, invited to submit a color slide of themselves in a pose that illustrated their special view of "happiness," eagerly did so, and then each youngster read for audiotaping a line that explained the message intended by the picture. For example, a picture of a girl cuddling a kitten was accompanied by the voiced message, "Happiness is having something to love that is your very own." The school glee club softly singing "Happiness Is" was recorded for background music. The resulting series of pictures and messages was featured at parent nights and other school meetings to great applause.

Teaching Aids

The use of teaching aids has increased enormously since the days when the slate was the only tool. In addition to the media already discussed, the teacher has radios, books, tape cassettes of visual and audio materials specific to health instruction, records, and a wealth of free or inexpensive teaching materials such as pamphlets, booklets, and article reprints. There are also visual aids such as scrapbooks, flannel boards, graphs, charts, posters, models, exhibits, and specimens, all of which can be used to actively involve the learner in many sensory experiences.

Because learning is more likely to promote positive health behaviors when the teaching activities engage the student emotionally and fully, teachers need to employ, as often as they can, techniques that are as close to real as possible. Models and mock-ups provide an artificial but realistic learning situation (e.g., the plastic head and torso for CPR practice). Drama forms such as sociodramas, skits, and plays also permit *action* on the part of the learner that reinforces desirable behaviors and attitudes. Exhibits of so-called health foods, quackish devices, or deceptive advertisements for "health" products can provide vital learning experiences for children.

A purely visual display using a pegboard, chalkboard, magnetic board, map, graph, cartoon, diagram, or other device may lack movement and auditory properties, but in many situations a simple display can bring a lecture or discussion point into focus better than more elaborate means. It cannot be said that any one medium is better than others; there are too many variables operating in the learning process. A teacher has to be competent in using them all and must choose the one best suited for the particular day, topic, and group of students. Each medium has advantages and disadvantages, but any one of them can be effective if used wisely and well. Some people learn more easily by hearing, some by reading, and others by watching or handling things. A wide variety of approaches and media should be provided so that each child experiences those which are most effective for him or her and also those which will reinforce what has been learned through their appeal to all the other senses.

LESSON PLANS THAT WORK

Hunter (1971) believes that there are three basic tasks in the teaching and learning process: (1) determining what is to be learned (2) determining what the learner will be doing to accomplish the desired learning, and (3) determining what the teacher will do to facilitate that accomplishment. These are tasks with which lesson planning is concerned. The lesson plan that evolves from and reflects the decisions relative to these three tasks should communicate what will be taught and how it will be taught.

Only twenty years ago we were still operating on the notion that teachers are born, not made. I knew it was a myth because I had seen too many bumbling beginners—including me—turn into reasonably decent teachers. I'd also seen a lot of charismatic teachers, pied pipers who looked wonderful to the kids. The pied pipers managed to produce some of the happiest illiterates in the entire school. Charisma is great, but it's neither necessary nor sufficient to be a good teacher.*

Lesson planning goes beyond the mere selection of subject matter, the teaching technique that will permit practice of the behavior specified in the objective, or how the lesson will be conducted. A lesson plan must be organized smoothly, logically, and concisely, clearly matching the intent of the proposed objective.

---

*Berges, Marshall: An Apple for this teacher of teachers Los Angeles Times, part 6, page 1, January 26, 1986. In Hunter, Madeline, 1986.

Lesson plans submitted by a student teacher must be more explicit and detailed than those prepared by an experienced teacher. The latter has had the time to learn what works and knows how children of a given grade or age group react to the health concepts proposed. Student teachers usually are required to present detailed daily plans specifying what will be taught and how it will be done. The following suggestions are made with the assumption that the reader is a prospective rather than an experienced teacher.

Ideally, a feasible and measurable objective, an outline of the key ideas, a brief plan of the activity, a list of resources that will be employed, and a culminating activity should be included. Student teachers should always consider the fact that whatever can go wrong may go wrong and should have a plan to cope with anything that might threaten successful achievement of the lesson.

Once the objective of the lesson has been determined, all the other decisions are directed accordingly. First, the subject matter portion of the objective needs to be elaborated and made explicit. This can be done by means of a list of key generalizations, or a brief outline. It need not be more than the "bare bones ideas" you intend to consider in teaching one lesson.

A lesson plan, in essence, is like a well-organized story. It needs an interest-capturing *beginning* (the initiating activity that links today's plan to yesterday's achievement and whets the appetite for what is to come next). Next comes the *body* of the story (the description of what the students will be doing to practice the skill as they deal with the subject matter).

Never assume that the students can carry out your plan without any effort on your part to provide them with the subject matter described. Indeed, the reverse is true. If the students can carry out your objective so competently that all you have to do is to arrange an opportunity that allows them to do so, there is no need for a lesson. In fact, what you have written in that event is an evaluation activity, not a learning opportunity.

Once you have decided on the subject matter you want them to learn, you must next decide the manner in which it will be provided them. Will you start the lesson by giving a short lecture, show them a film or a film strip that presents the information, ask them to report to you what they have learned by doing the reading you assigned for homework or employ another technique? Research shows that everyone, youngster or adult, learns new material most quickly and easily if it is introduced at either the beginning or the end of a lesson. What does this suggest might sometimes be the focus of the culminating activity?

Finally, a lesson plan has to have a good *ending* (the culminating activity that motivates the learner to summarize, draw conclusions, and makes him or her want to learn more about the subject). The quality of the culminating activity can make the difference between learning and confusion. Sometimes lessons never actually come to an end, but just stop when the bell rings. The learner never finds out why the day's activities took place or what any of it had to do with what had been presented previously.

The plan that follows could be used either as a learning opportunity or a lesson. It depends on the abilities and past learning experiences of the class. To achieve the objective, a primary student probably would first need to complete several enabling activities. Intermediate level students probably could bypass these and carry out the lesson in a single session. Study this plan. See if you can identify its unstated but implicit enabling objectives. What do the students need to be able to do before they can describe ways an individual can favorably affect and promote the health of others?

To develop one lesson absent the overarching logic of a stated framework of goals and a carefully designed scope and sequence plan is difficult to do effectively. However, an illustrative lesson on personal standards of behavior and their relationship to the welfare of others has been worked out, given these limitations. This topic is surely basic to desirable health behavior, although perhaps easy to overlook. This lesson illustrates the application of what the students have learned earlier about the ways in which personal actions can affect the well-being of others.

Outline of a Lesson

Objective: Describes ways an individual can favorably affect and promote the health of others.

Generalization: There are many ways by which an individual can contribute to the well-being of family, friends, and community. Choosing and carrying out a plan for some good action is an important step toward becoming the kind of person one admires.

Strategy: Using lecture-discussion and brainstorming to identify actions that can affect and promote the health of others.

Initiation activity: Introduce the concept of an individual's caring about the well-being of others by telling the story of Benjamin Franklin's plan for his day, as shown in his own diary. The question he posed to himself at the start of each day was, "What good shall I do this day?" Then he jotted down a proposed action. At the end of the day, in answer to the question, "What good have I done this day?" Franklin wrote a short description of the actions that he had taken that seemed to have been good ones.

Establish in brief discussion what Franklin probably meant by "good." Ask questions such as "What do *you* think 'good' means when used to describe an action?" or, "If no one ever did anything that was intended to help others, how could that affect your health and your family's health?"

Activity: Ask for volunteers to describe actions that young people or adults often take to help others and how these actions affect community health. If necessary, show pictures of helpful actions (e.g., a boy scout acting as school crossing guard or a candy striper reading to a young patient in hospital) in order to get the ideas started. Begin by asking the students to comment on what is happening in the picture and to speculate about the motives and the rewards of such actions, and lead them to think about actions they have noted themselves.

As each idea for a helping action is proposed, list the action on the chalkboard or on a transparency and ask the class to decide whether the action helped others at home, at school, or in the community. Then ask volunteers to tell about some action they have themselves taken that affected the well-being of another. Help each person to analyze how this made him or her feel as a result. Ask questions such as, "Did you do that because you wanted to or because it was required?" "Did you feel happy about what you had done?" "Would you do it again if you could?"

Culmination: When everybody who wanted to participate has been heard (and no one should be pressed to contribute unwillingly), ask the class to review the total list of actions that have been described and to speculate about what

kind is most often chosen. Are they most often for people at home, at school, or in the community? Then ask each child to think for several minutes and decide on something good that she or he can do during the next day. Ask each of them to write or dictate to a teacher's aide or older student a brief description of the action they chose and how, on implementation, it affected the well-being of others, to be handed in at the next class meeting. Allow those who prefer to present their action in the form of a drawing or poster. Devise some means of sharing the products of the assignment among the class members and help them to draw some conclusions about the whole experience.

Now that you have read the plan, decide whether students might be better equipped to participate effectively in the brainstorming that would be required if they had first completed lessons based on objectives like the following.

1. Define the meaning of "good actions."
2. Differentiate between actions that might enhance and those that might detract from the health of others.
3. Identify actions an individual could take that might promote community health.
4. Explain ways such actions contribute to the well-being of others.

Are there other objectives that might be necessary for younger children? How could you be sure if the students in your class were ready to deal with the principal objective of the lesson as it is? Chapter Seven considers some ways to measure readiness by means of pretests and other measurement techniques.

Every lesson needs to be planned. Whether a teaching plan is broad, as in the case of a learning opportunity, or specific, as for a lesson, it should be based on a measurable objective that is attainable by the students for whom it is intended; it should focus on process rather than information; it should be learner-oriented; and it should come to a meaningful ending.

SUMMARY

Application of the concepts, skills, and techniques discussed in this chapter depends on the depth of one's understanding of their interrelationships and their dependence on the ability to apply what was considered in the two preceding chapters. In order to develop effective teaching and learning plans you must first have studied the sources of a health curriculum (i.e., the learner, the community, and its body of knowledge); determined what the scope and sequence of the curriculum are to be; defined its goals; and based upon data obtained from the sources, inferred sets of feasible objectives by grade or level (i.e., primary, upper elementary, and middle school) to form a framework for the teaching-learning plans that might facilitate their achievement.

Chapter Five has dealt with the final step in the curriculum planning process, which has to do with *how* the goals and objectives might be implemented effectively. Three fundamental problems must be solved. For any particular group of students, these are: first, deciding what is to be taught and learned; second, what the learner is to be doing in order to achieve the instructional objectives; and third, what the teacher will do in order to help the learner to do so.

A number of propositions have been discussed as considerations basic to lesson planning. Some of these are as follows:

Health behavior is the result of decisions, whether conscious or subconscious in nature.

Problem solving and decision making are skills with lifelong utility and total transfer to other situations.

Emphasis on process rather than information is essential in planning active teaching strategies.

Thinking skills can be taught and learned but cannot be fostered by telling and reciting activities.

The more senses involved in a learning experience, the greater its effectiveness as a teaching strategy.

Active participation in learning activities heightens the impact and increases the rate of learning.

Intellectual skills must be practiced if they are to be mastered.

The best teaching technique is the one that provides the greatest number of concurrent positive outcomes, matches the objective, is perceived as satisfying, and fits the abilities of the students for whom it is planned.

Health education in schools tends to be evaluated on the basis of what is offered students in its name, rather than in terms of its philosophy and purposes as proposed by its specialists. We hope that you will perceive your health teaching assignment as an expression of trust. Any one course in health education can contribute only partially to the long-range goals set by the school. However, creative, thoughtfully conceived health lessons can make a difference in the life style choices of students and can often change those of their parents as well.

Lesson plan for health education*

Teacher _____ **Unit** _____ **Date** _____

Specific objective for this lesson

Initiation

(Your plan to make a transition from a hypothetical previous day's accomplishment and to initiate today's learning activities; not what you plan to *say* but what you plan to *do*)

Content	Estimated time	Materials (fact-finding sources)	Plan of action	Special class arrangements
(Stated as generalizations that structure the subject matter of the lesson, or an outline of the subject matter relevant to the lesson objective)	(Based on your *own previous practice in preparation for* this assignment)	(Actual materials you will be using, such as books, pamphlets and films—*not* pencils, erasers, chalk, etc.)	(What the students will be doing, explained step by step)	(Will they be seated in usual order? In small groups? Moving about?)

Culminating activities

(How you will terminate the lessons so that students know what they have learned and how this relates to what is to come next)

Anticipated problems (what might go wrong?)   **Possible solutions (what could you do if something goes wrong?)**

For example: No one in the class has done the homework necessary to carry out your plan.

For example: Give in-class time to do this, or switch plans to an activity that does not depend on that material.

*Use this guide only as a structure for the presentation of your lesson plan. Do not attempt to fit your plan into the blank spaces.

QUESTIONS AND EXERCISES

Discussion questions

1. If you were asked what the content of health teaching should include during elementary school grades, what areas would you list? How would that list influence the lessons that you might plan?

2. In what situations would choice of a vicarious teaching technique have advantages over directly experienced activities?

3. Why is it essential that children comprehend the purpose of any values-clarifying activities? How could you determine whether or not they have in fact understood that purpose?

4. If you were limited to but one of the senses as your means of communicating with your students, which would it be and why?

5. What do you see as the advantages, if any, of buzz sessions over brainstorming as a means of quickly generating a number of good ideas relative to a health issue?

6. Suppose that your class wanted to visit a nearby health facility, but for several good reasons it could not be arranged. Suggest other ways that you could satisfy that interest, but without the expense and other problems involved in making off-campus visits.

7. Health teaching in elementary schools is most often integrated with science courses, and sometimes with mathematics or physical education. Suggest some ways that, whatever scheduled instruction was provided, you could add to the curriculum by integrating certain objectives with other host subject areas, such as reading, writing, art, and history.

Exercises and problems

1. For each of Bloom's categories of cognitive objectives, write one instructional objective for an age group of your choice, employing as a behavior one of those defined on pp. 123-124. Next, for each of those objectives, suggest a teaching technique that would best implement that behavior.

2. Develop a health lesson for a specified elementary grade that includes each of the following components:
   a. An instructional objective
   b. A brief outline of the content to be taught
   c. An initiating activity
   d. A description of the principal activity required of the students.
   e. A culminating activity
   f. A list of possible problems that could interfere with the conduct of the lesson, along with ways that these could be quickly solved.

3. Exchange plans with a fellow student. Read the other's plan and judge its clarity (if you could not carry out the plan without asking for more information, it's not clear enough). Write your comments and questions directly on the plan and return it to the author for study and any necessary reworking.

4. For a given general objective, develop an outline of the related subject matter in two formats, as follows:
   a. Traditional outline form, main points and subpoints adequate to describe the content for a learning opportunity.
   b. A list of generalizations that express all of the key ideas implicit in the objective.

5. Select or develop an affective objective that interests you and work out a lesson plan for its implementation, just as for the cognitive objective in exercise one. Be ready to explain your plan to the class.

SUGGESTED READINGS

Andrews R and Hearne R: Effects of the primary grades health curriculum project on student and parent smoking attitudes and behavior, J Sch Health 54(1):18-20, 1984. Report of an experimental study of primary school students' knowledge and attitudes regarding positive health behavior. The effectiveness of a standard teacher/textbook approach was compared to the PGHCP experimentally-based curriculum in health education. Results showed that the experimental group evidenced significantly more positive attitudes toward good health practices and more negative attitudes towardsmokingthandidthecontrolgroup.Experimental group children also demonstrated significantly greater levels of knowledge about good health, the body systems, and the effects of smoking than did control group children. Moreover, although parents of children in both groups reported that they had changed their smoking habits as a result of their children's health program, the number of those changing was significantly greater among those with children in the experimental group.

Bailey G: How to improve your presentations by keeping your mouth closed, Perform Instr J 23(3):27-28, 1984. Silence is one of the most important of the nonverbal communication cues used in teaching. This paper describes nine categories of silence uses ranging from set and closure signals to humorous silence, which is so effectively used by comedians. Silence works just as well in the classroom to relieve tension or emphasize a point. Silence is probably used more often as a means of restoring order or calling the group to attention than for any other purpose.

Bennett, W: What works: schools without drugs, Washington, DC, 1986, US Department of Education. A 78-page booklet providing a synthesis of the most reliable and significant information currently available regarding substance abuse (drugs and alcohol) by children and youth. The purpose of the book is prevention, not cure. Includes fact sheets on categories of drugs, their effects, and suggested preventive actions that can be taken by parents, schools, students, and communities. Ideas for teaching activities suitable for use with elementary children are described and information regarding hot lines, related catalogues of materials, and other resources and readings is provided.

Eddy J, St Pierre R, and Alles W: A reexamination of values clarification for the health educator, Health Educ 16:1, 1985. Excellent analysis of educational problems and concerns associated with certain uses of values clarification activities. A series of seven guidelines are proposed by which to direct their proper use. Recommends that values-clarifying activities be incorporated into the curriculum only when chosen and implemented in a systematic, preplanned, and educationally sound manner.

Goodlad, J: A place called school, New York, 1984, McGraw-Hill. Described as providing a more comprehensive view of U.S. schools than any guide previously published, Goodlad's study is based on data gathered nationwide over a period of several years. Over a thousand classrooms, 1,350 teachers, 8,624 parents, and 17,163 students were involved. The book is as easy to read as it is absorbing to those interested in what the schools are doing today. Chapter 7, ''What Schools and Classrooms Teach,'' and Chapter 4, ''Inside Classrooms,'' may be most relevant to the content to this chapter.

Harrington, D, editor: Early adolescent helper program, J of Experiential Educ 9:2, 1986. Describes an innovative experiential program designed to involve early adolescents (ages 11 to 14) in active, responsible ''grown-up'' roles as tutors, counselors, helpers, or interns. Students serve as interns (helpers) in child care or senior citizen centers after school at least twice a week. In school they participate in a seminar that combines relevant information with practice in problem solving, decision making and work-readiness skills. They also serve as helpers by tutoring their peers or younger children, by serving as museum guides, by reading stories to children at public libraries, by assisting at playgrounds, and in many other ways.

There are problems that must be anticipated and worked out with these young people. Rules and limits, as well as responsibilities and consequences, must be spelled out. Assignments must be flexible and there must be support for failure. Progress will result, as experience has shown, as self-confidence and competence grow. Information about the way to start such a program in a school or agency can be obtained by writing or calling the Early Adolescent Helper Program at the address shown in the article.

Lovett Z and Webbing J: A bridge between teaching and learning, Educ Horizons 60(3):119-121, 1988. Explains a form of mapping and facilitating the organization of information. At the center of the "web" is the main idea, theme, or topic of interest. The technique can be used with all students, regardless of the level of their skills. Even first graders can develop webs of information by using magazines or text books, listening to teachers and other speakers, by brainstorming, or by using other sources of information as means of identifying or discovering information related to selected main points.

Travis HR: Sexual responsibility: examining relationships, Health Educ 17:4, 1984. Planned as the last lesson in a unit on human sexuality education designed for sixth graders, this describes a session dealing with moral aspects of human sexual behavior. Earlier lessons had covered topics such as male and female physiology, sexual intercourse, birth, and birth control. Some of these topics were discussed with the sexes separated; the others were conducted with the members of two classes assembled together.

The techniques employed included buzz groups, lecture-discussion, and Socratic questioning. The dialogue is provided in considerable detail; the plan is structured as an introduction, a series of discussions following short lectures, and a somewhat formal concluding statement. The lesson was provided by a health science associate professor at a nearby university, but the plan could easily be implemented by a classroom teacher.

REFERENCES

Bandura A: Social learning theory, Englewood Cliffs, NJ; 1977, Prentice Hall.

Blackwood, PE: Science teaching in the elementary school. In Hollson M: Elementary education, New York, 1967, Free Press.

Bloom BS et al: Taxonomy of educational objectives: handbook I: cognitive domain. 1956

Bloom BS, Hastings G, and Madeus G: Evaluation to improve learning, New York, 1981, McGraw-Hill.

Bruner J: The process of education, Cambridge, 1960, Harvard University Press.

Combs A: What the future demands of education, Phi Delta Kappan 62:369, 1981.

Conrad D and Hedin D: National assessment of experiential education: summary and implications, J Experiential Educ Fall 1981, p 16.

Feldman RD: What are thinking skills? Instructor and Teacher 8:95, 1986.

Goodlad JI et al: A place called school, New York. 1984, McGraw-Hill.

Hunter M: Teach for transfer, El Segundo, CA, 1971, TIP Publications.

Hunter M: Great teaching is like conducting a symphony, Education, UCLA Graduate School of Education, Fall 1986.

James T: Learning as practice in theory, Phi Delta Kappan 62:185, 1981.

Kierstead J: Direct instruction and experiential approaches: are they really mutually exclusive? Educ Leadership 42:8 1985.

Kolbe LJ et al: Propositions for an alternate and complementary health education paradigm, Health Educ 12:3, 1981.

Mickler ML: Interviews with Ralph W Tyler, Educ Forum 50:1, 1985.

Moyer J: Child development as a base for decision making, Childhood Educ May/June 1986.

Parcel G and Barnowski T: Social learning theory and health education, Health Educ 12:3, 1981.

Parker PF and Rubin LJ: Process as content: curriculum design and the application of knowledge, Chicago, 1966, Rand McNally.

Resnik H: From social studies to social science, Learning 13:3, 1985.

Wales CE, Nardi A, and Stager R: Decision making: new paradigm for education, Educ Leadership 43:8, 1986.

White J: Decision making with an integrative curriculum, Childhood Educ 62:5, 1986.

CHAPTER 6

Health Education Evaluation

When you finish this chapter you should be able to:

- **Distinguish between the goals of evaluation and measurement.**

- **Compare the uses of formative evaluation with those of summative evaluation.**

- **Explain the interrelationships among objectives, learning opportunities, and evaluation procedures.**

- **Describe the ways that changes in learner knowledge, attitudes, and practices can be assessed.**

- **Apply evaluative criteria to the analysis of health teaching resources and materials.**

What does the word *evaluation* mean to you? Does it arouse unpleasant feelings of anxiety, stress, or expectation of criticism or failure? Perhaps you equate it with marking a score sheet and the effect that analysis of those marks can have on a course grade. Since you are a student at this time, your reactions may reflect both descriptions. Notice that the first is largely emotional and experience related, but the other confuses evaluation with measurement.

Generally, evaluation is a means of making an informed decision about a performance, person, or program. The fundamental activity involved is collecting information. It is the ends that are sought that differentiate between evaluation and measurement. Measurement in education is concerned with description and comparisons of individuals (Wolf, 1987). The goal of evaluation is always the same, whatever the object of scrutiny—to appraise something according to a specified standard.

Evaluation is not limited to whatever terminal procedure a teacher employs to assign a final grade to a student. That is **summative** evaluation. There is also **formative** evaluation, the ongoing process of which is begun before instruction (pretesting) and is continued throughout the course. Formative evaluation may be the more worthwhile means of promoting desired growth or change in ability and knowledge, because it gives the students feedback about their progress at a time when they can best use it. Summative evaluation procedures are designed to elicit evidence of the end product of the course—the total change that has occurred due to instruction. Final grades can not be appraised fairly by means of a single test or procedure, but must represent a synthesis of significant observations and data of several kinds obtained by measurement (Scriven, 1967).

PURPOSES OF EVALUATION IN SCHOOL HEALTH EDUCATION

Ideally the purposes of evaluation in school health education include the following:

1. To determine present health knowledge, attitudes, and practices as a basis for defining objectives for future instruction.
2. To identify and diagnose sources of learning difficulties.
3. To assess the effectiveness of teaching materials and strategies.
4. To appraise the total health curriculum.
5. To provide continuing information about student achievement.
6. To improve counseling effectiveness.
7. To test the relevance of evaluation procedures to the stated course objectives.
8. To provide a basis for necessary modifications or improvements of all aspects of the school health program.

The focus of this chapter will be delimited to evaluation of the learners, the effectiveness of the teacher, and the quality, utility, and appropriateness of the health teaching materials and resources employed in the classroom. Evaluation of these elements of the teaching-learning task is essential at every level of implementation, whether it be the classroom, the program, or the curriculum, and whatever the age group for which a plan is designed and implemented. If health instruction is to keep pace with the unending changes in society and in science, evaluation activity must be continuous and unending.

EVALUATION IS MORE THAN MEASUREMENT

A primary difference between evaluation and measurement is that the first is concerned with quality or value, while the second is concerned only with quantity. Evaluation is far broader in scope, and its outcome has far more weight in making decisions about the object of interest. Cryan (1986) discusses the difference between the two in these words:

Measurement is only part of the evaluative process, and testing is only one way of measuring certain characteristics. Because evaluation is continuous, comprehensive, and integral to the process of instruction, it must represent a variable set of procedures that are carried out daily as well as periodically. Those procedures accomplish purposes of: 1) preliminary diagnostic judgments to identify individual and group needs; 2) ongoing formative judgment of student and teacher progress toward instructional goals, and 3) concluding summative judgments of overall performance.

Popham (1981) says that measurement is *status* determination, whereas evaluation is *worth* determination, as is implicit in the word itself. Evaluation is a comprehensive process, including both qualitative and quantitative descriptions of student behavior, as well as value judgments about that behavior. Evaluating health teaching and learning requires systematic assessment of the *total* performance of a student (quality of classroom participation, level of motivation evident, and ability to apply learned health concepts and information in solving real or hypothetical health-related problems). Although both formative and summative evaluation procedures are employed during the course of study, the formative is given the most attention, but always for feedback purposes rather than for ranking or grading.

RELATIONSHIP OF EVALUATION TO INSTRUCTIONAL OBJECTIVES

An evaluation activity or procedure, as an integral part of the instructional process, theoretically represents one side of an equilateral trian-

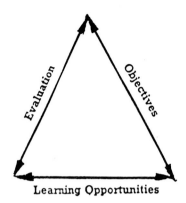

gle, the other two sides being a given measurable objective and the learning opportunity designed for its appropriate practice. The dynamic interrelationships among them are not mutually exclusive. Each of these components affects and is affected by the other two. For example, just as objectives serve as guidelines to the development or selection of appropriate learning opportunities, so also do they suggest valid evaluation activities. There must be consistency between the two. On the other hand, evaluation yields information about the learner's performance, and at the same time tells us which learning opportunities are working and even which objectives need to be revised or tossed out. Finally, learning opportunities often lead unexpectedly to new insights relative to student interests, community needs, and the like, which motivates the creation of new objectives.

These three components of the total process of teaching and learning might also be expressed by means of three interrelated questions. (1) Where do we want to go—the objective; (2) How can we get there—the learning opportunity; and (3) How far have we come—the evaluation. Specification of clearly stated objectives is an essential step in planning instruction in which evaluation is not only a means of measuring progress but also a contributing factor in the instructional process (Bloom, Madaus, and Hastings, 1981).

If the stated objectives are the *real* objectives, it is impossible to separate them from planning for evaluation. Implicit in a measurable objective is the activity that is acceptable as evidence of its mastery. If the objective proposes that the student should be able to distinguish between illness and wellness, then the evaluation procedure must provide some means whereby the ability to do precisely that is elicited. Some instructors find it easier, in fact, to decide what they will accept as evidence that the student has learned what was taught, and *then* choose the cognitive skill that fits that expectation. Teaching strategies or learning opportunities are the means by which the teacher helps the student to build a bridge of competence between "cannot do it" and "can do it."

An objective specifies a process and some content to be learned. A lesson plan is designed to provide opportunities to practice that skill in connection with that content, until everyone in the class has mastered the objective. For example, if the objective stipulates that the learners will be able to explain *relationships* between certain environmental conditions and the health and safety of the community, it is neither fair nor logical to give them a test designed to measure the ability to name *sources* of pollution, to cite laws expected to prevent certain environmental problems, or to select from a list of federal and state agencies those charged with protection of the environment. Can you suggest objectives that would match the purposes implicit in the above three test problems?

WHAT CAN BE EVALUATED BY TEACHERS?

The problem of evaluation in health teaching is more perplexing than in most other school sub-

jects because its desired outcomes are often not easily measured in the classroom. Tests of many kinds can provide data regarding growth in knowledge, but gains in information are not always transferred to the actions and attitudes that are the most important goals of health teaching. There is a wide difference between what a person knows and does, as most of us will admit. Moreover, what can be taught in elementary schools is severely limited in several ways—by the amount of time that is available, the interest of the teacher in teaching about health, and the amount and quality of professional preparation for the task the teacher has had, whether preservice or inservice.

Elementary teachers are expected to appraise their students' performance subsequent to instruction, at least with regard to increases in knowledge. Positive shifts in health attitudes, correction of misconceptions, and evidence of new or reinforced desirable health practices are also hoped for. It is relatively easy to measure changes in knowledge, but it is possible to ascertain, to some degree, resulting changes in the other dimensions of health behavior as well. What children are thinking and feeling can't be measured as directly as knowledge, but a great deal can be inferred about these less quantifiable attributes from what children say and do. Among the ways these kinds of data can be gathered are: (1) direct observation, (2) interviews, (3) checklists, (4) questionnaires (these can be read to young children or administered to those with reading skills), and (5) samples of their work, drawings, and the like.

Hochbaum (1981) reminds us, however, of the many influences on health behavior other than those associated with education, most of which are outside the classroom and therefore outside a teacher's ability either to control or to counteract. In fact, some of those influences are not easily controlled by the individual who experiences them. He says, "Social, economic, political, physical, environmental and a multitude of other conditions may render the chosen behavior possible and easy, or make it difficult or impossible.''

The Learner

Evaluating health knowledge. In planning instruction it must be decided what should be measured and how it will be assessed. The set of abilities or responses a teacher is willing to accept as evidence of a student's achievement becomes an operational definition of what she or he views as important, whatever the stated objectives may have been. Health knowledge is the aspect of health instruction that is easiest to measure so knowledge tests are those most depended on by teachers. Although possession of information does not guarantee that its owner will use it, neither can it be denied that it is basic to making a reasoned choice.

Carlyon (1979) believes that it is unrealistic and absurd to expect more from health education than from any other discipline offered in the schools; no one would try to teach children everything they need to know about mathematics or a language by means of a crash course once or twice during the public school years. He explains:

As I understand it, health instruction curriculum shares the overall goal of the entire school curriculum, which is to help students become knowledgeable, critical, independent learners. Health curriculum, more than the rest of the curriculum, focuses on knowledge, critical abilities, and learning skills related to normal growth and development and maintenance of well-being. It is assumed that people thus equipped are more likely to live healthful lives than those who are not.''

Ways of constructing your own knowledge tests or identifying reliable standardized instruments are described in the next chapter. Remember that well-designed paper and pencil tests are not limited to the assessment of factual information but can be effective in measuring the ability to apply that information as well as in assessing attitudes and practices.

Evaluating health beliefs and attitudes. The first step here is to try to distinguish between attitudes and beliefs. Attitudes usually are defined as being based on beliefs, and most people differentiate between the two. Green et al. (1980) define a *belief* as a ''statement or sense, declared or implied, intellectually and/or emotionally accepted as true by a person or group.'' Conviction about their truth is what is significant about beliefs. Those teaching about health need to find out what students believe about it because it often reflects misconceptions, misperceptions, or outdated concepts.

Unfortunately, evaluation of health beliefs is difficult. There are several methods for doing so, all of which are subject to errors of perception and interpretation. The teacher can simply *ask* the student what his or her attitude is toward some health-related issue. However, although no one should know the answer better than the respondent, self-report is not dependably accurate. The individual may want to conceal a negative attitude and so says something that is not exactly true. The answer may reflect a belief rather than an attitude, or it may be influenced by what the student has learned is approved rather than reflect the real attitude. Moreover, what many people *think* is their attitude toward something is often not their real attitude at all, although they may be quite sincere in their answer, for example, the individual who compliments a woman by saying that she thinks like a man.

A teacher can obtain information about students' attitudes from their peers, parents, or other adults who know the students well. Of course, parents are understandably reluctant to report negative attitudes, and studies show that few parents can reliably report their child's actual attitude.

Health belief checklist

	Very important	Important	Fairly important	Not important
I believe I should				
Eat three meals a day				
Have my teeth checked by a dentist at least twice a year				
Have breakfast each morning				
Eat eggs and bacon each morning				
Be happy all the time				
Like myself				
Enjoy simple pleasures like food and nature				
Never snack between meals				
Accept disappointments calmly				
Show love of other people				
Trust my friends				
Feel responsible for other people				
Be able to laugh at myself when I am wrong				
Be glad if I am the largest person in the room				
Face problems and try to solve them				
Respect the differences I see in others				
Stand up for my ideas				
Not push others around				
Tell an adult when I don't feel well				
Take medicine when I don't feel well				
Do some strenuous exercise every day				

Modified from Nolte, AE and others: Instructor 81(1):47, 1971.

A person's attitudes can be inferred from her or his reactions to issues and people. Observation can provide clues to attitudes, although the interpretation of observations, like beauty, depends a great deal on the eye of the beholder. In addition, a teacher must be cautious about making judgments about a child's attitudes based on his or her own attitudes.

Beliefs and attitudes also reflect values. Popham (1975) says that a value is a shared preference for broad constructs or concepts such as justice, honesty, and health. If it is known what children already believe and value relative to health and health practices, then not only can appropriate learning opportunities be arranged, but their effectiveness in changing misconceptions can also be appraised.

Typically, written health attitude tests ask

HEALTH EDUCATION

Good	___ :	___ :	___ :	___ :	___ :	___ :	___ :	___	Bad
Fair	___ :	___ :	___ :	___ :	___ :	___ :	___ :	___	Unfair
Clean	___ :	___ :	___ :	___ :	___ :	___ :	___ :	___	Dirty
Fast	___ :	___ :	___ :	___ :	___ :	___ :	___ :	___	Slow
Hard	___ :	___ :	___ :	___ :	___ :	___ :	___ :	___	Soft
Sharp	___ :	___ :	___ :	___ :	___ :	___ :	___ :	___	Dull
Strong	___ :	___ :	___ :	___ :	___ :	___ :	___ :	___	Weak
Sad	___ :	___ :	___ :	___ :	___ :	___ :	___ :	___	Happy
Nice	___ :	___ :	___ :	___ :	___ :	___ :	___ :	___	Awful
Useless	___ :	___ :	___ :	___ :	___ :	___ :	___ :	___	Useful

the respondent to indicate feelings or opinions relative to specified health practices or issues. Most such instruments are designed in the form of answer-completion tests, checklists, or self-report devices such as Likert or Semantic Differential scales. Few, if any, standardized attitude tests that are appropriate for use with elementary school students are available. However, the previous example of a checklist regarding health beliefs (Nolte et al., 1971) could be used with young children as a pretest for health teaching and modified to serve as a summative test. Its authors do not claim that any of the items represent absolutes, nor do they specify which of them need to be interpreted or discussed further with the children.

The semantic differential test of meaning. Considerable use has been made of the semantic differential testing technique developed by Osgood, Suci, and Tannenbaum (1957) in studies of children's attitudes toward health (Thygerson, 1977). A scale is used to measure the connotative meanings of concepts, as revealed by the respondent's rating of them on the basis of sets of bipolar adjectives. Connotative meanings reflect the attitude of the student toward the concept. Thus a student might be asked to rate health education or another such concept on a form like the one in the following box. The respondent is instructed to check the space that corresponds most closely to his or her feelings about the concept.

Although some of the sets of adjective appear to be totally irrelevant, a response is to be given for each, based on a quick reaction to the words themselves in association with the concept. If the student believes that health education is extremely useful, a check should be made in the space closest to that adjective. A mark next to the opposing adjective records a negative attitude. The middle space allows a neutral feeling to be expressed, and the remaining spaces are used to indicate varying degrees of positive or negative feelings about the concept.

One way of scoring that is frequently used is to allot each position a certain number of points, the highest possible being seven points, neutral being four points, and the lowest rating being one point. Notice that the pairs are not always set up with the positive rating in the same place, so that the first score point for any pair of adjectives may be either seven or one. In the sample scale, the most positive attitude would yield 70 points, the most negative attitude 10 points, and a neutral attitude 40 points.

The questions below ask about different people you don't know. Circle the word that shows what you think about a person.

YES = The person probably smokes
MAYBE = Not sure if the person smokes
NO = The person probably does not smoke

YES MAYBE NO Greg has many friends. Do you think he smokes?
YES MAYBE NO Cheryl almost never looks good. Do you think she smokes?
YES MAYBE NO Raymond is a very good runner. Do you think he smokes?
YES MAYBE NO Linda is not healthy. Do you think she smokes?
YES MAYBE NO Keith usually feels healthy. Do you think he smokes?
YES MAYBE NO Tony has a hard time when he runs. Do you think he smokes?
YES MAYBE NO The other kids don't like Valerie. Do you think she smokes?
YES MAYBE NO Jimmy is the best-looking boy in the class. Do you think he smokes?

Adapted from An Evaluation Handbook for Health Education Programs in Smoking, Centers for Disease Control, Atlanta, 1983.

There is no right answer in this situation, but there is a positive direction. All the interpretations of the sets of adjectives are based on extensive analyses conducted by Osgood and his colleagues (1957). The scales permit comparisons between individuals and groups relative to their attitudes toward specified persons, concepts, or issues. This test can be used to see how similarly one individual perceives a number of related concepts, and to measure changes in attitudes after a course in health education. Even young children can be asked to respond to a scale like this, either verbally or by checking spaces. For elementary school children it may be wise to limit the possible intervals to five, however.

A major advantage of the semantic differen-

tial assessment of affect or meaning is that the sets of adjectives are not based on obvious or seemingly relevant comparisons, so the responses are less vulnerable to faking.

Likert scales. The Likert scale is probably the most widely used among available affective scales. Typically, the Likert scale offers the respondent a five-point rating scale ranging from strongly agree (SA), agree (A), uncertain (U), disagree (D), and strongly disagree (SD), relative to a series of positive or negative statements. With young examinees, only three (e.g., yes, maybe, and no), or two (yes or no) ratings may be elicited. The scoring scheme depends on the number of ratings in the scale and awards the most points to the most positive response to positive statements and the most negative response to negative statements. The major advantages of the Likert scale are its relative ease of construction and scoring and the reliability of its results. Following is a scale constructed for use with elementary students that is focused on their attitude toward smoking

Evaluating health behavior. Health behavior has to do with the actions customarily taken by an individual that have an impact on personal and community well-being. A goal of health education is to promote desirable behaviors and practices (personal health care actions that may not always be consistent but that are at least the result of decisions one way or another), either through change or by reinforcement of existing desirable patterns. This is not easy since 1) behaviors can only be assessed at a given point of time, and 2) only certain health practices can be observed at school. And nobody knows if what was observed was typical or if it will be different if noted under other circumstances. As in the case of attitude assessment, if the only feasible ways of determining a person's health-related behavior are self-reports and questionnaires, the results may be biased due to conscious or unconscious "bending" of the truth. The respondent may report a behavior that reflects what is the best behavior rather than the usual behavior. The response may be slanted for a number of reasons, for example, knowledge of best behavior, desire to appear to good advantage in the instructor's eyes, prior experience, or even for fun or to shock the teacher (Veenker, 1985).

Certain informal procedures can be used to supplement information gathered through structured means. Casual but direct observation of student behavior in the classroom, cafeteria, or school grounds can yield information to be recorded in health records in anecdotal form. Making such notations is easier and more efficient when a checklist or other such form has been prepared for this purpose.

A weakness inherent in some techniques for appraising behavior is their dependence on verbal descriptions of actions. Words do not mean the same thing to all people or even to the same people at all times. For example, self-report instruments typically ask the respondent to judge the frequency of specific health behaviors. The individual may be asked to indicate whether between-meal snacks are eaten (1) often, (2) frequently, (3) sometimes, (4) seldom, or (5) never. Only the last of these frequencies is dependably interpreted the same way by everybody. One person's "often" may be another's "frequently" or vice versa. "Sometimes" may mean once a month to Tom and once a week to Joanne. Unless the directions for each alternative are carefully written to ensure uniformity of interpretation, it is impossible to draw any valid conclusions from the answers; yet it is difficult to construct such an unambiguous instrument that is comprehensive enough to be useful and at the same time feasible in terms of the time needed to administer it.

Another common problem is the irrelevance of what is measured to the actual concern, that is, health behavior. *Knowing* what to do is not evidence of application, yet overemphasis on content is reflected in the measurement techniques used in many classrooms. An analysis of typical teacher-made tests revealed that 8 out of 10 measured knowledge of specific facts only (Burns, 1968). Even though questions may offer choices among several possible health actions, the correct answers are designed to reflect knowledge primarily. It cannot be otherwise if the intention is to evaluate retention of factual material covered in the course.

Finally, because health behavior does not begin or end in the classroom, and because certain kinds of behaviors cannot be evaluated during the school year ages, the outcome of some instruction may not be demonstrated for many years. Ironically, it is even possible that the most significant impact on health behavior may never be recorded. For example, how do you measure the amount of undesirable behavior that never happened because health instruction reinforced health practices learned at home or prevented the later emergence of some that were potentially harmful?

It is probable that what can be learned about children's health behavior is more useful and meaningful as the basis of decisions relative to the health content and teaching techniques employed, than as evidence supportive of the effectiveness of health instruction. Veenker (1985) says that it is not knowledge but the many factors and forces in school, home, and community life that determine the kind of health practices an individual follows. To claim that any change is directly and solely attributable to a course in health education is foolish. Teachers can accomplish wonders in the little time allotted for their efforts, yet they cannot and should not be expected to counter the many forces that promote negative health behaviors in our society. Hochbaum (1982) agrees, saying:

In school health education, for example, the appropriate criteria [of effectiveness] are certain cognitive and affective changes in children and in some cases in their parents and other significant persons. While these are already well accepted objectives there is always the lingering notion that the "real criteria" are to be found in actual behavioral change. This poses unrealistic demands on available evaluation methods . . . It may, moreover, infuse in the health educator a sense of failure and futility, when the expected behaviors do not occur, while in reality he or she may have succeeded supremely well in accomplishing all that education can accomplish: create conditions favorable to the desired behaviors though without assuring the emergence of such behaviors.

EFFECTS OF EVALUATION ON THE LEARNER

Evaluation can have both positive and negative effects on the learner. A good evaluation activity can be as much of a learning opportunity as it is a procedure for the appraisal of results. Look at any textbook or curriculum guide that lists ideas for learning opportunities and notice how many of them are in fact evaluation activities. The principal difference between the two is in the assumptions on which each depends. The assumption underlying a learning opportunity is that the students *do not* know the subject matter and part of the plan has to provide for its provision in some manner. The assumption of the evaluation activity is that the learner *does* know the information needed to carry it out, and that it has been learned as an outcome of earlier experiences in the classroom. Moreover, it is expected that the student has also had practice in dealing with it as specified in the objective.

An evaluation activity (where *activity* refers to the use of a realistic problem as a means of assessing ability) requires the learner to apply this new information in a new, hypothetical situation. As a result, skill in problem solving is reinforced, information about the problem is reinforced or even added to, and the learner does not have to be told where her or his strengths or weaknesses lie. Motivation to learn is increased when evaluation is used either to estimate progress or to gauge total achievement following a series of lessons.

If evaluation is seen as a threat, it can have negative effects, not only on present learning, but also on the students themselves, because it influences their attitudes toward health education as a course and the promotion of health as a valued pattern of behaviors. For example, the pressure of test taking, particularly when the results are used to determine positions on a grading scale, may be motivating for a few. For others, the result may instead be frustration, dependence on test-taking tricks, cheating, and what is the worst perhaps, feelings of defeat and apathy.

Testing procedures must be planned carefully, so that the effect will be positive in as many ways as possible. After administering a test, it helps to go over it, item by item, and allow the students to give their reasons for having answered any item differently from what you have intended to be the correct response. Often you will discover that another answer was just as good or that the item was so ambiguous in meaning that other answers are just as acceptable as the "right" one. This can be painful for you if you wrote the test, but it is worth it. All of your students will have learned the correct answers, which ones they missed and why, and where to focus further study. If there was any difference in opinion regarding certain items, the issue has been faced and resolved on the spot. You will feel satisfaction in knowing that learning has been the outcome, even more than assessment. You will have earned your students' respect by your willingness to accept criticism and deal with it fairly. And it is a quick way to evaluate the test itself and improve it for the next application.

EVALUATING THE CURRICULUM PLAN AND THE TEACHER
Evaluating the Curriculum Plan

The curriculum plan in a school or district is the result of a great many decisions, made by administrators and teachers, that specify how health education will be organized, how much time it is allotted, what subject matter it will include or omit, at which grades it will be taught, whether specialists or special resources will be provided, a statement of the system of beliefs about health education as a basic course of study, and more. Some of these elements are written, others are specified as part of school administration. All of these should be reviewed continually and revised as needed as means of assurance that the plan reflects the state of the art and not some outdated no longer adequate curriculum.

A handbook prepared for state policy makers detailing recommendations for school health education (Education Commission of the States, 1981) suggests standards by which programs may be examined. Many of the above problems are addressed directly in this document. Another publication, *How Healthy Is Your School?* (Nelson, 1986) contains a wealth of material for the evaluation of the school health program, including ways of assessing student achievement and the curriculum.

Most often, health teaching in elementary schools is integrated in organization. As such it works quite well in effecting cognitive and affective changes that influence children's health behavior. Direct teaching is even more successful, but whichever plan is specified for a school, evaluation must be an ongoing part of it.

The processes of evaluation are much the same whether they appraise the learner's progress or the success of a lesson, unit, or entire curriculum. The only real difference is *what* is being evaluated and whose values determine the criteria to be applied. Any appraisal technique can yield data that are useful in making a formative evaluation of organized programs of instruction. Indeed, formative evaluation provides the best perspective from which to view instructional programs. Most subject areas have goals and objectives that are not fixed but change over time. Valid summative program evaluation is therefore difficult and maybe too late. Nor is it possible to evaluate a program without considering the skill and interest of the instructor and the characteristics of the student who is being taught.

Parts of the plans made for the curriculum are often specified in formal documents termed ''frameworks'' or ''guides.'' Goodlad's recent study of schooling in the United States (1984) found that those prepared at state or district levels were of minimal effectiveness. However, those curriculum guides developed for the guidance of teachers in specific subjects were quite good. He reports:

Three of our seven states produced subject-oriented guides intended to be helpful not just to local districts, but to individual teachers. Indeed, some of these could be used with very little modification or extra effort, as frameworks for entire courses. However, there were no trends in our data to suggest that teachers in the 18 schools we studied in these three states, more than teachers in the other 20 schools, perceived their curriculum guides as useful. Overall, teachers in our sample viewed state and local curriculum guides as of little or moderate usefulness in guiding their teaching.

Written curriculum plans differ considerably in what is provided to guide the process of instruction. There is wide variation in the specificity of the plans. Some focus on content, others on choices among student activities; some are suggestive (''the teacher might''), while others are prescriptive (''the teacher must''). Guideline questions for describing the kinds of decisions suggested as appropriate for more specific plans such as curriculum guides follow:*

1. Does the plan provide the outline for organization and sequence of the course or curriculum area?
2. How specific is the treatment of subject matter (unit topics, daily topics, specific examples, etc.)?
3. Does the plan include specific activities for students? If so, are the activities described in sufficient detail to suggest what the student is actually to do and the related cognitive process? What is the general emphasis in types of activities described?
4. Does the plan give specific activities or methods for teachers? What is the general emphasis in types of activities?
5. Does the plan specify the materials to be used in instruction? Are there descriptions of what is to be done with the materials?
6. Are there any explicit statements about the nature of learning and the conditions under which it occurs (e.g., statements about motivation, learning environment, maturation and capacity, cognitive processes)?
7. Are there any explicit views on the structure of the subject matter? Are the criteria for selecting and organizing subject matter and materials given?
8. Is there a statement of objectives or desired results of instruction? To what

degree of specificity have these been developed (course, unit, or activity)?
9. What are the suggested purposes for evaluating students? What evaluation methods are recommended? Are the specific procedures given? Is there a proposed schedule for evaluation? What suggestions are provided for the analysis and use of the evaluation?

Payne (1969) adds that two evaluative criteria are essential in appraising curriculum plans: clarity of meaning and internal consistency. An important check on internal consistency is to compare the stated objectives with the learning opportunities and evaluation procedures provided for their implementation. Clarity depends on the care with which these facilitating activities (both for learning and evaluating) have been described. Where this important quality is neglected, it is not possible to judge the validity of any curriculum decisions.

Evaluating teacher effectiveness

Evaluating teacher effectiveness has been the purpose of a vast amount of research (AERA, 1986). No one has yet been able to devise an evaluation scheme that is not plagued with faulty assumptions as well as uncontrolled or uncontrollable sources of error that threaten the reliability of any conclusions that might be drawn from the obtained data. In general, three approaches have been employed. These include: (1) psychometric analysis of the relationship between measures of teacher behavior based on comparisons between pre- and post-test scores on standardized achievement tests, (2) systematic observations of teacher behavior, testing its consistency with specified criteria of acceptable performance; and (3) self-reports obtained by means of structured interviews or questionnaires.

Most state-wide studies of teacher effectiveness are based upon the first of these

---

*From Payne A: The study of curriculum plans, Washington, DC, 1969, National Educational Association.

approaches. Typically, mean scores on standardized achievement tests obtained in individual school districts are compared with their previous scores and also with other districts. Any difference, however slight statistically, is by inference used as irrefutable evidence of the quality of teaching for that year, in that school district. Some monumental assumptions are never admitted, the least of which is the assumption of common curriculums.

Individual teacher performance has tended to be based almost entirely on the observations noted by a busy administrator during a routine, quick visit to a randomly selected class. Any growth in teaching effectiveness has largely depended on a teacher's self-motivated efforts to discover better ways of achieving course objectives.

Currently, however, taxpayer dissatisfaction with the quality of public education has resulted in "back to basics" and accountability demands. And this in turn has sparked increased attention to the quality of education in individual schools and districts, as well as to the specification of criteria defining teacher competencies upon which appropriate inservice development programs can be based. For example, educators in Orange County, Virginia, have replaced annual teacher evaluations with professional growth assessments tied to comprehensive master teaching training programs. Instead of focusing on identifying the 2% of the teaching staff deemed incompetent, full attention is given to the other 98% to improve their instructional effectiveness (Edwards, 1986).

The first step in this process was the identification of 15 performance indicators applicable to all teaching situations and content areas. These were stated in terms specific enough to serve as guides but flexible enough to allow for individual teacher style and creativity. The 15 key teacher behaviors, described as "Procedures for Effective Teaching" (PET) include:*

1. A model of courtesy is exhibited.
2. Positive associations are used with enthusiastic or humorous statements.
3. The teacher circulates among students inviting participation.
4. The teacher mediates or redirects incorrect responses.
5. Students are asked to describe the learning objectives.
6. Concrete examples are used to link learning objectives to prior learnings.
7. Guided practice with teacher-shaped responses is used.
8. The teacher monitors student readiness to proceed to independent practice.
9. Student independent practice without grades is used to determine the success of instruction.
10. Questioning techniques are used to assess fluency and stimulate divergent thinking.
11. Transition strategies for group and class changes are established.
12. Expectations of behavior and routines are explained.
13. The teacher anticipates student behaviors instead of reacting to them.
14. Non-verbal communication techniques are used to encourage appropriate behavior.
15. The teacher makes a statement to the whole group and then directs it to an individual.

Ample time and opportunity for success are provided, in that teachers are given five years and thirty observations in which to demonstrate and assess their proficiency with all the performance indicators. The observations are made by individuals who are themselves classroom teachers. Selection of the teaching skill to be demonstrated, the day, and the class to be visited is up to the teacher to be evaluated. The observers are directed to document only the teaching strengths present during the visit. Subsequent reports of the visit are reviewed by the teacher and observer for completeness and

*Edwards CH Jr.: An effective teaching approach to teacher evaluation and staff development. ERS Spectrum (Arlington VA: Educational Research Service) 4:2, 1986.

accuracy before they are submitted to the school administrator.

A broader study of teacher effectiveness evaluation standards is reported by Johnson and Orso (1986). A survey of evaluation instruments used in large school systems in each of the 50 states was undertaken and 48 systems in 48 states responded. Analysis of these instruments yielded a group of categories of teacher behaviors and criteria for their evaluation that were common to all of them.

Five categories of behavior were identified as follows: (1) instruction, (2) classroom management, (3) professional responsibilities, (4) personal characteristics, and (5) interpersonal relations. Ten criteria are listed relative to the first four of these categories, and five for the last. For the category of instruction the following were criteria commonly specified in all of the instruments studied, along with the percentages of systems that specified them:*

1. Employs a variety of instructional media and instructional techniques (100%).
2. Implements the district's instructional goals and objectives (100%).
3. Provides for attention to individual differences (100%).
4. Evaluates students effectively and fairly on a regular basis (93%).
5. Shows written evidence of preparation for classes (78%).
6. Is knowledgeable of subject matter being taught (76%).
7. Reviews test results with students (53%).
8. Motivates students (53%).
9. Actively involves students in learning (44%).
10. Provides positive reinforcement whenever possible (44%).

Examples of the other criteria for other categories include: for classroom management, "establishes an environment conducive to learning" (100%); for professional responsibilities, "participates in professional development activities such as workshops, courses, other school visits, etc." (80%); for personal characteristics, "uses clear speech" (53%); and for interpersonal relations, "establishes positive relationships with students, parents, and community" (78%). It was concluded that, important as instruction skills are, teachers have difficulty in instructing effectively unless these other categories of teacher behavior are mastered as well.

Probably the most reliable gauge of a teacher's effectiveness is whether or not the instruction has enabled most, if not all, of the students to demonstrate successful achievement of the course objectives. Theoretically, most students can master every educational objective identified by the teacher and students as worthy of achievement. Bloom, Madaus, and Hastings (1981) believe that, for most students, aptitudes are predictive of the *rate* of learning rather than of achievement potential and that, with enough time and appropriate help, the grade of A could be earned by 95% of students. They also suggest that a teacher's effectiveness needs to be evaluated on the basis of the ability to present, explain, and order the elements of the learning task so that mastery is the outcome for all students. Such an outcome may not be acceptable in most schools because many people are conditioned to the system in which the full range of grades, A to F, is expected, and a teacher who rewarded 95% of the students with an A would be regarded with suspicion and disapproval. Nonetheless, it certainly is an ideal toward which teachers should aspire. We will discuss this suggestion further in the section on grading in the following chapter.

The following self-evaluation checklist has been suggested for the elementary teacher's use as criteria for effective teaching of any sub-

*Johnson NC and Orso JK: Téacher evaluation criteria. ERS Spectrum (Arlington, VA: Educational Research Service) 4(3):33-36, 1986.

Checklist for teachers*

Yes   No

____ ____ I encourage students to express different ideas and values.

____ ____ I encourage students to explore their ideas and values.

____ ____ I prepare for the wide range of ideas and values students may express.

____ ____ I select learning opportunities to stimulate student curiosity.

____ ____ I select a wide variety of resources and materials for student use.

____ ____ I support the right of a student to express an idea or value which may not be universally accepted or agreed upon and with which I may not agree.

____ ____ I provide opportunities for students to use and apply the facts and information they gather.

____ ____ In health education, I emphasize the idea of a variety of practices followed by different groups of people.

____ ____ I encourage students to explore and examine a range of ideas and practices.

____ ____ I encourage students to examine the results of taking certain actions regarding health.

____ ____ I am a continuous learner along with the children.

____ ____ I involve children in the process of learning.

____ ____ I am more interested in how children react and behave than I am in how many facts they know as the result of health instruction.

____ ____ I use varied cultural backgrounds and experiences in positive ways as I teach.

____ ____ My instruction is organized around specific objectives.

____ ____ I use some kind of planning system to help me use time more effectively.

____ ____ The methods of teaching I choose focus upon the students and not on myself as the teacher.

____ ____ My health teaching focuses upon the total child, his or her actions, his or her feelings, and the context in which he or she lives, as well as his or her physical well-being.

____ ____ I use characteristics of the children in the teaching-learning process.

____ ____ One of the criteria I use in choosing teaching methods is based on what I hope to accomplish.

____ ____ When children are immersed in the learning process, I observe their reactions.

____ ____ I provide opportunities for students to bring their own experiences into the learning process.

____ ____ I help children clarify their responses to questions rather than declaring them right or wrong.

____ ____ I provide opportunities for children to assume responsibility in accomplishing specific learning opportunities.

____ ____ Children in my class are aware of the actions they are taking in trying to accomplish health objectives.

____ ____ I am aware of the strengths and weaknesses of the children in my class.

____ ____ I know the varied cultural and ethnic backgrounds of the children in my class.

____ ____ I have identified the varied occupations of the childrens' parents.

____ ____ I am aware of the health problems the children may have or may encounter in others.

____ ____ I know the variety of religious backgrounds represented by the children in my class.

____ ____ I vary class organizational patterns for instructional purposes by using individual, small-group, large-group, or other patterns.

____ ____ I involve children in teaching others who may be younger than themselves.

____ ____ I help children feel that they are worthwhile as individuals.

____ ____ I keep up with recent professional literature that will assist me in teaching.

____ ____ The children in my class are aware that I do not know all the answers.

---

*Modified from Nolte, AE, et al: Instructor 81(1):47, 1971.

ject. Obviously, the desired answer in every instance is "Yes."

Evaluating Teaching Materials and Resources

Textbooks. A textbook can be a valuable resource for teaching and learning if it is accurate, up to date, and written at the vocabulary and reading level of the students for whom it is intended. Education in the United States traditionally is so textbook-oriented that everybody—teachers, students, and parents—seems to feel more secure about the quality of instruction if there is a book from which information can be drawn and assignments made. Goodlad (1984) found that, in the classrooms observed across the country, textbooks continue to be the most common medium for teaching and learning. However, since health education is so dynamic a field, even the newest text will be out of date in some respect the very year it is published.

The first step in evaluating a textbook is to check its publication date. If more than 5 years have elapsed since it was copyrighted, it has been at least seven years since it was written. Unless it is entirely concerned with relatively timeless facts, there is likely to be newer information now. For example, physiological facts such as the names of bones or body parts are not likely to change, whereas theories or current information about nutrition or health promotional techniques or practices may have changed considerably. Even when it is new, a textbook can never be regarded as the best or only source of information, but only one among many to be investigated.

The next step is to examine the table of contents to see if the book is over-concerned with human physiology and anatomy or focuses on causes and prevention of diseases and disorders rather than the promotion of a healthful life

style. Does the list of chapter topics approximate the scope of the curriculum framework adopted by the school or district? If the book is to be useful, the content should be compatible both in content and philosophy of health education with accepted best practice.

A continuing problem in every discipline is that some children cannot read at the level expected for their age and grade. In such situations it is possible to secure texts prepared for younger students or specially written for slower readers. One health educator, when transferred to an inner-city school, found that his accustomed use of the textbook as a data source for his students was hindered by the number of non-readers (many of them recent immigrants) in his classes. To solve the problem, he first identified sections of the book that seemed to be the most clearly and simply written, as well as the best suited to his objectives. He tape recorded those sections, speaking as clearly and carefully as he could. Then, as each section of the book was needed to help meet the objec-

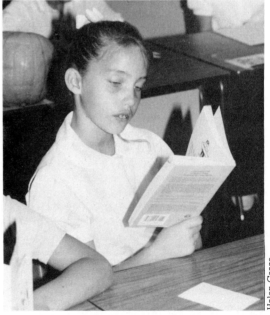

Helen Cease

SAMPLE CRITERIA

A. Suitable material meets all of these criteria

	Yes	No
1. Is appropriate to the course of study	___	___
2. Is a reinforcement of other materials	___	___
3. Is significantly different	___	___
4. Is impartial, factual, and accurate	___	___
5. Is up-to-date	___	___
6. Is non-sectarian, non-partisan, and unbiased	___	___
7. Is free from undesirable propaganda	___	___
8. Is free from excessive or objectionable advertising	___	___
9. Is free or inexpensive and readily available	___	___

B. Pamphlets

	Excellent	Good	Fair	Poor
1. Readability of type	___	___	___	___
2. Appropriateness of illustrations	___	___	___	___
3. Organization of content	___	___	___	___
4. Logical sequence of concepts	___	___	___	___
5. Important aspects of topic stand out	___	___	___	___
6. Material directed to one specific group such as teachers, pupils, or parents	___	___	___	___
7. Reading level appropriate for intended group	___	___	___	___
8. Based on interests and needs of intended group	___	___	___	___
9. Positively directed in words, descriptions, and actions	___	___	___	___
10. Directed toward desirable health practices	___	___	___	___
11. Minimal resort to fear techniques and morbid concepts	___	___	___	___
12. In good taste; avoids vulgarity, stereotypes and ridicule	___	___	___	___
Total rating	___	___	___	___

Adapted from Osborn BM, and Sutton WF: J Sch Health 34(2):72, 1964. Copyright 1964, American School Health Association, Kent, Ohio 44240. Copies of the sample criteria rating scale to evaluate health education materials were distributed throughout Los Angeles County. Additional copies are not available for mailing. Anyone who desires to use this scale is most welcome to reproduce it singly or in quantity through the courtesy of the Tuberculosis and Health Association of Los Angeles County.

Continued.

SAMPLE CRITERIA—cont'd

C. Posters

	Excellent	Good	Fair	Poor
1. Realistic and within experience level of students	___	___	___	___
2. Appeals to interest	___	___	___	___
3. Emphasizes positive behavior and attitudes	___	___	___	___
4. Message clear at a glance	___	___	___	___
5. Little or no conflicting detail	___	___	___	___
6. In good taste	___	___	___	___
7. Attractive and in pleasing colors	___	___	___	___
Total rating	___	___	___	___

D. Recommended for use
1. For use by:
   a. pupils___   b. teachers___   c. parents___   d. adults___
2. Appropriate grade level:
   a. primary___   b. elementary___   c. junior high school___
   d. secondary___   e. college___   f. adult___

E. Not recommended for use
Why not?_____

Date: Evaluated by:

tives, he helped his students follow each word in the text by eye, as the ear heard it. The students were elated by their success in understanding the new material and the language. They were learning to read, learning to listen with comprehension, and learning about health practices at the same time.

Supplementary teaching materials. A wealth of written materials, produced by voluntary health agencies, industrial organizations, public health agencies, and other health-concerned groups is freely available for classroom use. The problem is not how to find enough current pamphlets, booklets, and other supplementary printed matter for health teaching, but how to select the most relevant and appropriate from among them. Often a school or district has an established policy that teachers must follow in choosing materials for use in their classrooms.

Where no clear-cut guidelines exist, the criteria in the preceding box for the evaluation of such printed materials can be applied.

Audio-visual media. Audio-visual media such as films, filmstrips, slides, transparencies, records, and tape recordings should be previewed before use with your students. Factors or qualities that should be noted include the time needed for the effective use of the medium, any advertising copy associated with the material that may be unacceptable for use in the school because of district policy governing commercial promotions, its appropriateness for the particular students (including vocabulary, subject matter, and relevance to the students' present needs and abilities), its relationship and potential contribution to the course objectives, its scientific accuracy, and the key points conveyed or illustrated.

AN ANALYSIS CHECKLIST FOR AUDIOVISUALS WHEN USED AS EDUCATIONAL RESOURCES

Title _____

Distributor _____ Loan/Rental Terms _____

Media Type

____ 35mm Slides   ____ Video Tape   ____ 16mm Film   ____ Film Strip

____ Slide/Tape   ____ Audio Tape   ____ 8mm Film   ____ Other

Evaluation Instructions

Listed below are general criteria to be used in analyzing and rating audiovisuals. Please read each element below each of the four dimensions listed: content, technical production, format, and characterization. Select one of the numbered descriptors that best describes your interpretation of how well each of the elements was used in the production. Place that number in the lined space to the right of each element. A space is provided for listing subtotals of each dimension as well as space for circling the final overall rating. Please note the following example.

Example	**Answer**	**Item code**	
Are the facts and ideas worth stating? . . .	Ex. 3	3 = Excellent	1 = Average
		2 = Good	0 = Poor

Content: (Based upon proposed course or curriculum and the following additional criteria, is significance of content given primary importance?)

1. Are the facts and ideas worth stating? . . . . , . . ____
2. Does the production indicate research practices of high standing? . . . . ____
3. Apparent usage of grammar/spelling . . . . ____
4. Accuracy of content . . . . . . ____
5. Viewer appeal . . . . ____
6. Writing style . . . . ____
7. Does audiovisual elicit or exude undue biases? . . . . . ____
       SUBTOTAL ____

Technical Production (Based upon the following are basic production elements used effectively in the audiovisual production?)

1. Unity . . . . ____
2. Center of Interest . . . . ____
3. Variety . . . . ____
4. Cohesiveness . . . . ____
5. Conflict . . . . ____
6. Climax . . . . ____
7. Resolution of climax(es) . . ____
8. Pace . . . . ____
9. Warmth and Emotion . . . . . ____
10. Establishment of authoritativeness . . . . ____
11. Harmonious blending of all parts of the production? . . ____
       SUBTOTAL ____

Reprinted with permission from *Health Education*, Aug/Sep, 1986, p. 32. *Health Education* is a publication of the American Alliance for Health, Physical Education, Recreation and Dance, 1900 Association Drive, Reston, VA 22091.

Continued.

AN ANALYSIS CHECKLIST FOR AUDIOVISUALS WHEN USED AS EDUCATIONAL RESOURCES—cont'd

Characterization: (Based upon the following criteria what was the overall quality and approach of announcers, cast, or crew?)

1. Voice Quality . . . . ___
2. Fluency . . . . ___
3. Informative . . . . ___
4. Intimacy . . . . ___
5. Creativity . . . . ___
6. Interest . . . . ___
7. Terseness (Concise, avoiding wordiness) . . . . ___
                    SUBTOTAL   ___

Format: (Based upon the intended use of the audio-visual do design elements do what they are set up to do?)

1. Use of special effects . . . . . .   ___
2. Does film create proper mood? . . . .   ___
3. Length of production . . . . . .   ___
4. Volume levels of music, characters, special effects .   ___
5. How do audiovisual materials compare with similar A/V of this type? . . .   ___
                    SUBTOTAL   ___

Overall Rating

Please circle the total number of points which indicates your total overall rating.

Excellent: 75-99+
Good: 50-74
Average: 25-49
Poor: 0-24

SUMMARY

Evaluation is a word used in education to describe what is happening during the process of appraising the worth of the products, procedures, people, and materials involved in schooling. Measurement is the part of that process concerned with gathering specific information quantifying specified aspects of the object of interest. Measurement is often mistaken for evaluation because scores on tests or rating scales are cited as an index of student performance. But a score, however high or low it may be, does not tell us anything about the worth of a performance. It simply reports a measurement. It is status determination.

This does not mean that values are not operating in any way when measurements are designed and applied. Very few measurements are absolute, and even so, only at a given point in time (e.g., age, weight, height). And, the measurement possibilities may be of the either-or kind, but somebody's values influenced the decisions required in designing the instrument, as did those of the people up and down the line who approved its application.

Surveys show that at the elementary level, less emphasis is placed on measurement per se than on evaluation activities. Teachers of children in the primary grades report that observation and interaction are their favored evaluation techniques. Among experienced teachers at the primary level, about two thirds say that they have gained a general feel for their students

PACKAGING

___ ___ Packaging (Is complete, detailed, objective information about the
Yes No program readily available for the purposes of identification, catalog-
         ing, and selection?)

___ ___ Reference Users Guide (Does a reference user's guide accompany
Yes No the audiovisual materials?)

Intended Audience(s): Who is the programming, in general, geared for?

_____ _____ _____

___ ___ Does the audiovisual reach its intended audience?
Yes No

Intended Utilization
___ As integral part of curriculum (Course Requirement) _____
___ As a supplement to regular curriculum (course supplement for whomever is
    interested)
___ For remedial instruction (course supplement for weak students)
___ For advanced study (course enrichment for students with special inter-
    ests)
___ For special project _____
Frequency of utilization per quarter/semester (estimate) _____
Sections of the curriculum _____ Quarter/Semester _____
Comments: (continue on reverse, if necessary) _____
_____
_____
_____
_____

Recommendations:
___ No action   ___ Loan/Rent   ___ Purchase   ___ Revise   ___ Withdraw
                          Reviewer _____
                          Department _____

                          Date _____

Reprinted with permission from *Health Education*, Aug/Sep, 1986, p. 32. *Health Education* is a publication of the American Alliance for Health, Physical Education, Recreation and Dance, 1900 Association Drive, Reston, VA 22091.

abilities within the first week or two, or within the first month to nine weeks (Salmon-Cox, 1981).

What should be remembered is that neither evaluation nor measurement is adequate in describing the quality of a performance or product. Evaluation is not as comprehensive as it must be, without measurement, and measurement cannot be substituted for the insightful observations and interpretations of behaviors that cannot be measured but must be inferred.

For the teacher who must make decisions about lesson planning during the course, and who must assign a letter grade symbolizing the learner's success, it is essential that measurements and observations be frequent, and that the student receive immediate feedback from the results. The younger the child, the more dependence on evaluative observation of behavior and products of learning, and the less dependence on paper and pencil testing. Cryan (1986) has some very nice suggestions. He says that one should evaluate children's behavior first by describing how it fits with what is reasonable to expect. He recommends that you observe, interview, interact, take notes, and write down your goals for their learning. He also recommends that you use your own collected information as the true picture of the child's performance, and measure specific behaviors only when it is necessary to diagnose entering ability or when transitions to more complex material are required. To reduce both your own and the child's anxiety level, he advises keeping the extent of "testing" to an absolute minimum. Finally, Cryan warns against what Goodlad calls "CMD" (Chronic Measurement Disease), preoccupation with pulling up plants to look at them before the roots take hold. He reminds us that learning will develop its roots if the conditions provided for learning and the kinds of learning supported are as important as what is being taught.

QUESTIONS AND EXERCISES

Discussion questions

1. Why is it more difficult to evaluate the effectiveness of health education than of most other school subjects?

2. Differentiate between the purposes of formative and summative evaluation procedures. If you were required to limit your evaluations to one of the two kinds, which would you choose and what would be your reasons for that choice?

3. Some educators are willing to stipulate in advance of instruction that a certain amount of achievement of an objective will be adequate evidence of its success, for example, "By the end of the course, the student will be able to state at least three reasons why cigarette smoking is dangerous to one's health." In this event, is the focus on measurement or evaluation?

4. Can absolute mastery of the objectives defined for health instruction be a reasonable goal if the objectives themselves are in all ways feasible for the students involved? Explain.

5. Knowles (1977), a physician whose pronouncements derogating the value of school health education are often quoted by those wishing to do the same, said that "school health programs are abysmal at best . . ." and, "there are no examinations to determine if anything's been learned." If you were asked to respond to such an accusation by describing what an appropriate evaluation plan should cover, what would you propose? List the procedures you would recommend be adopted, and briefly describe the kinds of things that should be evaluated.

6. What might be some difficulties you would encounter if you were forced to develop an evaluation plan based on objectives stated too ambiguously to provide any guidance, such as, "knows," "understands," "appreciates," etc.? How might you resolve this problem?

7. If you were asked to describe an effective way to appraise the health beliefs of primary school children, what would you recommend, and why? Would your answer be different if the problem involved middle school children? In what way?

8. Should a summative evaluation activity address primarily cognitive outcomes, or should equal emphasis be given to assessment of changes in attitudes or behaviors? What is your rationale for your answer?

9. If a teacher employs a wide range of measurement techniques during a semester course, and determines the course grade on the basis of all of the resulting scores, summarized and weighted carefully, is the final outcome an evaluation or is it measurement?

Exercises

1. For each of the following situations decide whether the action involves measurement or evaluation, and explain why it is so.

a. A principal wishes to select an elementary health textbook series that will provide a comprehensive view of the subject matter, that is up to date, and that fits the increasing level of reading skills and vocabulary expected at successive grades. A teacher committee is asked to analyze three available series and submit their recommendations relative to the best choice among them.

b. A teacher gives a standardized knowledge test as a means of determining the relative background in health information of each individual in the class before instruction, so that plans can be tailored to class needs.

c. As the school year comes to an end, a teacher reviews the complete record of each student, looking at knowledge test scores, quality of participation, growth in problem-solving skills, change in attitudes as revealed by both observation and measurement techniques, and a host of other significant data accumulated during the past year's activities.

d. To demonstrate individual differences in physical growth rates, a teacher determines the height and weight of each sixth-grade student during the first week of school and again during the final week. The change in the two sets of figures is announced and a chart constructed to show comparisons.

2. Select a health-concerned pamphlet, booklet, textbook, or any other material prepared for use in elementary health education teaching. Adapt any of the guidelines proposed in this chapter appropriate for the purpose of evaluating its utility and acceptability. Prepare a brief report of the results of your analysis, and include the set of criteria you applied.

3. Obtain a copy of a recent district curriculum guide prepared for the elementary health instructional program, kindergarten through grade 7. Apply Payne's questions to the analysis of the plan as proposed. How well does it adhere to the criteria implicit in those questions? On a scale of one to ten, how would you rank the document for its adequacy of description? What are its strengths and what are its weaknesses in your view?

4. In association with a classmate, choose an instructional objective listed among those in the guide as the focus of this exercise. Decide, between you, who will develop a learning opportunity that would provide appropriate practice for the objective, and who will design an evaluation strategy that would allow the students to demonstrate mastery of the objective. Each of you must work independently, so that neither knows what the other is planning. When the proposals are finished, study the results together. Would completion of the learning opportunity have prepared the learners to fulfill the requirements of the evaluation activity? Does each plan match the intentions of the objective? What are your conclusions? Have you been measuring or evaluating the outcome of this exercise?

REFERENCES

American Educational Research Association: Handbook of research on teaching, ed 3, 1986, Macmillan (edited by MC Wittrock).

Bloom BS, Madeus GF, and Hastings JT: Evaluation to improve learning, New York, 1981, McGraw-Hill.

Burns R: Objectives and content validity and tests, Educ Technology 8(23):18, 1968.

Carlyon WH: The seven deadly sins of health education. Paper presented at Patient Education at the Primary Care Setting conference, Minneapolis, April 5-6, 1979.

Cryan JR: Evaluation: plague or promise? Childhood Educ 62(5):344-350, 1986.

Education Commission of the States: Recommendations for school health education, Report No 130, Denver, Colo, 1981.

Edwards CH Jr: An effective teaching approach to teacher evaluation and staff development, ERS, Spectrum 4:2, 1986.

Goodlad JI: A place called school, New York, 1984, McGraw-Hill.

Green LW et al: Health education planning: a diagnostic approach, Palo Alto, Calif, 1980, Mayfield.

Hochbaum GM: Behavior change as a goal of health education, Eta Sigma Gamman 13(2):3, 1981.

Hochbaum GM: Certain problems in evaluating health education, Health Values 6(1):14, 1982.

IOX Associates, Evaluation handbooks for health education programs, Culver City, Calif, 1983.

Johnson NC and Orso JK: Teacher evaluation criteria, ERS Spectrum 4(3):33-36, 1986.

Knowles, J. The responsibility of the individual. *Daedalus*, 106 Winter, 1977, pp. 57-80.

Martin E and Stainbrook GL: An analysis checklist for audiovisuals when used as educational resources, Health Educ 17(4):31-33, 1986.

Nelson S: How healthy is your school, New York, 1986, NCHE Press.

Nolte AE et al: Values for your children. Instructor 81(1):47, 1971.

Osborn BM and Sutton WF: Evaluation of health education materials, J Sch Health 34(2):72, 1964 (adapted).

Osgood CE, Suci GJ, and Tannebaum PH: The measurement of meaning, Urbana, Ill, 1957, University of Illinois Press.

Payne A: The study of curriculum plans, Washington, DC, 1969, National Education Association.

Popham WJ: Educational evaluation, Englewood Cliffs, NJ, 1975, Prentice Hall, Inc.

Popham WJ: Modern educational measurement, Englewood Cliffs, NJ, 1981, Prentice Hall.

Salmon-Cox L: Teacher and standardized achievement tests: what's really happening? Phi Delta Kappan 52:9, 1981.

Scriven M: The methodology of evaluation. In Perspectives of Curriculum Evaluation, Chicago, 1967, Rand McNally & Co.

Thygerson AL: Task analysis: determining what should be taught, Health Educ 8(2):8, 1977.

Veenker C Harold: Evaluating health practice and understanding, Health Educ 16(2):80-82, April/May, 1985.

Wolf R: The nature of education evaluation. In Educational evaluation: the state of the field, International J Educ Research 11(1):7-19, 1987.

SUGGESTED READINGS

Iwanicki E and McEachern L: Using teacher self-assessment to identify staff development needs, J Teacher Educ 35(2):36-41, 1984. Thought-provoking and challenging paper. Asserts that relevant staff development needs can best be identified and appropriate services planned by reviewing improvement areas noted by teachers participating in self-assessment activities. Implications of the differences among an individual's open self, secret self, blind self and undiscovered self are explored. Possible self-assessment techniques for collecting information about these 4 aspects of the self, grouped into three basic strategies, (i.e., individual, feedback, and interactive assessments) are listed and discussed.

McKenzie J F. A checklist for evaluating health information, J Sch Health 57:1, 1987. Easy-to-use checklist items providing immediate feedback on the accuracy of consumer health information provided in the media. Structured analysis of the qualifications of the author or institutional source of the information and of the value of the information itself.

Miller D and Davis L: An evaluation of the Beltman traffic safety program for children, Health Educ 15:5 1984. Study of the effects of a multi-media traffic safety teaching kit (Beltman) applied experimentally to 550 kindergarten, first, and second-grade children in 28 classes. Teacher evaluations of the programs were positive and enthusiastic. It was concluded that, combined with parental involvement, the program can affect knowledge of safety significantly, and promote more consistent use of seat belts by children experiencing the program.

Nelson S: How healthy is your school: guidelines for evaluating school health promotion, New York, 1986, NCHE Press, National Center for Health Promotion. A manual prepared under contract with the School Health Initiative of the Office of Disease Prevention and Health Promotion, Department of Health and Human Services. Describes methods, resources, and a basic evaluation framework for systematically identifying, planning, implementing, and assessing school health programs from policy level to practice. Includes a wealth of forms, checklists, inventories, and other instruments for the assessment of school health facilities, services, and curricula, as well as student health knowledge, attitudes, and practices. Invaluable resource for teachers and school administrators.

Results of the School Health Education Evaluation, J Sch Health (entire issue) 55:8, 1985. Collection of 14 articles and 8 evaluative comments from the field regarding the design, methods, and findings of the School Health Education Evaluation, (SHEE) conducted between 1981 and 1984. Includes descriptions of the methods used in the design and implementation of the study, the criteria and procedures involved in the selection of the four curriculums studied (The School Health Curriculum Project; Health Education Guide; Project Prevention; and 3 Rs and High Blood Pressure), and the processes involved in developing an evaluation instrument to be used in the assessment of student outcomes in grades 4 through 7. Results showed that health education works, that it works better when there is more of it, and that it works best when it is supplemented with broad scale administrative and pedagogic support for teacher training, integrated materials, and continuity across grades. The concluding comments from the field are well worth reading for their further insight and suggestions for future investigations.

Shapiro P et al: Student evaluation: a change of focus needed, Educ Canada 26:2, 1986. The concept of accountability has led to overemphasis on summative practices and dependence on standardized tests and final examinations. Evaluation should be viewed as ongoing, not terminal. Rather than being judgmental, as is the case with summative evaluation, the purposes of student evaluation should be formative and developmental if the outcome is expected to fulfill the demands for accountability.

CHAPTER 7

Designing Classroom Tests and Evaluation Activities

When you finish this chapter you should be able to

- **Define the meaning of key measurement terms.**

- **Design a test blue print.**

- **Develop a functional set of test specifications.**

- **Identify ambiguities or other common errors in proposed test items.**

- **Construct an achievement test appropriate for use with a specified age group of elementary children.**

- **Explain ways differing referencing frameworks affect the meaning of course grades.**

Just as evaluation is not limited to measurement, measurement is not limited to testing; yet very probably most people think of *test* as a word that is synonymous with both of those terms. Tests have been used to assess achievement and competence as long as there have been teaching and learning. The most frequent use of educational tests has been to assess the learning status of individual students in order to make instructional and other decisions concerning those students. Predominantly, the tests used as means of determining course grades and endorsing promotion to the next grade are teacher-made. This means that every teacher needs to know how to plan a test, prepare valid test items, and correctly interpret scores resulting from administration of tests. It isn't easy. And it is sometimes an anguishing responsibility. Whether a test is a good and fair assessment of learning or one that is ambiguous, poorly planned, or otherwise inadequate, can result in the difference between a satisfied, motivated learner and one who is frustrated and apathetic about the whole business of schooling.

Elementary teachers need to be just as knowledgeable about test construction as any other teacher. The Goodlad study (1984) found that test taking in early elementary grades accounted for 2.2% of total class time, and that upper elementary grades spent 3.3% of their time in test taking. That may not sound like very much testing activity until you learn that even junior high or middle school students spent 5.5% of class time and senior high school students only a bit more than that (5.8% of class time) in testing.

It is not possible within the purview of a text concerned with health teaching to provide much more than a brief overview of the concepts and skills involved in educational measurement. We hope that if you are not lucky enough to have been provided at least a semes-ter's course work in this important aspect of your teacher preparation program, you will do some independent reading in one of the very good texts available to you, for example, Ebel and Frisbie (1986), *Essentials of Educational Measurement;* Wiersma and Jurs (1985), *Educational Measurement and Testing;* Mehrens and Lehmann (1984), *Measurement and Evaluation in Education and Psychology;* or one of the most enjoyable reads you will ever experience in a textbook, Popham's (1981) *Modern Educational Measurement.*

Because measurement people employ a great many terms not common to other fields of education it seems worthwhile to introduce and explain some of them before we begin. We will limit the definitions to those for reliability, validity, content validity, objectives-referenced, norm-referenced, achievement tests, and standardized tests.

Reliability refers to the extent to which a test is consistent in measuring what it measures, or its stability over time. The longer the test and the more representative the items, the greater its reliability.

Validity refers to the extent to which a test actually measures what it purports to measure, or more precisely, the extent to which interpretation of its measures fits its purported purpose. A test that is not reliable can never be valid, although a test can be reliable without content validity.

Objectives-referenced tests are those used to ascertain the extent to which an individual's score compares with the maximum possible as a measure of the performances proposed by a set of objectives.

Norm-referenced tests are those used to measure a student's performance relative to that of other students taking the same test.

Criterion-referenced tests are those used to measure a student's status in relation to a set of clearly defined behaviors. In contrast to norm-referenced tests that emphasize relative comparisons among those examined, criterion-referenced tests are *absolute* measures, designed to determine, as precisely as possible, what an examinee can or cannot do, without reference to the performances of others (IOX, 1983).

Achievement tests are sets of items or questions representative of the knowledge or skills associated with a given content area or discipline and designed to measure a student's comprehension of that knowledge or competence in those abilities.

Standardized tests are instruments commercially prepared and scrupulously validated by experts in measurement and the subject matter of concern. Such tests are supported by manuals detailing uniform procedures to be followed in administering, scoring, and interpreting the results. Scoring is typically objective and established norms are provided (Mehrens and Lehmann, 1987).

FUNCTIONS OF CLASSROOM TESTS

Ebel and Frisbie (1986) believe that the primary function of teacher-made tests is to provide precise measures of achievement that can be used to report learning progress to students and to their parents. Surely this is true. Scores on a good test do provide a teacher with quantitative evidence on which grades can be defensibly based, and students do want to know what grades they have received. For several years, Middleton was charged with responsibility for teaching health to all of the seventh grade students in a junior high school. This meant that every day she met five or six separate groups—some thirty classes each week. Grades were not a requirement of this staggering work load; merely a "pass" or "fail" notation was called

for. But after a few years, the plan was changed. Students were not happy with just "pass" as recognition of their work, nor were their parents. A passing letter grade communicates much more about the learner's effort and ability than the word "pass," especially when all that "pass" tells you is that the student did not fail. A good grade is a source of pride and pleasure. More than that, as a matter of record, it can be an asset long after school days are over.

Assessment of achievement and awarding of grades should not be limited to analysis of scores on tests, yet alternatives to testing should be used with care and with full realization of their shortcomings. Observations, however specific and objective, have value in assessing achievement, but they are not adequate as replacements for *good* classroom achievement tests. Imperfect as tests may be, they are typically more reliable, objective, and valid than the alternatives tend to be (ratings of classroom performances, evaluation of written work and projects, structured observation of behaviors and attitudes reported in anecdotal records, etc.).

Expectation of testing, particularly among upper elementary and middle school students, prompts review and sharpened attention to important aspects of what has been studied and what is to be covered in the test. Just the experience of *being* tested—working through the questions, and receiving feedback on its results—adds significantly to every student's store of knowledge, whatever the prior level of achievement may have been.

Finally, and not least among the functions of testing, is its influence on and contribution to the quality of planning for the teaching it requires. In order to construct an acceptably valid test you have to think carefully about your goals and objectives *before* you plan either your lessons or your tests. When you know what you want your students to be able to do after your instruction, lesson planning is much easier and test questions simply have to match your objectives.

KINDS OF ACHIEVEMENT TESTS

Ebel and Frisbie (1986) categorize achievement tests broadly, by the type of test-score interpretation they yield, as content-referenced, group-referenced (norm-referenced), or criterion-referenced. Because teachers are typically concerned with their students mastering specific content and skills, content-referenced tests would appear to be appropriate for both student and teacher needs. A content-referenced interpretation is made when the performance level of individuals is compared with an explicit content area, without regard to how other examinees have scored. A special kind of content-referenced interpretation is termed *objectives-referenced*. When the test items adequately correspond to the instructional objectives of interest to the test user, scores can be interpreted in terms of mastery of these objectives. The use of instructional objectives as guides to valid evaluation has already been discussed in Chapter Four. Scores on teacher-made tests, whether interpreted in relation to mastery or not, are usually also ranked in grades.

PLANNING TESTS

Ideally, test construction is based on a set of specifications established as the first step in the total process. Decisions must be made and explicitly set down as guides to the development of the instrument regarding: the kinds of items to be used; the number of items of each kind; the kinds of tasks the items will require; the level and range of item difficulty; the time the test will take for completion; and the

amount of direction that will be necessary. Few of these are mutually exclusive. The decision shaping one aspect of the test is influenced by decisions made about others. For example, the number of items in a test depends somewhat on the amount of time available for its administration. The kinds of items used depends on the maturity and cognitive skills of the examinees. The areas of content chosen for emphasis depend on what has been studied during the period for which the test is being constructed. The level of difficulty (whether the items can be answered correctly by only the better students or by most of the students) depends on whether the purpose of the test is to rank-order the examinees according to their scores, or to determine the number of students whose achievement approaches mastery, and so on.

CONSTRUCTING TEST BLUE PRINTS

Often two-way grids, sometimes called test blue prints, are employed as preliminary plans for test construction. The purpose of the grid is to guide the format of a completed instrument, not to summarize. In a typical grid, the content to be covered is listed at the left in a column, and cognitive behaviors or objectives are listed across the top in a row. For example, the left hand column for a test in health education might list the content areas, with cognitive behaviors such as Bloom's (1956) knowledge, comprehension, application, and perhaps analysis as well, set across the horizontal axis. A content outline has been adapted from an existing health textbook designed for upper elementary school students. Items are assigned to each of the columns and rows as illustrated in Figure 7-1. Notice that the content dimension covers the total scope of health; hence such a test would be summative in purpose. Formative tests would be limited to one or two of the listed

FIG. 7-1

	Number of Test Items for Each Cognitive Level				
	Knowledge	Comprehension	Application	Analysis	Total
Content Areas					
Growth and development	2	2	1	0	5
Consumer and Personal health	3	2	0	1	6
Physical fitness	2	2	2	0	6
Nutrition	3	2	1	0	6
Safety and First aid	2	2	1	0	5
Mental and Social health	2	2	2	1	7
Environmental and Community health	2	1	1	0	4
Diseases	2	2	1	0	5
Drugs	2	3	1	0	6
TOTAL	20	18	10	2	50

content areas; more items would be allocated to each; the test would be shorter; and less time would be needed for its administration and scoring.

A grid of this kind can serve as a guide to the kinds of items needed at a given grade level, and can reveal the balance, or lack of it, among the items planned for each content category. Another technique used in developing test specifications for norm-referenced measures is to list only the content categories along with the number of items intended to be provided for each. The list could similarly be limited to the set of objectives employed in the instruction, and items allocated to measurement of their achievement (Popham, 1981).

In the simplest situation, where instruction has been based on a single textbook designed for a specified grade, the book's section headings may well provide a usable list of topics as outlines of the content. Given that the sections are about equal in the importance given them, items could be constructed on the basis of topics systematically selected from that list.

PREPARING TEST ITEMS

Once the specifications are determined, appropriate items have to be constructed. "Appropriate" is a word often used in this context but less often explained. It stands for the degree to which the tasks implicit in each test item match the content or objective they are supposed to elicit. The decisions made so far only serve as guidelines to the listed aspects of test construction. Still to be decided is which kind of test will be developed, for there are generally only two been made, the items particular to the kind of test chosen must be written. And this is a task fraught with difficulty and pitfalls.

First, what are the kinds of tests between which you can choose? Written tests are usually categorized as either **free response** or **structured response,** sometimes instead as **essay** or **objective,** or as Popham (1981) prefers, as **constructed** versus **selected.** A free-response or constructed item is one that requires examinees to use their own words to respond in writing to a relatively small number of questions. The results are judged more or less subjectively depending on the form. The test requiring the most subjective analysis is the least structured of all, the essay test.

Tests referred to as having structured or selected responses, are those in which the students can only *select* an answer from a limited number of alternatives. They are asked to read all the proposed answers and then to check the one that either is the one correct answer or is the *best* among those offered. The score is obtained by comparing the responses to these kinds of items with a standard key.

Free response tests require recall of information in order to prepare an answer, whereas structured responses appear to depend more on a student's ability to recognize the correct answer among those provided, all of which seem plausible to one who does not have the needed information. When skillfully constructed, both kinds of tests demand recall and reasoning. Whether a given response represents rote recall or reasoning depends on how the student has been taught, not solely on how the question is written. When facts have been the focus of instruction, possession of facts will be the end product, and this limitation is perpetuated by fact-specific questions.

In general, the use of free-response tests is limited in the elementary grades to older children who have learned to read and write well enough to comprehend the questions and construct an answer in their own words. Structured-answer tests can be devised or are available in standardized form for use with nonreaders. Teachers or aides read the questions, and the students point to pictured alternatives or tell the teacher which answer is correct. The television series "Sesame Street" uses this sort of pictured format with great success.

Next, what are the mistakes to be avoided? Choosing between these two categories is relatively easy. So long as the test items are carefully designed, are relevant to the instruction and subject matter, and fit the format, you should be successful in developing a good test unless, in writing the items, you make what Popham (1981, p. 237) terms a "lot of dumb mistakes." Fortunately these are mistakes that can be avoided if you keep them in mind as you write your questions.

1. Unclear or inadequate directions. Don't assume that your students know exactly what you want them to do with each item or even that they know how to do it. Write the directions for answering each kind of item first, not last, and if possible try them out on a few students of the same grade level before you prepare the final copy of your test.

2. Ambiguity. Probably everyone has experienced the frustration that an ambiguous test item causes an examinee. For example, consider this true-false item: "When both parents are working, they often have difficulty with disciplining their children because they are seldom home at the same time." There are two "theys;" does either of them refer to the children, or do both of them refer back to "parents?" How can the respondent tell which meaning is correct? The item writer knows, but the respondent has to be a mind reader.

3. Specific determiners or unintended clues to the right answer. There are several ways that an item can unintentionally point to the right answer or at least delimit those that can be right. Some-

HEALTH KNOWLEDGE PRETEST FOR PRESCHOOLERS

This pictorial multiple-choice instrument has 45 items developed for use with 4-, 5-, and 6-year-old children. Face validity of the test was established through consensus of a ten member panel of experts. Items are based upon objectives inferred from wide review of health curricula and instructional materials appropriate for this age group. The test is group-administered and read to children by a teacher and aides. Each child has a booklet with the items as follows, and a crayon with which to mark the picture selected as the best or correct answer. The teacher reads the words that are provided above each set of pictures in the examiner's booklet.

Mark an X on the picture which shows the health worker who takes your temperature and helps you get ready to see the doctor.

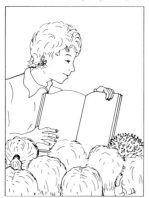 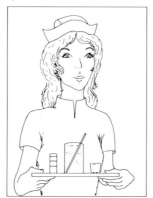 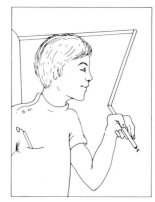

Mark an X on the picture which shows the health worker who you go to see when you are ill (sick).

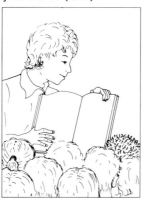 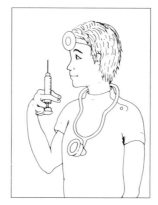 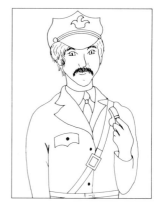

*Further information may be obtained by writing to the test author, Wanda Jubb, at 2867 Greystone Lane, Chamblee, GA 30341.
Reprinted by permission.

Mark an X on the picture which shows where garbage should be kept.

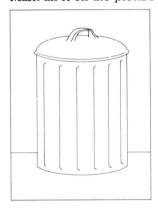 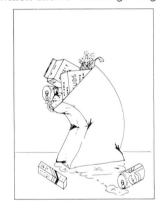 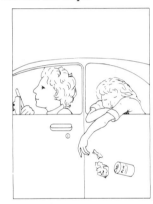

Mark an X on the picture which shows what you should drink to help your teeth grow healthy and strong.

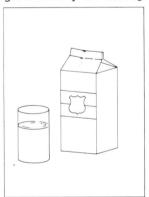 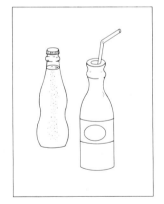 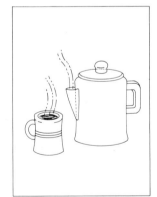

times only some of the distractors in a multiple-choice test fit the stem grammatically; sometimes distractors are irrelevant, illogical, or otherwise impossible, for example: ''Sleep is soundest during the: (a) first two hours; (b) before midnight; (c) after midnight; (d) last two hours; (e) after the first two hours. Only two of these alternatives fit with the last word of the premise, ''the.'' Some words, such as ''always,'' ''never,'' or ''all,'' typically seen in true-false items, are giveaways to experienced test takers who know that very few things are always or never anything. Another clue to the right answer is furnished when one statement is very much longer than the others, in the attempt to make certain that what has been said is absolutely correct.

4. Complicated sentences and unfamiliar vocabulary. Overlong statements may be perceived as clues that they are true, but the situation may simply be that the writer didn't know how to say what he or she wanted to say more succinctly. Overuse of unfamiliar or difficult words also tends to discourage the reader thereby motivating the choice of an answer that is simply a quick guess in order to get past the item and get on with the test. Try this one for example: ''True or False? Qualified physicians such as those specializing in healiocosmopathology have accomplished unusual cures with their methods of treatment.''

Some of these common mistakes are probably more easily avoided than others, but keep all of them in mind as you write each of your test items. The items you develop will vary according to the age and past experience of your students, of course, but because you have been their teacher and know what they have studied and can do, you will be better qualified than anyone else to write items that will be right for them.

Teacher-made tests and the kinds of items of which they are composed are nothing new to anyone who has attended school in this country. But this time you must approach testing from the other side of the desk. Therefore, review of the most often used kinds of teacher-made tests follows.

Free-Response Tests

Free-response tests are composed of essay and short-answer or completion kinds of items. *Essay* tests take much less time to prepare than do objective tests, but they require a great deal of time to score. Moreover, good essay questions are not all that easily written. They must ask the student to exhibit the cognitive skill or process that was stipulated in the objectives. If the behavior was ''explain,'' the question has to require explaining, not listing, comparing, describing, or any other behavior. The question has to be written in such a way that it cannot be answered by filling in memorized sections of the material provided in the textbook. Instead it must require application of what has been studied in a different context than as considered during the learning opportunities.

A poorly or carelessly constructed essay item is more likely to measure a student's ability to figure out what it means than her or his knowledge about the subject matter. An item such as, ''Discuss the importance of various locations of accidents,'' is not only impossibly global, but baffling as well. Does it mean that the respondent should itemize locations and describe their importance as factors in the incidence of accidents? What does ''importance'' mean? Should locations be ranked according to the probability of an accident occurring there? What is meant by ''discuss?'' How many is ''various?'' Is there a location where an accident could *not* occur? This item, taken from a teacher's manual for a health textbook, is so ambiguous that suggestions for its improvement are limited to tossing it out. A good way to ensure that every student will perceive the task similarly is to pose a problem situation and then ask a series of questions based on that situation. For example:

Accidents claim more lives of school children than all other causes of death combined. Explain how each of the following serves to prevent an accident: (1) traffic lights and reflectors, (4) safety rules, (5) fire drills, and (6) crossing guards.

An essay item structured in this way is more easily scored because the possibility of misunderstanding the question is minimized and the range of possible answers is delimited. Still, the student is given freedom in composing answers, and the requirement that knowledge about these factors be applied to the explanation of accident prevention among peers makes it meaningful and relevant to their own needs and interests.

Examples of other simply but clearly posed essay items are the following:

How a person grows and develops is influenced by two important factors: heredity (determined by the genes we receive from our parents) and the environment (physical, social, mental, and emotional) in which we live. Write a short paragraph that describes some important traits that make you different from other people but that can only be the result of your environment.

For each of the following foods, (1) name an acceptable substitute food that could supply the same nutrient, and (2) give at least two reasons why this kind of food is essential to a balanced diet: (a) whole milk; (b) meat; (c) oranges; (d) bread; and (e) spinach.

Essay tests are difficult to score and require a lot of time to do it. Moreover, the obtained scores are notoriously unreliable. Many biasing factors, some of them entirely unrelated to the quality of the answers, influence the judgment process. Some of these include whether a paper is read before or after a poor or excellent one; whether the handwriting is legible, the spelling correct, and the paper neat; how tired the teacher is when reading the papers; how the student perceived the meaning of the questions compared with the teacher's intention; how well designed and comprehensive the directions are; and what the teacher already knows about the student's past performances and personality. Some students are so good with words, and even with redirecting the discussion toward a related topic about which they know more that the reader is lulled into believing that the assigned topic has been addressed.

Teachers often vary in their evaluation of the same paper at different times. Astonishingly, research shows that the same paper can be awarded every grade from A to F depending on who reads it. And, in addition to its being laborious and time consuming to read a great number of essay papers, so few questions can be asked that the resulting sample of a student's achievement may not adequately represent his or her grasp of the material or the course. Given other essay questions, a student who has done poorly might have done very well, and vice versa.

The advantages of essay questions are that they give students an opportunity to show ability to analyze a problem and prepare a solution in their own words and at their own pace. Some students do not perform well when under pressure to read and answer a long list of questions, nor do they like to be restricted to a few prepared responses in choosing an answer.

Scoring is more likely to be consistent when a set of criteria for evaluating the answers can be predetermined. Papers should be read without knowing who has written them so that any subjective set toward their authors can be avoided. The answers to each item should all be read at the same time, and evaluated and scored relative to the performance of every examinee on that question. In this way a student gets credit for the quality of the answer to each question, rather than one score arrived at on the basis of some generalized accomplishment index based on a quick reading of all of the items at once.

Another technique is to skim all the papers quickly, sorting them roughly into piles labelled *excellent, good, fair,* and *weak,* or something similar. Next, each paper is carefully reread, with shifts made between the preliminary assignments to higher or lower ratings as seems more appropriate. Each paper is thus judged along with others that are similar in quality to see if it belongs in that category or if it should be rated higher or lower.

The evaluation of essay papers is even more complex when students are allowed to select from a list of alternative questions. In effect, each student has taken a different test. In addition, since it cannot be demonstrated that essay items are equally representative of the same amount and kind of learning, what happens is that not only different tests but different kinds of tests may have been assembled as a consequence of the choices. Certainly, there being fewer answers to any one of the items, there is less possibility of making valid comparisons among the few.

Short answer and completion tests are a more restricted form of the free-response test and may be better suited and easier for children whose writing skills are limited or not yet developed. Such an instrument can be duplicated and distributed to each child, or read aloud by the teacher for the entire class. In the same way, answers can be written by the individual students or agreed to in discussions by the total group. Short answer tests are composed of specific questions that can be answered with one word or a very short statement, for example:

Meat and nuts are foods representing which class of nutrients? _____
What most often causes tooth decay? _____

A direct question is better for short answer items than an incomplete statement, especially when used with young children, because they are used to that format. In addition, it forces the teacher to prepare items that have one and only one right answer. Incomplete sentences invite ambiguity because the author, knowing the word wanted, assumes that everyone else will think of that word and no other. In actuality, there may be several alternative words that would finish the statement just as logically, even if differently.

Completion items are similar to short answer questions but usually are written as incomplete sentences rather than as questions, for example:

Pathogens (germs) that cause diseases such as colds, measles, and flu are called _____.
Blood vessels that carry the blood away from the heart are termed _____.

The blank should be placed at the end of the statement, otherwise the student may have forgotten what was wanted by the time the entire statement has been read. Limit the blanks to one or at most two in any one item. Make the blank long enough to permit the word to be written legibly, and as nearly as possible equal in length to the others. When one blank space is noticeably different, it provides a clue to the expected answer.

The advantages of the short-answer and completion tests are that they can be more easily and quickly scored, and a great many more questions can be asked than is the case with essay questions thus providing a better sample of a student's knowledge and comprehension.

The learners still have to produce their own answers, and must recall the information needed to do so. Because these kinds of items must be so specific, they are best used in testing factual material such as dates, definitions, and terminology and are not useful in appraising problem-solving skills.

How accurate the answers to these kinds of free-response items can be depends on the way they are written. Teachers sometimes unwittingly reward rote recall and penalize creative thinking when only one answer is accepted—the one that uses the words from the text. An example of this is, "There are more than _____ bones in the human skeleton." The answer wanted is 200, but actually *any* number less than 200 would be correct. Some other weaknesses to guard against in constructing items include overemphasis on trivial information, for example, "Your hair grows about _____ inches a month," or "The current population of the world is in excess of _____," or calling for inconsequential words such as, "The first teeth to _____ are called baby, or primary teeth." Another pitfall is that the desired answer may be factually incorrect, as in "Good dental health is ensured when we visit our dentist _____ times a year." Good dental health cannot be ensured by *any* means, and, although biannual visits generally are recommended, people vary in their needs, and unexpected problems often occur.

No item should omit so much that it is incomprehensible as a statement, for example, "Most microbes can be killed by _____, by _____, and by _____." Without the missing words "sunlight, dryness, and very high temperatures," the item is a guessing game, not a test of knowledge.

Short answer tests should not be scored solely by comparison with a prepared key. Keys need to be supplemented with a qualified scorer's ability to judge whether a different answer is equally appropriate and correct.

Structured Response Tests.

Tests that require the student to choose among already prepared alternative answers to questions are usually termed *objective*, although actually only the scoring procedures are objective. Subjective judgment is always involved in devising the questions, and it influences the selection of the material for which it is considered important to test, as well as the choice of the right answer. The most commonly used objectively scored tests are the binary-choice (so called because they offer only two choices) such as true-false, right-wrong, yes-no, agree-disagree, etc., multiple choice, and matching item tests.

True-false tests. The true-false test item is simply a statement that the student reads and judges to be one or the other. It might be described as a two-response multiple-choice item, although the opposing statement (that the statement is or is not true) is unstated. Such an item can be written in a slightly different form so that the correct answer is yes or no, right or wrong, agree or disagree.

Another variation is to require the student to explain *why* an item is false, or to correct any item that has been judged false in part or entirely. This is supposed to minimize the effect of guessing but it costs a great deal of teacher time in order to evaluate the correctness of the explanation, and in effect changes the test from structured to a combination structured and free-response style.

True-false items are those most often chosen by teachers for their tests and quizzes. They appear to be easy to write but actually the creation of concise, unambiguous items that are unmistakably and unarguably either true or false is not easy at all. Critics of the true-false

---

ITEM-WRITING TIPS OR GUIDELINES

1. Keep the word length of all items as even and short as possible.
2. Select statements that are representative of important ideas or generalizations.
3. Make certain that each item is true or false beyond question.
4. Construct about the same number of binary response items of either kind.
5. Write statements as clearly, concisely, and simply as possible.
6. Paraphrase rather than copy statements verbatim from the book.
7. Do not use a negative as means of altering statements. If the negative is essential to a true statement, underline or capitalize the word, and <u>never</u> use double negatives.
8. Don't try to trick the examinee into giving a wrong answer.

---

format hold that, with only two alternative answers, anybody can get 50 percent of the items right without knowing anything at all about the subject matter. This is true only if you have but one item to answer. The longer the test, the less the possibility that guessing has much effect. For example, it has been shown that chances are only 2 in 100 that a person who has guessed blindly on a 15 item test will get 80% or more of them correct. On a 25 item test, there are only 2 chances in 1000 of getting 80% or more correct by blind guessing, and the odds drop to 3 in 100,000,000 of getting all 25 right (Nitko, 1983). Don't forget that if there is a 50% chance of getting an item right by chance, there is also a 50% chance of getting it wrong.

Ebel has long championed the use of true-false tests as means of measuring a wide variety of meaningful propositions far beyond trivial or single fact-related information. The rationale for this belief is summarized in the four statements that follow:

1. The essence of educational achievement is the command of useful verbal knowledge.
2. All verbal knowledge can be expressed in propositions.
3. A proposition is any sentence that can be said to be true or false.

4. The extent of students' command of a particular area of knowledge is indicated by their success in judging the truth or falsity of propositions related to it (Ebel, 1979, and Ebel and Frisbie, 1986).

He held that if true-false items are held in low esteem, it is not because the binary-choice format is inherently limited to assessment of trivial information. Rather it is because the form is so often used ineptly by unskilled item writers.

There are the usual pitfalls into which the careless or inexperienced writer can fall. Often statements from the textbook are copied as is or doctored with a negative word to make them false; yet it cannot be assumed that every statement in the book is true. And even if true, such statements, taken out of context, may not be able to stand alone, as they must to be good true-false items. Also, this places too much emphasis on memorization, and the items picked in this way tend to focus on trivia. Words such as *always, never, all,* and *always* are often employed to make an item false, and students quickly learn to mark any statements with one of those words as false when they are guessing. They may also be tricked into marking a statement false when it is true for the same reason, because sometimes ''never,'' ''always,'' or ''all'' is correct. Another tip-off for the test-wise is the wordiness that sometimes accompanies true statements as the writer attempts to make them definitively so. If these kinds of items are frequent, test scores are more likely to reveal which students are practiced test takers than which of them are better prepared and more knowledgeable.

Another dubious practice is to use phrases like "the best way to," "the chief reason for," or "the best method of," which forces the student to make a judgment when the alternatives are unknown. The student has to ask, "the best way compared to what?" The most aggravating fault, from the students' point of view, is the attempt to trick them into missing the item, as in, "Walter Reed is the physician credited with the discovery that malaria is transmitted by mosquitos." The disease with which his name is associated is not malaria, but yellow fever. Even the student who knows that, may miss it in the pressure to read and react to a long list of true-false statements.

The purpose of a test is to find out how much the student knows; it is not a contest to find out whether a clever use of words can trick students into making a mistake.

Ambiguity is a frequent fault in item writing. For example, look at this statement: "The best way to help a drowning man is to jump into the water and save him." Certainly saving a drowning person is the best way to help him, but the student must weigh that part against the part about jumping into the water, which may or may not be helpful to either the victim or the would-be rescuer. Another foolish ploy is to make the correct answer depend on knowledge about some unessential word, as in the statement, "The cochlea is a part of the inner ear." This item does not test anything other than knowledge about the anatomy of the ear; to answer, the student has to possess knowledge about the cochlea, which has little to do with

health behavior or knowledge except in a trivial way.

These are some of the weaknesses in test construction to keep in mind when writing true-false items or any structured test problems. Actually the distractors in a multiple-choice or matching-item test are simply a cluster of true-false items related to the same premise or stem. It follows that each distractor in a multiple-choice test must be written with attention to the same guidelines as in the case of the true-false item.

As in the case of any test, true-false tests can be read to young children, whose responses are verbal or recorded by simple marks such as plus or minus signs. The distinguishing characteristic of true-false statements designed for young children is the simplicity of the language and concepts with which they are asked to deal.

Multiple-choice tests. A multiple-choice item consists of an incomplete statement or question called the **stem** and, at the elementary level, usually no more than three or four alternatives from which the student is directed to choose either the correct or best answer that fits the stem. When incomplete statements are used, the responses (called **distractors**) are written so that they fit into and complete the sentence, for example, "If you are nearsighted, you can see objects near you (1) better than those far away; (2) less clearly than those far away; (3) as well as those far away." Or, an item can ask the student to indicate the best of several proposed answers, for example, "What is the best time to brush your teeth in the morning? (1) as soon as you get up, (2) while you are bathing and dressing, (3) after you have eaten your breakfast."

An advantage of the multiple-choice item is that the desired choice does not have to be the one answer deemed true, although it does have to be defensibly best among the alternatives provided. It can be constructed to call for problem-solving skills such as interpretation, analysis, application, and other cognitive processes, as well as simple recall of information. Construction of this type of test is perhaps the most time consuming. In a very real sense, each item represents three or four questions, depending on the number of distractors. A 50-item multiple-choice test is the equivalent of a 200 item true-false test when there are four distractors. As a result, since there are more questions, the potential reliability of the test is increased. Of course, reading time is also increased, which can lead the student to make errors even though she or he may have known the answer, because when the *best* answer is the correct answer, the student often chooses the first good answer without reading all of them. This problem can be dealt with most effectively by carefully constructing the instructions that precede multiple-choice items.

The most challenging task is to write three or four distractors that are so plausible that only an individual who really knows the answer can choose among them with confidence. A distractor so unreasonable as an answer that no one chooses it is termed "non-functioning." In the following example, which distractor would you predict would seldom if ever be chosen? "Between 1975 and 1985, air pollution in major cities in the United States (1) was largely caused by automobile exhaust; (2) was the cause of 1 million deaths per year; (3) decreased; (4) increased in some places and decreased in others."

You must be careful to prepare distracters that sound logical, are similar in nature, and either complete a partial statement or answer a stated question. The stem must include enough of an incomplete statement (and all of a question) so that the alternatives that are to complete it or answer it are readably short, and about the same length. An example of a typical-ly inadequate stem is, "Aspirin is (1) harmless, (2) addictive, (3) harmful, (4) rarely overused." The stem is inadequate because it does not tell the examinee anything about the problem. As a consequence it is nothing other than a cluster of four true-false questions, each of which begins with the words "aspirin is." A better question might be, "The most likely effect of heavy overuse of aspirin would be (1) stomach ulcer and bleeding; (2) physical addiction; (3) tolerance, or the need to take more of the drug each time; (4) severe skin rash or loss of hair."

Frequently you will see options consisting only of "all of the above," "none of the above," or "A and B only." These may be alternatives worth the student's consideration, or they may simply be evidence of the difficulty involved in writing four good distractors. When "none of the above" is the right answer to such an item, and the student picks it, what has been revealed is that the individual knew that the others were wrong, but not whether he or she knew the correct answer, which leaves the teacher nowhere as far as knowing the status of student learning is concerned.

Another way to design the response pattern for a multiple-choice test is to develop distractors, all of which are correct but one. The examinee is to pick out the one that is wrong. This system potentially provides the teacher with a lot more feedback on the student's fund of knowledge. Can you see why?

A variation of the multiple-choice test is a combination of its usual form with a matching test. The same three or four alternatives are used in connection with a longer list of related items, for example:

Directions: Beside each of the substances in the following list, place the letter from the key that matches the nutrient it represents. You may use any item more than once.

Key: A—Vitamin, B—Protein, C—Carbohydrate, D—Mineral

Substances

1. Calcium   ____
2. Meat   ____
3. Niacin   ____
4. Sugar   ____
5. Milk   ____
6. Iron   ____
7. Thiamine   ____
8. Gelatin   ____

Matching-item tests. In another variation of a multiple-choice test, for each item in a list of terms, topics, or other elements, a word is chosen from another list that describes, defines, or somehow relates to it. Usually a list of terms is placed to the left and the list of alternatives to the right. The list of alternatives should be longer than the other so there is no automatic answer to the last item. For young children the second list should not be longer than five or six items, so the search for the matching answer each time is not complicated or long. For the student to quickly grasp the relationship of the items to the alternatives, all the elements in the first column should have some clear connection, rather than being an assortment of unrelated terms or objects. Finally, the directions should clearly explain the task. The following is an example of this type of test item.

Directions: Beside each item in column I place the number that is given for its function in column II.

I Organ	II Function
____ Heart	1. Excretion
____ Brain	2. Movement
____ Lungs	3. Structure
____ Skeleton	4. Digestion
____ Muscles	5. Circulation
____ Kidneys	6. Reproduction
____ Skin	7. Coordination
____ Stomach	8. Respiration
	9. Perspiration

Directions can be varied to say, "Draw a line connecting each item in column I with its function listed in column II." For the primary grades, matching tests can be developed in the form of pictures, real objects, or models. In the simplest form one item represents column I and three pictures or real objects are used in place of column II.

"Sesame Street" uses this technique in reverse with its singing game, "One of these things is not like the others," in which four or five pictures are shown, and the children try to discover which one is unrelated to the others. What they are doing is classifying, which is basic to conceptualizing. Matching tests are best used to measure growth in knowledge of factual information and of important terminology.

STANDARDIZED TESTS

Standardized tests are those whose validity and reliability have been determined by means of rigorous statistical and other procedures, and for which norms have been established (Mehrens and Lehmann, 1987). Norm-referenced tests are, by definition, a means of comparing one student's performance with that of others of the same age group or grade. The advantage of using standardized tests is that, used correctly, they are presumed to be valid, and can tell you how your students compare with others who have taken the test. A disadvantage is that the test may not be appropriate for your needs. It may not match the objectives that structured your teaching. Another problem is that any one test can only sample the entire domain of achievement items that might have been asked of your students. Consequently, any conclusions based on the resulting scores are likely to depend on too little information. For example, administration of one standardized test of health knowledge showed that nutrition was the content area in which students appeared to be weakest. This judgment was based on the fact that more people missed nutrition questions than those in any other of the areas tested. Still, since there were only five questions concerning nutrition, the possibility exists that five different questions might have yielded quite different results. The longer the test of any particular subject or sub-topic thereof, the more reliable and valid it will be.

How useful standardized test scores are to elementary teachers is debatable. Perhaps the question should be, what use do elementary teachers make of the information they receive as an outcome of standardized testing?

Salmon-Cox (1981) studied a group of 68 elementary school teachers in urban and suburban school districts who administered and received information from a published, standardized test of student achievement. She found that about half of them used the information only as a supplement to or in confirmation of what they already knew about their students through interaction with them, observation of classroom performance, and application of teacher-made tests. Generally, the teachers had more confidence in their own measurements and judgments than in standardized test scores when the results of the two appeared to be divergent. All of them believed that no single source of information about student achievement could be dependably employed as a summative assessment, especially not a standardized test.

EVALUATING TESTS

Textbooks on measurement provide many more suggestions for constructing good tests than can be discussed here. Remember that no test is so good that it does not need continual evaluation and revision to keep it up to date and as valid as possible. A practical way to do this is to study the results of every administration. If time is taken to tabulate the scores and responses to a multiple-choice test, analysis quickly reveals which distracters are not functioning. Let the children take part in this activity. Hand back the papers and have them, with a show of hands, tell you how many got each item right, and even how many picked each of the distracters. Any alternative not chosen by at least 3% of the class is not functioning and needs to be replaced. Another valuable source of information is a survey of the missed items. Which ones were missed by most of the respondents? Were those who missed a question the students whose test scores were highest or those whose scores were low? Which wrong distracters were selected most frequently as the correct answer? The answers to these questions tell the teacher a great deal about the item itself, and about the students' knowledge or lack of it regarding that item.

An instrument that has evolved and been improved as an outcome of this kind of scrutiny can be used with some confidence as a pretest, and can provide guidance to the development of lessons appropriate to the special needs of the students in a given class. And it can be used as a summative test to demonstrate the amount of change that has taken place as a consequence of the instruction. Don't forget, however, that a student who has done well on a pretest cannot show as much improvement as one who has missed most of the questions earlier. As a matter of fact, if a great many people do very well on a pretest administration of an instrument, it is too easy and should tell you that you are planning to teach what your students already know. This is a good thing to find out *before* you plan your semester's work. But, it means that a new test will have to be devised to match the changes you wish to make in your teaching plans.

EVALUATION ACTIVITIES

Measurement of the achievement of students should not be restricted to pencil and paper instruments, however valid and well designed they may be. Written tests have their special uses, but hypothetical situations requiring practical application of what has been learned are uniquely suited to health education, especially when comprehension, problem solving, and decision making have been the goals of instruction. In a sense, such evaluative means as these are criterion-referenced, in that students are required to show that they can or cannot demonstrate competence.

For example, in testing for comprehension, assume that the objective is that the student will be able to "Identify factors that contribute to the abuse of drugs." One way to evaluate that competence would be to divide the class into small groups of two or three. Then distribute cards, each of which lists one of the factors that have been identified in preceding lessons. Ask each group to plan a dramatization of their factor in operation. When the resulting skits are presented to the total class, they should be able to easily identify which factor is being shown. If the presenting group cannot do that, or the class cannot recognize what they are illustrating, you will know which factors need further study and how many students need more instruction. Another way to evaluate achievement of this objective is to develop a series of short stories about drug abuse or misuse and ask the children to suggest what the causative factor could have been in each case. The answers may vary because the factors involved in drug use problems are rarely one-dimensional. What is important is that the suggested causes are possible and relevant.

Comprehension of the key idea related to an

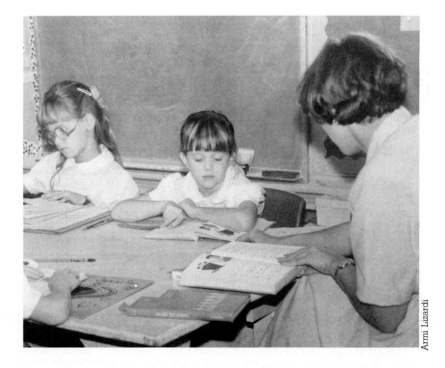

Armi Lizardi

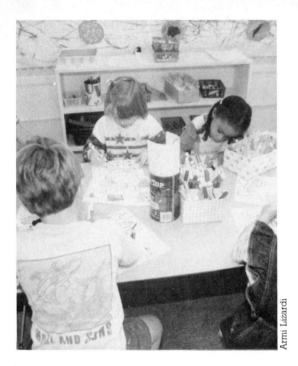

Armi Lizardi

objective such as, "Describes ways children resemble their parents," could be measured by asking each child to draw a picture that illustrates some ways in which a child resembles his or her parents. The special features illustrated can be labeled or highlighted by some means, and the pictures need not be restricted to humans. You will be able to see at once whether the concept of heredity has been understood.

Success in motivating understanding of the often trivial reasons why people begin to smoke and the forces that keep them smoking despite the publicity given the very real ill effects of the habit could be appraised by asking students to write a letter to a friend who has not yet thought of smoking. In the letter, they would be asked to tell that person why the decision not to begin smoking should be one that every young person ought to make.

Problem-solving ability can be appraised in many ways. Present the children with a health-related problem that elicits demonstration of competence in dealing with it. The examinee must either have the knowledge needed, or know how to find it, and know how to apply it in thinking about and working out a good solution. For example, if the objective specified that a student should be able to infer relationships between malnutrition and the growth and development of children, a description of a diet poor in protein and other nutrients can be presented. The task is to analyze that diet and predict what its effect would be on the development and well-being of children with no other foods to eat. Another approach to the same objective would be to describe a child with an existing nutrition-related health problem, and ask the students to suggest or infer which of the essential nutrients are probably lacking in the individual's diet and propose solutions to the problem that could be effected by the addition of specified nutrients to the daily diet.

Decision-making ability can be measured in many other ways, for example, if your objective is to have the students develop practical criteria to be applied to the selection of any health-affecting products, set up an exhibit of eight to ten kinds of toothpaste, soap, painkillers, shampoos, etc. (actual samples or empty packages of such products may be used), and ask the students to indicate which ones, if any, they would choose from each category, and to name the criteria they applied in making that decision.

Role playing can be used as effectively in an evaluation activity as in a learning opportunity. Health problems can be presented to small groups, who are to work out the solutions and then dramatize both the problem and the solution. The criterion of their success could be the ease with which their fellow students are able to recognize the problem being presented and to agree that the solution is a good one.

Any learning opportunity with which you are comfortable, or that you might see described in a guide or text, can be adapted for use as an evaluation activity. All you have to do is assume that the students have already learned what the learning opportunity purports to teach. This usually means that the information and skills needed to carry it out have been learned elsewhere or at another time. In fact, the majority of "learning opportunities" as written are based on the unstated assumption that the students already know what they need to know in order to carry them out.

EVALUATION OF AFFECTIVE OBJECTIVES

Health education objectives that specifically address the affective domain and are concerned with the development of positive health attitudes and values need to have matching evaluation activities, just as do cognitive objectives. Tyler (1973) suggests ways that this can be done. He says:

The definition of a value as an object, activity, or idea that is cherished by the individual which derives its educational significance from its role in directing his interests, attitudes, and satisfactions implies that an assessment should furnish opportunity for the students to make choices that can be perceived as connected to particular values. . . . Hence, the testing situation appears to require opportunities for choices, and for the student to state why he made those choices. . .

Perhaps the most direct evidence is obtained in group discussions, or informal interviews in which the choices are examined in various ways, and different alternatives are proposed. The feeling of the individual can be inferred from his voice, the content of his comments, and the persistence of the same choice in spite of questions regarding other alternatives. With good rapport, the student's report of how he feels about the choice is likely to be sincere.

Attitudes and cognitive changes often can be assessed simultaneously by means of evaluation activities. For example, student-created posters, pictures, and other artifacts reveal far more than knowledge, since they reflect attitudes and feelings about the worth and meaning of what is depicted. Behavioral choices reflect changes in attitudes, too. Once students have completed related learning opportunities, do they volunteer to participate in health-concerned community programs? Do they use seat belts without being reminded? Do they urge their parents and friends to do so? Do they often bring newspaper clippings to class that illustrate some of the health problems or issues that have been discussed? All these actions are indicative of success in the affective as well as the cognitive domains; yet these changes are more powerfully revealed unintentionally by means of evaluation activities than by scores on objectively scored tests.

Evaluation activities chosen for their relevance to actual health problems that students of any particular age group face every day or are concerned about, bring health education and health behavior to life. Reading about health in a book, and hearing about it from a teacher or visiting speaker is one thing, but using what one has learned as a consequence can be exciting and deeply satisfying even to young children. They discover that what they have learned works! On top of that, demonstrating competence in coping with a real health problem is a lot more fun than checking the right answer on a piece of paper.

GRADE, GRADING, AND GRADES

In the United States, the word *grade* is used in various ways in speaking about schools and school work. One sort of grade is a division or segment of schooling, representing a year's work. Most college students have completed thirteen of them—kindergarten and twelve more. *Grades* usually refers to test scores, or the marks given to completed assignments, such as written reports or projects. Grades of this kind are of a formative nature, and cumulatively serve as an important source of judgments about a student's overall performance and ability. Final grades are summative and become a part of a student's record, and form the primary basis of the decision to promote a student to the next grade. *Grading* has to do with ranking, is done by the classroom teacher, and reflects that person's judgment of a youngster's achievement as it relates to his or her capabilities.

The meaning of any grade given a student depends on the referencing framework within which it has been assigned. Commonly there are three of these: first, task-referenced or criterion-referenced, which is based on absolute standards of achievement; second, group or norm-referenced, which is based on relative standards in that the student's grade reflects her or his ranking compared with every one else in the group or class; and third, self-referenced, which reflects a comparison between a pupil's performance and the teacher's perception of that individual's capability (Nitko, 1983, p. 344).

Elementary school grading is more comprehensive in scope than grading at the secondary school level. Judgments are not limited to a single letter grade or percentage figure as a summation of a semester's work. Instead, elementary teachers are required to indicate a wide range of judgments based on observations of the child's social and personal development, study habits and attitudes, as well as her or his cognitive progress and achievements.

The responsibility of a teacher at every level of education is to take care that course grades indicate a student's competence relative to the instructional objectives that have structured the work. Only behaviors that reflect academic achievement should be used to determine grades. Grades must never serve as tools of discipline, or as rewards for pleasant personalities, good attitudes, or skillful apple-polishing.

To exclude such things as obvious effort and level of motivation, writing and speaking skills, and personality in making judgments about a student's academic progress is not an easy thing to do, yet accurate and meaningful grades depend on it.

The following was published more than twenty years ago but it is as meaningful today as then, and ought to be required reading for every teacher, every time grades are due.

Teachers should not be in a position merely to declare that students are improving or not improving. They ought to contrive situations in which they will be trying to find out whether improvement occurs and how much. In other words, they should approach the task of evaluation not with the arrogance of a judge, but with the humility of an enquirer. The proper frame of mind for evaluation is fear and trembling. Then, if everything turns out all right, the relief of the teachers should be even more stupendous than that of the students! (Diederich, 1964)

SUMMARY

Elementary teachers need to be as knowledgeable about test construction as those at any other level of education. Admittedly, the more advanced the grade, the more paper and pencil tests are employed in assessing classroom achievement. But objective tests can be and commonly are constructed and administered effectively at every grade, even pre-school (Jubb, 1983). The complexity of the items and the difficulty of the concepts being explored varies according to the age group concerned, but the principles of test construction stay the same.

UNIFIED SCHOOL DISTRICT – Kindergarten Progress Report, 19 ___ – _____ School Year

Pupil's Name: _____

Check ✓ or deletion (———) = Positive observation

READING READINESS

Recognizes capital letters:
Eval. 1 – A B C D E F G H I J K L M N O P Q R S T U V W X Y Z
Eval. 2 – A B C D E F G H I J K L M N O P Q R S T U V W X Y Z
Eval. 3 – A B C D E F G H I J K L M N O P Q R S T U V W X Y Z

Recognizes lower case letters:
Eval. 1 – a b c d e f g h i j k l m n o p q r s t u v w x y z
Eval. 2 – a b c d e f g h i j k l m n o p q r s t u v w x y z
Eval. 3 – a b c d e f g h i j k l m n o p q r s t u v w x y z

Associates consonant letters and sounds:
Eval. 1 – b c d f g h j k l m n p q r s t v w y z
Eval. 2 – b c d f g h j k l m n p q r s t v w y z
Eval. 3 – b c d f g h j k l m n p q r s t v w y z

Knows colors:
Evaluation 1 – Red Yellow Blue Orange Green Purple Brown Black White
Evaluation 2 – Red Yellow Blue Orange Green Purple Brown Black White
Evaluation 3 – Red Yellow Blue Orange Green Purple Brown Black White

	Eval. 1	Eval. 2	Eval. 3
Works from left to right	☐	☐	☐
Sees likenesses and differences	☐	☐	☐
Hears rhyming sounds	☐	☐	☐
Recalls parts of stories	☐	☐	☐

LANGUAGE – Oral and Written

	Eval. 1	Eval. 2	Eval. 3
Knows full name	☐	☐	☐
Prints first name	☐	☐	☐
Knows address (Street, City)	☐	☐	☐
Knows telephone number	☐	☐	☐
Knows birthdate (Mo., Day) and age	☐	☐	☐
Shares	☐	☐	☐
Follows series of 3 verbal directions	☐	☐	☐
Participates in discussions	☐	☐	☐
Expresses ideas clearly	☐	☐	☐
Participates in musical activities	☐	☐	☐

MATHEMATICAL READINESS

Recognizes numerals 1-20
Eval. 1 – 1 2 3 4 5 6 7 8 9 10 11 12 13 14 15 16 17 18 19 20
Eval. 2 – 1 2 3 4 5 6 7 8 9 10 11 12 13 14 15 16 17 18 19 20
Eval. 3 – 1 2 3 4 5 6 7 8 9 10 11 12 13 14 15 16 17 18 19 20

Counts to 50:

	Eval. 1	Eval. 2	Eval. 3
Is able to count to . . .	☐	☐	☐
Matches sets and numerals 1-10	☐	☐	☐
Matches sets and numerals 11-20	☐	☐	☐

Identifies geometric shapes
Eval. 1 – ☐ ○ △
Eval. 2 – ☐ ○ △
Eval. 3 – ☐ ○ △

PHYSICAL DEVELOPMENT

	Eval. 1	Eval. 2	Eval. 3
Controls pencil and crayon well	☐	☐	☐
Controls scissors well	☐	☐	☐
Ties shoes	☐	☐	☐
Throws a large ball	☐	☐	☐
Catches a large ball	☐	☐	☐
Skips	☐	☐	☐
Hops on one foot – Right	☐	☐	☐
– Left	☐	☐	☐

SOCIAL DEVELOPMENT

	Eval. 1	Eval. 2	Eval. 3
Shows self-confidence	☐	☐	☐
Displays self-control	☐	☐	☐
Accepts and respects authority	☐	☐	☐
Observes safety rules	☐	☐	☐
Plays and works well with others	☐	☐	☐

WORK HABITS

	Eval. 1	Eval. 2	Eval. 3
Has good listening skills	☐	☐	☐
Follows directions promptly	☐	☐	☐
Has good attention span	☐	☐	☐
Works well independently	☐	☐	☐
Finishes work promptly	☐	☐	☐
Cleans up after working	☐	☐	☐

Date of First Report: _____, 19___

Attendance Record:
Days present _____
Days absent _____
Days tardy _____

Teacher's Signature · · · · · · · · · ·

Date of Second Report: _____, 19___

Attendance Record:
Days present _____
Days absent _____
Days tardy _____

Teacher's Signature · · · · · · · · · ·

Date of Third Report: _____, 19___

Attendance Record:
Days present _____
Days absent _____
Days tardy _____

Teacher's Signature · · · · · · · · · ·

Placement Next Year: Grade _____

Teacher's Signature _____

Principal's Signature _____

UNIFIED SCHOOL DISTRICT

PUPIL PROGRESS REPORT

Grades 1, 2, 3

Year 19___ -19___

Pupil's Name _____

School _____ Grade _____

Teacher _____

To Parents/Guardians:

This report represents your teacher's best assessment of your child's progress in learning skills as well as his/her attitudes and behaviors. We would appreciate you complimenting your child for making improvements, as well as helping him/her in the areas which need improving.

Conferences with your child's teacher or principal will provide a common ground for your pupil's best development; please make an appointment which is convenient for both of you.

We appreciate your cooperation in helping to make your child's education as positive and successful as possible.

Warren Newman

Dr. Warren B. Newman
Superintendent

STUDENT RESPONSIBILITIES

I get enough sleep.

I eat a nutritious breakfast.

I attend school regularly.

I arrive at school and all classes on time.

I am considerate and courteous.

I respect the rights and property of others.

I follow classroom and school rules.

I have a positive attitude toward my school work.

I accept responsibility for my own learning.

I work well independently.

I have a special study area at home, well lighted and away from television and other distractions.

I keep necessary materials in my study area at home.

I schedule specific and regular study times at home.

I complete all school work on time.

I discuss my schoolwork and any problems I have at school with my parents.

UNIFIED SCHOOL DISTRICT
1986

BOARD OF EDUCATION

A REPORT CARD FOR PARENTS

Do I ...

send my child to bed at a reasonable time?

give my child a nutritious breakfast?

send my child to school on time?

demonstrate a commitment to the schools?

share responsibility for my child's education?

help my child follow through on homework assignments?

provide a special study area at home and insist on a regular time for homework to be done?

talk to my child about any problems he/she is having at school?

make my child feel important?

praise my child?

teach my child responsibility?

hug my child?

send my child to school neat and clean?

listen to my child?

encourage my child to do his/her best?

read to my child, visit the library, provide reading experiences in the home?

encourage my child to follow school rules?

Pupil Name _____

DESCRIPTORS MARKED (+) BEST DESCRIBE YOUR CHILD'S
PERSONAL STRENGTHS AS OBSERVED AT SCHOOL.

Your child is:

	Trimester		
	1st	2nd	3rd
Flexible..............			
Helpful...............			
Honest................			
Imaginative...........			
Inquisitive...........			
Respectful............			
Self-directed.........			
Tolerant of differences in others.....			

Your child demonstrates:

Ability to communicate feelings......			
Desire to improve.....			
Leadership............			
Positive self-image...			
Sense of humor........			

EXPLANATION OF SYMBOLS USED:

[+] shows strength   [√] needs to improve

[ ] satisfactory performance   [√] not graded at this time

PERSONAL AND SOCIAL DEVELOPMENT

Follows school routines and procedures..
Respects personal and public property...
Shows courtesy to adults and peers......
Cooperates with others..................
Follows through on responsibility.......
Demonstrates self-control...............

STUDY HABITS AND STUDY SKILLS

Listens attentively.....................
Follows directions......................
Manages time effectively................
Works independently.....................
Checks work carefully...................
Completes daily assignments on time)....

LANGUAGE ARTS

Reading

	Trimester		
	1st	2nd	3rd

Instructional level is:
 [Grade   1st   2nd   3rd]
 [Text level 2-9   8-11 10-12]
Effort..................
Uses word attack skills.
Understands word meaning
Comprehends what is read
Does competent follow-up.
Reads orally with fluency
Enjoys independent reading....
Applies reading skills to other subject areas....

Listening

Effort..................
Listens with understanding....

Communication (Oral and Written)

O W O W O W

Effort..................
Expresses complete thoughts.....
Uses correct grammar/mechanics.
Exhibits creativity....
Uses appropriate vocabulary.....

Spelling

Effort..................
Learns assigned words........
Applies spelling skills to written work.

Penmanship

Effort..................
Forms letters and numerals correctly..
Writes neatly..........
Applies skills consistently....

MATHEMATICS

Instructional level.....
 [Grade 1st, 2nd, 3rd]
Effort..................
Masters arithmetic facts......
Understands math concepts.....
Works accurately........
Applies problem solving skills....

SOCIAL STUDIES

	Trimester		
	1st	2nd	3rd

Effort..................
Contributes to discussions/class
 activities.............
Understands concepts taught....

SCIENCE/HEALTH

Effort..................
Contributes to discussions/class
 activities.............
Understands concepts taught....

FINE ARTS

Participates in activities.....
Exhibits creativity....
Appreciates works of others....
Uses appropriate arts skills...

PHYSICAL EDUCATION

Demonstrates sportsmanship.....
Participates in activities.....
Develops physical skills.......

*SPECIAL PROGRAMS _____

COMMENTS

ATTENDANCE

Days absent.............
Days tardy..............

PLACEMENT FOR NEXT YEAR: _____ Grade

_____   _____
Teacher Signature   Principal Signature

_____   _____
Parent Signature   Date

SCHOOL	MARK DEFINITIONS				

UNIFIED SCHOOL DISTRICT
Report Card
Grades 4 + 5

A	=	Excellent	O	=	Outstanding
B	=	Above average	S	=	Satisfactory
C	=	Average	U	=	Unsatisfactory
D	=	Minimum understanding	1	=	Above grade level
F	=	Failing minimum req.	2	=	At grade level
NM	=	No mark	3	=	Below grade level

STUDENT NAME	GRADE	ID	HOMEROOM	TEACHER	SCHOOL YEAR

MARKING PERIOD	STARTING DATE	ENDING DATE
2	12/01/86	03/13/87

	DAYS ABSENT	DAYS TARDY
THIS MARKING PERIOD		
THIS SCHOOL YEAR	4	

SUBJECT	MARK	COMMENTS
Reading	C+ 2	Needs to work accurately and carefully. Needs to make productive use of class time Homework is not regularly completed.
Language Oral & Written	C+	
Spelling	B- 2	Homework is not regularly completed.
Math	B-	Daily work is improving.
Social Studies	D	Needs to make productive use of class time Homework is not regularly completed. Needs to assume responsibility. Listening habits need improvement.
Science/ Health	F	Needs to make productive use of class time Homework is not regularly completed. Needs to assume responsibility. Listening habits need improvement.
Penmanship	S+	
Fine Arts	S	
Physical Education	S	
Citizenship	U	Progress is not commensurate with ability. Needs to make productive use of class time Listening habits need improvement. Needs to improve self-control.

It is probably safe to say that teacher-made tests constitute a primary source of information regarding a child's growing competence as a learner throughout his or her elementary school experience. Whether the tests constructed and administered by successive teachers are good, poor, or indifferent, can have a lot to do with the quality and rate of a child's achievement along the way. And wherever paper and pencil tests are scored and reported, they tend to have more influence on course grades and promotion recommendations than all other sources of performance data put together.

Test construction is a skill that must be learned like any other. Competence in teaching and command of the subject matter to be tested are essential elements of, but do not themselves assure competence in, test construction. What are the skills that teachers need if they are to be able to construct a good achievement test for their students?

At a minimum you need to be able to demonstrate basic test construction techniques. You have to know how to write test instructions clearly and concisely enough that students will be able to follow them easily and without error. You must be able to differentiate between what is worth knowing and what is trivial or irrelevant and strive to focus on the former at all times. You need to know how to design a blueprint and specifications for a test that will be balanced in content emphasis as well as appropriate to the abilities and experience of your class. You must be able to write clear and unambiguous items. You will need to have a working knowledge of the form in which each of the principal kinds of items is expressed, whether freeform or structured. And you must know which sort of item is best suited to measure achievement of the skills and information with which the class has been dealing, which means that not only do you need to know which kinds of items are best for a given purpose, but their limitations as well. You must be willing to revise, refine, and evaluate the success of every item before it is administered as well as again and again after use.

No less essential to the development of a good teacher-made achievement test is the desire to give the time and energy it takes to accomplish the many tasks associated with its evolution. It might be argued that all of this effort could be avoided if standardized tests were employed rather than teacher-made tests. Be sure that you are familiar with the strengths and limitations of standardized tests, and that you know how to interpret scores obtained from their administration properly.

Other measurement techniques, such as evaluation activities, require students to demonstrate, in contrived situations, competence in applying what has been learned. In this sense, the activities are criterion-related, for they are typically derived from the objectives of the preceding instruction and the student either can or cannot carry out the proposed tasks. The rigors of design and writing that typify paper and pencil tests are not such a problem in devising evaluation activities. If you can clearly communicate a learning opportunity in writing, you should have no difficulty in writing an evaluation activity. Ideally, both paper and pencil and situational evaluation activities will be employed in assessing student achievement.

Grades are the ultimate evaluation symbol, and it is the teacher who must analyze all of the obtained evaluation data and make the assignment. It is often difficult to make decisions about grades, but the more valid the tests and evaluation activities you have applied and recorded, the easier it will be to justify what you decide is the fairest representation of each student's achievement.

QUESTIONS AND EXERCISES

Discussion questions

1. A test can yield only a sample of what has been learned by a student, so at best it provides just or only an estimate of his or her achievement. Can a final grade be reliably based on tests alone, and if not, what supplementary evidence would be acceptable and how could it be recorded?

2. In your view, what is the best kind of instrument to be used in assessing achievement in health education? Would you favor one that requires the student to construct answers or one that allows selection of answers from provided alternatives. What aspects of a particular grade level would have to be considered in making a choice?

3. What are the principal advantages and disadvantages of evaluation activities as indicators of learning as compared to paper and pencil tests?

4. How might the validity of an otherwise well written and designed test be lessened by unconscious biases of the teacher who has written it? How could the risk of such an unwanted influence be diminished?

5. If you were able to obtain a standardized test that matched the objectives of the health instruction planned for the children in your class, when would you administer it and how could you best use its results?

6. What is the relationship between clearly stated and measurable objectives and the development of valid tests?

7. Many instructors use multiple-choice tests almost exclusively for several reasons, one of which is the fact that they can be machine-scored. What advantages do you see in giving students a chance to react to both free and structured response items?

8. Explain why reliability is a necessary condition of a valid test, whereas a test can be completely reliable without being valid.

Exercises

1. For health content area and a grade level of your choice, develop two or three examples of each of the following test items: essay, short answer, completion, true-false, multiple-choice, and matching items of at least five pairs. Which are the least time consuming in development? What difficulties did you encounter? How could you test the items for clarity and representativeness of the subject matter?

2. Construct a two-way grid and plan a 60-item instrument designed to assess a health science unit provided for a grade and level of your choice (primary, upper elementary or middle school). Make sure that there is a balance among the items specified for each of the columns, according to the scheme that you choose (e.g., as the horizontal axis is divided, whether by objectives, cognitive skills or whatever).

3. Choose a measurable cognitive objective from any published list proposed for elementary students, develop a problem-solving situation for its administration, and develop criteria for determining the quality or product of that activity. A criterion does not just describe *what* is to be measured but also *how* it is to be done. For example, you will often see suggestions that creativity, or thoroughness, or worthiness be measured, but no explanation to help you know how to do that or how the quality is to be defined.

4. Describe an evaluation activity that would be capable of eliciting both the cognitive and the expected affective outcome of a specified plan for health instruction.

SUGGESTED READINGS

Berk R, editor: Criterion-referenced measurement: the state of the art, Baltimore, 1980, Johns Hopkins University Press. Comprehensive assessment of the art of criterion-referenced measurement. Covers content domain specification, item generation, and item and test validity and reliability. Every chapter ends with guidelines for practitioners, which discuss the implications of the recommended strategies for tests developed by classroom teachers and other educational evaluators.

Bernstein L, Bellorado D, and Bruvald, W: Evaluation of a heart health education curriculum for preschoolers, parents, and teachers, Health Educ 17(3):14-17, 1986. Describes test constructed to assess knowledge gains made by 3- to 5-year-old children in preschool study of heart anatomy, physiology, and healthy habits related to nutrition and exercise. Procedures devised for effective administration of test items to so young a group of children explained.

Ebel R and Frisbie D: Grading and reporting Student Achievement (chapter 14), Essentials of educational measurement, Englewood Cliffs, NJ, 1986, Prentice Hall. Excellent theoretical and practical descriptions of problems and considerations involved in assigning grades.

Haney W: Testing reasoning, and reasoning about testing, Review of educational research 54(4):597-654, 1984. Brilliant review of the development of testing and the influence research on testing has had on education. Focuses entirely on standardized testing. Covers major applications, purposes, and formats, from Binet's early intelligence test to instruments in use today as in minimum competency testing, placement in EMR classes, and for college entrance. Concludes that the testing of reasoning should mean not just the measurement of cognitive abilities, but also the challenging of thinking by both those who take the tests and those who would use their results.

Kolstad R et al: Performance on three choice versus five choice multiple-choice items that measure different skills, Educ Research Q 10:2, 1985-86. A study of two patterns of choice selection, three versus five distracters for multiple-choice items, found that three choices were just as effective as five for knowledge items, whereas five choices were better for items that measure comprehension or application. Suggests that more items, hence greater reliability, could be attained by developing three-item multiple choice items for knowledge tests, thus saving a lot of time and lengthening the test without losing validity.

Patrick D et al: Measurement issues: reliability and validity, Baseline 1:9, 1985. Definitions of key terminology and practical guidelines for assessment of reliability and validity in health promotion programming and evaluation. Explanation of principal kinds of validity (content, criterion, and construct) and ways to establish each covered.

Shick J: Those tantalizing textbook tests, Health Educ 18(6):42-45, 1987-88. Describes technical errors commonly found in tests accompanying health textbooks designed for teacher use. Richly illustrated by examples drawn from published tests, the errors of each are identified and suggested revisions supplied. Well worth reading and applying to the selection or revision of any test item, whether published or devised by the teacher.

Solleder M: Evaluation instruments in health education: annotated bibliography of knowledge, attitude, behavior and school health program evaluation instruments for elementary, high school, college and non-student groups, Association for the Advancement of Health Education, An Association of the American Alliance for Health, Physical Education, Recreation, and Dance, Reston, Va, 1986, AAHE.

REFERENCES

Bloom BS, et al: Taxonomy of educational objectives, handbook 1: the cognitive domain, New York, 1956, McKay Co.

Diederich PB: The classroom teacher and the teacher-made test, Educ Horizons 43(1):20, 1964.

Ebel R: Essentials of educational measurement, ed 3, Englewood Cliffs, NJ, 1979, Prentice Hall.

Ebel R and Frisbie D: Essentials of educational measurement, ed 4, Englewood Cliffs, NJ, 1986, Prentice Hall.

Goodlad JI: A place called school, New York, 1984, McGraw-Hill.

IOX Assessment Associates, An evaluation handbook for health education programs in smoking, Culver City, Calif, 1983, p 20.

Jubb W: The development of an instrument to assess health knowledge of children prior to first grade, Evaluation Instruments in Health Educ, 1986, AAHE.

Mehrens W and Lehmann I: Measurement and evaluation in education and psychology, ed 3, New York, 1984, Holt, Rinehart, & Winston.

Mehrens W and Lehmann I: Using standardized tests in education, ed 4, New York, 1987, Longman.

Nitko A: Educational tests and measurements: an introduction, New York, 1983, Harcourt, Brace, Jovonavich, Inc.

Popham J: Modern educational measurement, Englewood Cliffs, NJ, 1981, Prentice Hall.

Salmon-Cox L: Teachers and standardized tests: what's really happening, Phi Delta Kappan 62:631-34, 1981.

Tyler R: Assessing educational achievement in the affective domain, Measurement in Education, National Council on Measurement in Education, Spring 1973.

Wiersma W and Jurs S: Educational measurement and testing, Boston, 1985, Allyn and Bacon.

PART TWO

Content and Practice

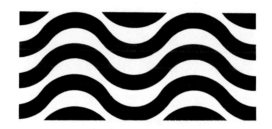

Chapter 8. Preventing Criticism or Controversy in Health Teaching

Chapter 9. A Scope and Sequence Plan for Elementary School Health Instruction

Chapter 10. Content Appropriate for Primary Level Students

Chapter 11. Primary Level Teaching Activity Ideas

Chapter 12. Content Appropriate for Intermediate Level Students

Chapter 13. Intermediate Level Teaching Activity Ideas

Chapter 14. Content Appropriate for Middle School Students

Chapter 15. Middle School Teaching Activity Ideas

CHAPTER 8

Preventing Criticism or Controversy in Health Teaching

When you finish this chapter, you should be able to:

- **Explain why the potential for controversy and criticism exists in health teaching.**

- **Analyze opposing points of view concerning controversial issues in health teaching.**

- **Synthesize a plan for deterring criticism when teaching health in the classroom.**

- **Describe methods for establishing policy guiding choices among materials and curricula that may be subject to criticism.**

Elementary and middle school teachers must be aware of the possibility of conflict about the subjects being taught. Although it is always important for a teacher to exhibit professionalism and responsibility, it is essential when teaching in areas of potential conflict and controversy. Sexuality education, including topics related to family life, human reproduction, sexually transmitted disease, including AIDS, are among these. However, controversy is not limited to this area of the health curriculum but also exists in others such as drug use and abuse, consumer health, and nutrition. Recent potentially controversial topics in health education include death and dying, divorce, abortion, violence, child abuse, and suicide. Controversy can arise anywhere, even in teaching the correct method for brushing teeth. Although dentists agree that a toothbrush should be used and their only debate is on the method of using it, Middleton was approached by a well-meaning individual who thought that sticks were the best tool for cleaning teeth. What would you say to this individual if he were the parent of one of your students? A good teacher must be tolerant and respectful of a parent's concern and point of view. In this case it would be helpful to point out that the toothbrushing method being taught is that outlined in the curriculum approved by the school board. It could be suggested that he teach the stick method to his child at home but that, if he can convince the school board that the stick method should be a part of the curriculum, then it would be taught to the other children in the class as well.

It is impossible for any health education program to meet the needs and expectations of every parent or group. Therefore controversy, or expression of opposing views, is highly possible, if not inevitable. It must be recognized that controversy surrounding all or part of a health education program is not always bad for the program. Effectively managed, controversy can result in a stronger program that is more widely accepted and endorsed. But it also can destroy part of a program or the entire program. The key ingredient for success in handling controversy is parental involvement and support.

REASONS FOR CONTROVERSY

The reasons for controversy are certainly as varied and complex as society itself. Several issues in the schools are outlined in this chapter, many of which concern sexuality education, since this is the most difficult and significant controversial area. However, this emphasis does not negate the importance of controversy in other areas such as child abuse, drug abuse, suicide, violence, and death and dying. Community members might be equally concerned about education in these areas, and teachers must be aware of possible conflicts involving values when such subjects are taught.

Sexuality Education in the Schools

Many opposed to sexuality education in the schools are concerned that schools intend to take over the role of the parent as the primary sex educator. Proponents claim there is no basis for this fear, and that the schools would serve as a supplement to the education received at home. Gordon (1981) supports this view, saying:

The *primary* responsibility for educating children about sexuality from birth to adulthood always has been, and must remain, in the home. Parents provide love, warmth and caring that are the foundation of many future values and attitudes concerning sexuality; and family life is strengthened by parents who take an active role in communicating with their own children.

Unfortunately researchers have found that peers often rank first as the source of information about sex, and, as can be imagined, the information from peers is often distorted. In a study of 1,152 teenagers, Thornburg (1981) found that the sources of sexual information after peers, in order of frequency, were literature, mothers, schools, experience, fathers, physicians, and religious leaders. Clearly parents, schools, and religious leaders all should have a greater influence than this study indicates if they are to help children become responsible and sensitive adults in regard to sexuality.

Teaching about Values

The single most controversial issue revolves around how morals and values should be handled in the classroom. A value is a preference for an idea, thing, or behavior held by individuals and groups. It is a belief that a certain idea or behavior is ''right,'' at least for that individual or group. The problem is the lack of agreement regarding which values are right for all of society. Although some values are generally accepted, diverse opinions exist in many areas of education. It is therefore difficult for a teacher to know how to address health-related ideas and behaviors in controversial areas.

There are two basic approaches to handling values regarding sexuality education in the classroom. One is to avoid dealing with values at all, to teach only the biology of human reproduction, and refer all other matters to parents. Many schools adopting this approach as a way to avoid controversy have been criticized and accused of teaching students the ''how'' of reproduction but giving them no direction and setting no limits (Dickman, 1982). It is, however, an approach commonly employed in schools throughout the United States.

The other approach involves a methodology that ''helps children clarify for themselves what they value. This is very different from trying to

persuade children what they value'' (Rath, Harmin, and Simon, 1966). Children are encouraged to investigate the values held by their family, religion, and culture and to use this information in deciding for themselves what they value. McNab (1982) explains, ''The task of the sexuality educator is to present accurate information about sexuality so that individuals, based upon their cultural, religious, ethnical, and familial upbringing, can make responsible decisions regarding their own sexuality.'' Scales (1983) also believes that the examination of values, in addition to factual information, is essential to sexuality education, and he adds another dimension, that of skill development. Increasing communication and decision-making skills of young people helps them deal not only with sexual matters but also with all aspects of life. Young people practiced in these skills will have an increased ability to make decisions such as what to wear or where to go and how to resist peer pressure and say no when that is what they believe is right.

The decision of how to teach about values in the classroom is made by the district. A teacher should never impose a value system on children. Ideally, a school district should determine which are the *fundamental* values regarding sexuality education on which most community members can agree. If such a list is formulated in a district, then a teacher is provided with written guidelines to the value system held by the district and community regarding sexuality education. Such a document provides the teacher direction and parameters for teaching in this controversial area. The following list is an example of fundamental values regarding sexuality that might be adopted by a school district:*

---

*Modified from Scales P: Family Relations **32:**287, 1983.

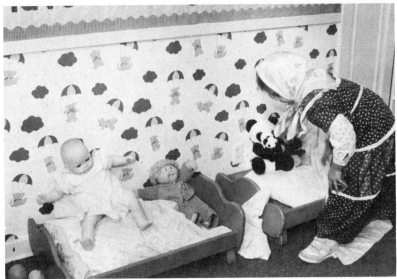

Armi Lizardi

1. Sexuality is more than the biology of reproduction; it involves attitudes, practices, and responsibilities as a sexual being.
2. Knowlege and information about sexuality are important through life.
3. It is important to examine one's own values in the area of sexuality and to respect the differing values of others.
4. Self-esteem is essential in making healthy and responsible decisions about sexual matters.
5. Each sexual decision has an effect or consequence for which responsibility must be taken.
6. Given its medical, psychologic, and social ramifications, adolescents are not usually ready for sexual intercourse.
7. It is wrong to exploit or to force someone into an unwanted sexual experience ("it is okay to say no").
8. It is beneficial when children can feel comfortable discussing sexual matters with parents and other trusted adults.

9. Parenthood requires many responsibilities that adolescents are usually incapable of assuming.

Other values that Scales listed are appropriate for district staff and community members to consider when establishing a sexuality program:*

1. Parents are the primary sexuality educators of their children, and schools and churches should supplement this role.
2. School districts should involve parents and other community members in planning sexuality programs.
3. Participation in sexuality programs should be voluntary.
4. School districts should use trained teachers who exhibit the highest standards of professional ethics and participate in regular continuing education programs.
5. In our society a wide range of values and beliefs about sexuality is to be expected.

---

*Modified from Scales P: Family Relations **32:**287, 1983.

Sexuality Education Fostering Sexual Activity

It is a commonly accepted fallacy that, if children are not told about sex, they will not become sexually involved. Proponents of sexuality education say that the reverse is actually true: the more information an adolescent has, the less likely he or she is to become sexually active at a young age (Gordon, 1981). In addition, teaching children the skills and knowledge necessary to abstain from sexual activity is important in reducing the teenage pregnancy rate. It generally is agreed that children need a source of sexual information other than peers to be sure that they receive accurate information.

AVOIDING PROBLEMS WHEN TEACHING SEXUALITY EDUCATION

First and foremost, elementary school teachers must remember that they are employed by a school district and must follow the guidelines established by the district. Some teachers who have problems in sensitive areas of the health curriculum have taken things into their own hands "for the good of the children." One example is a teacher suggesting to students that they "forget" to take home a letter notifying the parents of an upcoming lesson if they think their parents might object. Another is a teacher who decides that the approved text leaves out too much important information and brings in unapproved materials to help the children "really" understand the process of reproduction. In situations like these, the actions of a teacher can jeopardize an entire program or wipe out a long-established one. In the long run, it is the children who are deprived of the education they need.

Several other situations are discussed in the box (1 on pp. *208-210)*. These situations offer sound and practical advice to the classroom teacher of any subject, not only sexuality education. Unfortunately these experiences are not unusual. Indeed it is easy to see that many parents have a legitimate concern. Teachers, administrators, and all health professionals need to ask themselves if they are part of the solution or the problem.

Meeting the Challenge of AIDS

"Does AIDS hurt?" asks a second grade student. Such questions are more and more commonplace in today's elementary school classroom. Teachers, parents, and administrators are faced with the challenge of educating young children about how to prevent HIV (the virus which causes AIDS) infection. Teaching children how to avoid contact with a deadly virus should not be controversial. However, because the way that HIV spreads most often involves sexual contact, teaching about AIDS prevention is controversial.

Currently, educators, public health officials, and policy-makers are scrambling to appropriately address the AIDS crisis. Grady (1988) recommends that the three following components are essential for any effective school program:

- A physician-consultant who is knowledgeable about AIDS
- A policy concerning attendance of HIV-infected students (including those with ARC or AIDS and those without symptoms)
- Appropriate educational programs for school health professionals, teachers and school staff, students, parents, and others concerned with the problem of AIDS.

Grady goes on to emphasize that an AIDS policy must be established with the involvement of medical personnel, school nurses, administrators, teachers, parents, students, custodians, and public health officials. He urges that mechanisms for action when HIV is detected in a student or a school health worker must be in place

EASY WAYS OF GETTING INTO TROUBLE WHEN TEACHING SEX EDUCATION

During my career as a health educator I have observed or have had related to me numerous stories of problems teachers have encountered while teaching sex education. Without exception these teachers have been well meaning and have had the best interest of their students at heart. Poor judgment on their part, however, has often resulted in placing their sex education programs in jeopardy; many supporters of sex education have become nonsupporters because of incidents involving poor judgment. It is the hope of this article that such errors can be minimized by calling them to the attention of present and future teachers of sex education. The list offered here is by no means complete as teachers are constantly finding new ways to get into trouble. Here are a few easy ways of getting into trouble teaching sex education.

1. *Teaching sex education with inadequate background.* Sex education is one of the few areas where teachers are actually held accountable for what they teach. Teachers of almost any other subject area can have some poor days of teaching and as long as they maintain order it is unlikely they will ever be chastised for their teaching. Let teachers of sex education make an error and you can bet they will hear of it. It isn't that they shouldn't be held accountable, because they certainly should, but that such accountability is rare in education and a major challenge for sex educators. There are few nondedicated teachers teaching sex education for long, as it is a great deal of hard work. It requires a thorough background in the subject matter—university courses, seminars, and/or a great deal of solid reading. Making content errors in this subject will quickly result in lack of credibility with students, parents, colleagues, administrators, and will certainly draw the fire of the anti-sex education group.

2. *Keeping your principal or administrator in the dark.* It is imperative that your principals and administrators be apprised of what is happening in your classroom. If you really wish to get into trouble with administrators put them through a couple of late night phone calls from irate parents concerning sex education material or projects which they know nothing about. It is highly likely you will also be blessed with a call from that administrator. Keeping the appropriate administrator up to date, for some, will mean just a statement that you are now studying sex education. For others it will mean detailed lesson plans from which you are not to deviate.

3. *Giving "secret" lessons.* Another surefire way to get into trouble is to have secret lessons with your students. Just make a statement such as "Today's lesson is just between you and me—it is our little secret" and you can be certain many parents will hear of it. You have no business teaching material that you cannot defend.

4. *Violating district or school policy.* This is clearly a violation of your responsibility as a teacher. Curriculum guides are set up to give you parameters to work in, and in a general sense reflect the wishes of the community. You should stay within those parameters no matter what "you know is good" for your students. If you don't agree with the curriculum you should certainly work to change it, and a great many curricula need improvement. Until you get it changed, however, you are legitimately bound by contract to reflect the existing curriculum.

*From Gilbert G: Health Educ **10**(5):31, 1979.

5. *Using poorly constructed home made materials.* Parents especially do not find a poorly constructed penis model or free hand drawings of genitalia amusing. Remember that you are dealing with their children. Giving a homework assignment of freehand drawings of the male and female genitalia may seem innocuous, but many a parent has noted that their daughter drew an erect penis and wondered where she got her model image. Using anatomical drawings is certainly a legitimate exercise, but have them duplicated for your students.

6. *Using questionable language.* Slang terminology is often all students know of reproductive anatomy and physiology. Students should not be reprimanded for using such terminology unless they use it on purpose to create a disturbance, but they should be tactfully taught the correct terminology. Teachers who feel they must use such terms generally to "get on their level" may soon be on their level equally unemployed.

7. *Not previewing films or materials.* There should be a district committee to approve films, and you are courting disaster if you use films not on the approved list. It is always wise to preview films, but in sex education it is essential. I will never forget an acquaintance of mine who was not teaching health education by choice, and consequently used a large number of films. He ordered the district approved-for-high-school film, "The Story of Eric" (an excellent film on Lamaze childbirth), for his class. As the film progressed he was not prepared for the scene of actual childbirth. He jumped in front of the projector, and his class witnessed a childbirth in vivid color on his white shirt! He had not previewed his film and was not trained or willing to discuss childbirth.

8. *Not being prepared for opposition.* Most programs that are properly established suffer little opposition, as the vast majority of Americans support sex education, but numerous programs have been attacked. All teachers should be able to verbalize the need for sex education when called upon and should anticipate such encounters. Do not respond with hostility or contempt. Parents will have honest questions and they deserve sincere well-documented answers.

9. *Teaching by the joke.* Several instructors have gotten into trouble by telling or allowing students to tell "off color" jokes in the classroom. Teachers telling inappropriate jokes can give the sex education classroom an improper atmosphere for such an important subject. One local high school teacher got into trouble by leaving his classroom for a long distance phone call. In his absence a student leader was left in charge, who allowed jokes to be told. It was an all male class and the jokes soon got off color and deeper in raw sexual expressiveness. One male not accustomed to hearing women discussed in such terms left the room in tears.

10. *Setting unrealistic goals.* Many programs have been set up with goals and objectives to eliminate VD, divorce, etc. Such programs are doomed to failure. A good example of this is when a program sets out to lower the VD rate. When a good sex education program is established, the VD rate often goes up! The reason for this increase is that people recognize signs and symptoms and go in for treatment. At a later date the rate may go down.

Continued.

11. *Forcing teachers to teach sex education.* Mandating that all teachers should teach sex education is ludicrous. Forcing teachers to teach in any area they don't wish to teach is unwise. Such action frequently leads to poor quality education, and in sex education that can lead to disaster. Many teachers will never be comfortable teaching sex education. Such unwilling or embarassed teachers can easily be turned to an anti-sex education position by such forced compliance.

12. *Letting personal bias overly influence teaching.* Everyone knows what normal sexual behavior is—it is the way *they* behave. This erroneous belief of major consequence is often carried into the classroom and can be devastating. The advocate of open marriage, marriage at all costs, or any other particular lifestyle has no business preaching it in the classroom. We are all biased. Recognize that bias and be careful not to try to convert your students.

13. *Using inappropriate guest speakers.* The selection of guest speakers must be done with great care. Inviting right-to-life groups to class with brutal pictures can be a traumatic experience for students. Certainly the anti-abortion groups should have the right to express their point of view, but you as a teacher have the right and responsibility to screen how it is done. Inviting homosexuals to a junior high or high school class is another example of an easy way to get into trouble. Certainly they should have the right to express their opinion, but the problem thus created might jeopardize a total program.

14. *Citing personal sexual experience.* It seems hard to believe that teachers need to be reminded that this is not okay, but it still occurs. Do not let students push you into revealing your personal life. It simply has no place in the classroom.

15. *Using nonapproved questionnaires of students' sexual experiences or attitudes.* It may seem to you that finding out what is actually going on with your students is a good place to start your program, but your principal or administrator is likely to think differently. Remember that such questionnaires may be construed as a reflection of the performance of the school or district as a whole. Be certain to clear all such questionnaires beforehand. They may provide useful information, but be careful they don't cost you your job or hurt the reputation of your school.

16. *Leaving nonapproved reading matter out for public view.* It is of course appropriate for you as a teacher to read anything you wish, but remember that the district has approved materials for use with students. Do not leave nonapproved matter out where a student might pick up or where an outsider might view it. There is an excellent paperback on birth control and STDs (sexually transmitted diseases) entitled *Intercourse Without Getting Screwed* which is a valuable resource. Many parents, however, may not find the title amusing if they happen to walk by and view it on your desk.

Please ask yourself if you are unnecessarily endangering your sex education program. Sex education is far too important to be eliminated or watered down because of mistakes in judgment. Remember, sex education is one of the few areas of education where teachers are truly held accountable for their teaching. Making errors in teaching history, English, or any other subject seldom results in chastisement, but make an error in teaching sex education and you may be looking for a new line of work.

before the need arises. This is certainly sound advice, and most school districts nationwide do have policies in place regarding HIV-infected students or school personnel.

There is still, however, concern and controversy about the education aspects of AIDS prevention particularly regarding elementary school students. Even though the vast majority of elementary school students do not engage in high-risk behaviors for contracting HIV, programs specifically designed to be age-appropriate and to help keep them HIV-free are necessary. The U.S. Centers for Disease Control (CDC, 1988, p.4) recommend that:

School systems should make programs available that will enable and encourage young people who **have not** engaged in sexual intercourse and who **have not** used illicit drugs to continue to—
- Abstain from sexual intercourse until they are ready to establish a mutually monogamous relationship within the context of marriage;
- Refrain from using or injecting illicit drugs.
    For young people who **have** engaged in sexual intercourse or who **have** injected illicit drugs, school programs should enable and encourage them to—
- Stop engaging in sexual intercourse until they are ready to establish a mutually monogamous relationship within the context of marriage;
- To stop using or injecting illicit drugs.

Certainly all parents, educators, and public health officials agree that it is in the best interest of children and young people to abstain from sexual intercourse and from injecting drugs. Such responsible behavior prevents the spread of the HIV virus, prevents teenage pregnancy, and promotes a healthier, drug-free lifestyle. Why then is there controversy around AIDS education? The fact is that despite the rational reasons for saying no to sex and drugs, many young people engage in these risky behaviors.

Therefore, public health officials at the CDC, (1988, p.4) further recommend that school systems:

. . . provide AIDS education programs that address preventive types of behavior that should be practiced by persons with an increased risk of acquiring HIV infection. These include:
- Avoiding sexual intercourse with anyone who is known to be infected, who is at risk of being infected, or whose HIV infection status is not known;
- Using a latex condom with spermicide if they engage in sexual intercourse;
- Seeking treatment if addicted to illicit drugs;
- Not sharing needles or other injection equipment;
- Seeking HIV counseling and testing if HIV infection is suspected.

The ultimate questions for educators and parents are: How should specific information be presented to students? At what age should it be provided and by whom? The answers to these questions need to be carefully considered by communities and schools. Some suggestions are offered below.

AIDS-Related Content

For children at the primary level, ''AIDS education'' consists of health education. It does not need to, nor should it be, explicit. It should be age-appropriate and consistent with the developmental level of the child. AIDS education should be woven into a planned comprehensive health education program in the elementary school. Although a detailed explanation of HIV contraction is not appropriate at the primary level, basic health concepts can serve as building blocks for later AIDS education. Concepts such as these should be emphasized: there are health helpers in our communities; good hygiene practices include washing hands and covering sneezes; avoiding contact with people sick with a disease that you can catch is wise; and it is important to get proper medical help when you are sick. By laying a careful foundation of understanding of basic hygiene, we can give our young children the tools they need for later, more sophisticated explanations of AIDS and other health issues (Quackenbush, 1988). The CDC (1988 p. 51) does delineate some specific content for the primary level:*

- AIDS is a disease that is causing some adults to get very sick, but it does not commonly affect children.
- AIDS is very hard to get. You cannot get it just by being near or touching someone who has it.
- Scientists all over the world are working hard to find a way to stop people from getting AIDS and to cure those who have it.

Largely, the elementary teacher needs to be able to answer questions about AIDS that will undoubtedly arise in his or her classroom. In order to respond to students appropriately, teachers must understand established district guidelines. Also, teachers must be comfortable enough with basic content about AIDS to adequately answer questions while keeping in mind that the underlying theme is to allay excessive fear.

For students in upper elementary and middle school, the content addressed becomes more specific. However, "AIDS education" is still best taught within a planned comprehensive health education program. The CDC (1988, pp. 5-6) recommends the following information be included in the curriculum:*

From Centers for Disease Control: Guidelines for effective school health education to prevent the spread of AIDS; MMWR 1988:37 (Suppl. no 5-2).

- Viruses are living organisms too small to be seen by the unaided eye.
- Viruses can be transmitted from an infected person to an uninfected person through various means.
- Some viruses cause disease among people.
- Persons who are infected with some viruses that cause disease may not have any signs or symptoms of disease.
- AIDS (an abbreviation for **a**cquired **i**mmuno**d**eficiency **s**yndrome) is caused by a virus that weakens the ability of infected individuals to fight off disease.
- People who have AIDS often develop a rare type of severe pneumonia, a cancer called Kaposi's sarcoma, and certain other diseases that healthy people normally do not get.
- About 1 to 1.5 million of the total population of approximately 240 million Americans currently are infected with the AIDS virus and consequently are capable of infecting others.
- People who are infected with the AIDS virus live in every state in the United States and in most other countries of the world. Infected people live in cities as well as in suburbs, small towns, and rural areas. Although most infected people are adults, teenagers can also become infected. Females as well as males are infected. People of every race are infected, including whites, blacks, Hispanics, Native Americans, and Asian/Pacific Islanders.
- The AIDS virus can be transmitted by sexual contact with an infected person; by using needles and other injection equipment that an infected person has used; and from an infected mother to her infant before or during birth.
- A small number of doctors, nurses, and other medical personnel have been infected when they were directly exposed to infected blood.
- It sometimes takes several years after becoming infected with the AIDS virus before symptoms of the disease appear. Thus, people who are infected with the virus can infect other people—even though the people who transmit the infection do not feel or look sick.
- Most infected people who develop symptoms of AIDS only live about 2 years after their symptoms are diagnosed.

• The AIDS virus cannot be caught by touching someone who is infected, by being in the same room with an infected person, or by donating blood.

The important theme for students in upper elementary and middle school involves understanding the nature of viruses in general and the HIV virus specifically. This is fundamental to understanding the risk of HIV infection and the importance of preventive measures.

Meeting the challenge of AIDS presents educators with the most difficult task they will ever face. It is the task of saving the lives of their students.

Schools and Drugs

Educating students to adopt responsible, non-abusive behavior related to drugs has long been a topic in elementary health education. There is renewed concern about drug abuse. Today drug education programs, more often called prevention and intervention programs, are becoming important elements in elementary and middle school curricula across the nation. In 1986, the U.S. Department of Education circulated the document *What Works: Schools Without Drugs* throughout the educational community and to every school in the country. A forward in the document by Nancy Reagan urged that we "go further still by convincing [our children] that drugs are morally wrong." This document helped to launch the battle to rid schools and communities of illicit drugs and alcohol abuse.

The controversy related to drug education in schools in the past has often focused on the concern that education about drugs would encourage student experimentation. While this is still a concern for many educators and parents, the thrust of educational efforts has changed. Very few programs involve in-depth studies of all the various drugs of abuse and their effects. Current programs focus on helping students to enhance self-esteem and to develop skills to refuse drugs.

Following the guidelines outlined in *Schools Without Drugs* (1986), many schools have implemented programs that involve the community and law enforcement. The document recommends that school districts set specific policies to clarify rules regarding drug use and to include strong corrective actions. Teachers in elementary schools have the responsibility to understand and enforce the policies that are established by district officials. Additionally, care and sensitivity need to be given to the fact that many students come from homes where drugs are in use. The educational process should not promote guilt and fear among young people living in a home where parents use alcohol or other drugs. Teachers should be aware of possible difficulty that students in these situations face. These difficulties can range from uneasiness in hearing that their parents are involved in a behavior that is "wrong," to abuse situations related to drug use by parents or siblings. At all times it is the responsibility of the teacher to be sensitive to these situations and to be prepared to refer students if necessary.

Search and seizure of student lockers and desks is becoming more and more common in schools across the country. In the effort to rid our schools and communities of drugs, teachers and administrators have found themselves in the uneasy position of enforcer. Controversy over Fourth Amendment rights has taken search and seizure questions to the Supreme Court. A summary of the decisions regarding this issue follows (United States Department of Education, 1986, p.24):

What legal standard applies to school officials who search students and their possessions for drugs?

The Supreme Court has held that school officials may institute a search if there are "reasonable grounds" to believe that the search will reveal evidence that the student has violated or is violating either the law or the rules of the school.

Do school officials need a search warrant to conduct a search for drugs?

No, not if they are carrying out the search independent of the police and other law enforcement officials. A more stringent legal standard may apply if law enforcement officials are involved in the search.

How extensive can a search be?

The scope of the permissible search will depend on whether the measures used during the search are reasonably related to the purpose of the search and are not excessively intrusive in light of the age and sex of the student being searched. The more intrusive the search, the greater the justification that will be required by the courts.

Do school officials have to stop a search when they find the object of the search?

Not necessarily. If a search reveals items suggesting the presence of other evidence of crime or misconduct, the school official may continue the search. For example, if a teacher is justifiably searching a student's purse for cigarettes and finds rolling papers, it will be reasonable (subject to any local policy to the contrary) for the teacher to search the rest of the purse for evidence of drugs.

Can school officials search student lockers?

Reasonable grounds to believe that a particular student locker contains evidence of a violation of the law or school rules will generally justify a search of that locker. In addition, some courts have upheld written school policies that authorize school officials to inspect student lockers at any time.

Individual teachers should not take search and seizure tactics into their own hands. Any such action should be handled by administrators under the direction of the elected school officials. Policies and guidelines regarding these procedures must be established by local school boards of education.

EFFECTS OF CONTROVERSY ON SCHOOLS

Schools are run by school boards that are elected locally and are ultimately responsible for everything that happens in the district. In the United States the greatest amount of authority for education rests on the shoulders of local officials. Certainly each school board must adhere to state mandates and laws, and "strings" usually are attached to state and federal money. But for the most part school districts are run by the community.

This local autonomy in the educational system of the United States can be positive in effect in that a school board can implement programs uniquely suited to the children in that specific district. Parents can have easy access to the board members because they are members of the community and often neighbors and friends, particularly in smaller school districts. However, this easy access to school board members sometimes results in drastic program changes as a result of controversy. Many times a program change is needed, but in other cases a vocal minority of the community can effect changes in school programs that do not represent the wishes of the majority. Most proponents of sexuality education have found that the majority of people in the community favor such a program; however, often this positive preference is not communicated to the school board. A small but vocal and zealous group can pack a board room and make demands, which can be overwhelming for board members. If policies have not been established for making changes in the school curriculum, the school board may be persuaded to act on the concerns of a minority group without receiving input from other representatives of the community. For example, in one district a film was being considered for the sixth-grade family life unit. Before recommending the film the health education committee (which consisted of teachers, administrators, and a school nurse) wanted to show it to the sixth-grade parents. Eight hundred parents viewed the film and expressed their opinions on its possible inclusion in the program. Eighty-five percent of the parents surveyed approved of the film, so it was used in the unit. After a few apparently successful years of using the film, suddenly it was banned by the school board. On Monday night the board met, as usual, but instead of the usual 10 to 20 persons, the relatively small room was packed. A vocal group of about 50 people demanded that the film be dropped from the sixth-grade family life program because they objected to one frame of the film and one sentence of the sound track. The school board panicked and voted to drop the film from the program that night. There was no policy requiring that such changes be reviewed by a committee of advisers representing a cross section of community members, and there were no community representatives as voting members of the health education committee. Thus the result of controversy, in a district serving over 20,000 students, was that 50 people effected a change that did not represent the desire of the majority of parents surveyed.

CONSTRUCTIVE WAYS OF DEALING WITH CONTROVERSY

The fear of opposition to educational programs and materials is very real to district administrators, teachers, and board members. However, it is highly unlikely that opposition to some programs or materials, not only those for sexuality education, can be entirely avoided in a district.

The way to deal with controversy is to know how to manage it, not to avoid it. Scales (1980) said, "It is apparent that moral conflict and political authority are at the heart of sex education controversies. Managing discontent, rather than trying to stifle it, is the key to success." This can be applied to all curricular controversies. The following sections offer suggestions to school district officials concerned about controversy.

Become Informed

Keeping apprised of the issues and concerns common to both national and local political efforts is essential for the school. It is naive to think that local communities are not affected by national issues. How other districts handle conflicts associated with these issues can be helpful in determining policies.

Review Current Policies

School policies are written procedures that have been adopted by the school board and must be followed by district employees. The district should have an explicit policy for the selection of materials, development and implementation of curriculums, how complaints are handled, and how teachers are selected to teach sensitive topics. If policies do not exist or are vague, a process for their development should be outlined. Examples of policies regarding selection and reconsideration of materials used in the classroom are given in the box on p. *(216)*.

Set Up a Curriculum Advisory Committee

The most productive vehicle for support of all educational programs, particularly those which are controversial, is a curriculum advisory committee. Such a committee is usually comprised of representatives from the school district and community who recommend guidelines and

The School System's Policy on Materials Selection

The school system's policy on materials selection should include the following:
1. A statement on the school system's philosophy of resource and material selection
2. A statement on the legal responsibility of the governing board and the delegation of authority to district personnel
3. A description of resources and materials covered by the selection policy
4. A listing of criteria for selection of all resources and materials
5. A statement that all items will meet established criteria
6. Procedures for selection

The School System's Policy on Reconsideration

The school system's policy on reconsideration should include the following:
1. A statement that the procedure applies to all requests for reconsideration (including those from school personnel and school board members)
2. The name of the person to whom the request for reconsideration should be directed
3. An explanation of the use of the request for reconsideration
4. An explanation of the reconsideration committee: names of members, how and when they are chosen or elected, length of terms, and so on
5. An outline of the process used by the reconsideration committee with an indication of how long the process takes
6. A statement about the status during the reconsideration process of the resource being questioned
7. Criteria for the reevaluation of resources and materials
8. A statement that the decision reached by the committee is to be based on the established criteria
9. A statement indicating to whom the decision of the reconsideration committee is communicated (that is, the school board and the superintendent)
10. A statement of whether the decision relates to one grade level, one school, or the entire district
11. A statement of whether the same resources or materials will be reconsidered more than once during a specified time period
12. A provision for appeal of the decision

Modified from Parker B: Exec Educator **3**(8):24, 1980.

execute subsequent board policies for the use of specific teaching methodology and materials. The committee should have the authority it needs to be effective. Hot issues should be discussed by the representative committee, rather than in a forum open to the entire community. There should be a specific policy on the way issues are brought to the committee.

It is essential that all segments of the community are represented in the committee, including parents and other interested citizens. It is wise to involve parent-teacher groups in this effort, such as the National Congress of Parents and Teachers (NCPT), which has been participating in health education efforts throughout the United States since 1898 (Carlyon, 1981). Any vocal minority that may be opposed to certain educational programs or materials also should be represented. As Wagman and Bignell (1981) said:

Most concerns about sex education stem not from opposition to sex education itself, but from a lack of understanding and/or mistrust of the particular program being presented by the school. If parents have been involved in program development, they will be more likely to trust the program.

This is true of all health education programs, not only those for sexuality education.

Be Consistent and Calm

Once a policy has been agreed on, it should be followed consistently. If the process used to develop the policy included wide representation from the community, school personnel, and students, it should be sound. Policies should be flexible and changeable, but not at whim nor without due process. Be calm and avoid shouting matches with concerned individuals. It is important to understand that they have a right to their point of view. Stay calm by standing firm on the policy established. Explain that any change in policy must follow certain procedures.

Hire Trained Personnel

For potentially controversial subjects (such as sexuality education, AIDS education, drug education, and death education) qualified teachers should be hired or trained. Teachers should not be forced to teach these subjects if they do not desire to do so, nor should they teach in these areas if they are not adequately prepared.

Inform Rather Than Advertise

The community must be kept apprised of the programs and stands the district takes, but this is not the same as looking for attention. Informing parents of the sexuality education curriculum and urging them to review materials is one thing; issuing a press release announcing a new and wonderful comprehensive sexuality education program is quite another.

All state laws must be adhered to regarding notification to parents about sensitive topics taught in schools. This usually involves a letter to the parents explaining the program and inviting them to review the materials used. Most states allow students to be removed from classes if the parent wishes. No matter what the state law is regarding notification, every *effort* should be made to inform parents and to *remove* a child from a class if the parents request it.

SUMMARY

Controversy exists more often in health education than in other subjects because there are so many different groups and individuals in the community interested in the health of children. Controversy is possible in many areas of the health education program, but it is most pronounced in sexuality education and AIDS education. The reasons for controversy are varied. Many parents are concerned that the school is trying to take the place of the parent as the primary sex educator. Additionally, there seems to be some confusion about how to teach about values and morals. And, some parents and community members are concerned that teaching sexually explicit information will lead to more sexual experimentation among adolescents. Studies show the reverse, however.

Schools in the United States are run by school boards, elected locally by the community. This local autonomy allows school board members to tailor educational programs to the needs of the children in that community. Parents and community members usually have easy access to school board members, which can have both positive and negative effects. It is possible for special interest groups to influence school boards to act in ways that do not represent the desires of the majority of community members. Fear of opposition and conflict on the part of school administrators and board members can severely hinder the educational process. The key to success in controversial situations is to manage discontent rather than stifle it, which can be done in the following ways:

a. Being informed about issues that may be controversial.

b. Making certain that policies exist about textbook adoption, ways to handle complaints, development and implementation of a curriculum, and selection of teachers for sensitive subjects.

c. Setting up a curriculum committee that is representative of the entire community and has authority to make decisions and recommendations that will be sincerely considered.

d. Being consistent in following established policies.

e. Being calm and considerate when dealing with individuals whose opinions differ from yours.

f. Hiring trained personnel whenever possible.

g. Keeping the parents and community adequately informed.

Teachers often have problems in controversial areas because they do not follow district guidelines. Actions of well-meaning teachers may jeopardize or destroy programs. Basic professionalism in teaching is essential.

QUESTIONS AND EXERCISES
Discussion Questions

1. Why does controversy arise more often in the elementary school curriculum in health education than in math or reading?

2. Many people believe that sexuality education is the responsibility of parents rather than the school. Does sexuality education belong in the schools? Defend your point of view with specific arguments. Is AIDS education more easily defended? Why or why not?

3. What approaches do school districts take regarding teaching about values and morals in sexuality education? Why is it preferable for a school district to have outlined a set of fundamental values in sexuality education?

4. What is meant by the statement, ''AIDS education at the primary level is actually good health education?''

5. School administrators and school board members often are fearful of opposition to certain school programs. Why is it important for these officials to learn how to manage discontent rather than stifle it? What are the practical ways to prepare for managing opposition? Be specific in these suggestions.

6. Why do teachers have problems when teaching in controversial areas? Explain a potential problem and speculate on its ramifications.

7. Take a moment to consider the possible concerns of community members if you were to teach a lesson on AIDS, death, violence, child abuse, or drug abuse. What reasons for controversy in these areas could you list? Are there any similarities between these areas and sexuality education? What conflicts regarding values in these areas might exist?

Problems and Exercises

1. Interview a proponent and an opponent of sexuality or AIDS education in the schools. Then write a report presenting both views. Be objective in your report. Ask yourself, "Did I learn anything from this encounter? Am I able to accept an individual's right to have a point of view that is different from my own?"

2. Find out what laws exist in your state, and local school district regarding the teaching of human reproduction, AIDS, drugs and alcohol, and death. Are there any policies on the selection of teaching materials in the district? What procedures are followed to add or drop teaching materials from the school curriculum?

3. What laws or policies exist in your state and local school district regarding HIV-infected students or school workers?

4. Attend a school board meeting. Familiarize yourself with the protocol of the board and the items that are handled in a meeting. At what point in this meeting could a community member voice a concern about teaching materials or curriculum issues? Does the school board have a curriculum committee to which these questions are referred? If so, who serves on that committee, and how does it handle various issues?

5. Assume that your principal has chosen you to teach sexuality education that includes an AIDS education unit in the school. What steps should you take to ensure that you do not have problems? Plan a parent meeting where you will explain the program.

6. Describe how to handle an irate parent who has demanded an explanation for a search of his/her child's locker.

7. Rewrite Gilbert's article (1979) on pp. *(000-000)*, changing the sensitive area addressed, for example, "Easy Ways of Getting Into Trouble When Teaching Drug Education."

REFERENCES

Carlyon P: The PTA's health education project and sex education in the schools, J Sch Health **51**(4):271, 1981.

Centers for Disease Control: Guidelines for effective school health education to prevent the Spread of AIDS, MMWR 1988;37 (Suppl no S-2).

Dickman IR: Winning the battle against sex education, New York, 1982, SIECUS.

Gilbert G: Easy ways of getting into trouble when teaching sex education, Health Educ **10**(5):31, 1979.

Gordon S: The case for moral sex education in the schools, J Sch Health **51**(4):214, 1981.

Grady MI: Helping schools to cope with AIDS, Med Aspects Human Sexuality Jan 1988.

McNab WL: Do's and don'ts in teaching sexuality education, Health Educ **13**(6):31, 1982.

Parker B: Leadership: political battles offer you the challenge of a lifetime, Exec Educator **3**(8):24, 1980.

Quackenbush M and Villarreal S: Does AIDS hurt? educating young children about AIDS, Santa Cruz, 1988, Network Publications.

Rath LE, Harmin M, and Simon SB: Values and teaching: working with values in the classroom, Columbus, 1966, Charles E Merrill Publishing Co.

Scales P: Barriers to sex education, J Sch Health **50**(8):337, 1980.

Scales P: Sense and nonsense about sexuality education: a rejoinder to the Shornacks' critical view, Family Relations **32**(4):287, 1983.

Thornburg HD: Adolescent sources of information on sex, J Sch Health **51**(4):274, 1981.

United States Department of Education: What works: schools without drugs, 1986.

Wagman E and Bignell S: Starting family life and sex education programs: a health agency's perspective, J Sch Health **51**(4):247, 1981.

SUGGESTED READINGS

Centers for Disease Control: Guidelines for effective school health education to prevent the spread of AIDS, MMWR 1988;37 (Suppl no S-2). (A booklet released by the U.S. Public Health Service to help school personnel develop prevention programs. Content guidelines are provided for students in grades K through 12.)

Dickman IR: Winning the battle against sex education, 1982, A SIECUS Publication. (A booklet that is a complete guide for setting up sexuality education programs that meet the needs of children and are accepted and supported by the community)

Fitch JA and Gobble DC ed: Controversial issues, Health Educ **13**(6), 1982. (A special issue on controversy in health education, internal and external to the profession)

Fulton GB: Sex education: some issues and answers, J Sch Health, May 1970. (Discussion of the issues and organizations opposed to sexuality education a decade ago; extremely useful in comparing present with past issues)

Hallenbeck M: How to serve successfully on a textbook selection committee, Am Sch Board J, Aug 1980. (Suggested guidelines and policy tips for selecting books for schools)

Morris BM: The real issues in education as seen by a journalist on the far right, Phi Delta Kappan, May 1980. (Excellent discussion of the issues and concerns of the new right as seen by one of their members; "must" reading to understand this position)

Park JC: Preachers, politics, and public education: a review of right-wing pressures against public schooling in America, Phi Delta Kappan, May 1980. (Comprehensive discussion of the workings and constituency of the new right; addresses implications to education)

Parker B: Your schools may be the next battlefield in the crusade against "improper" textbooks, Am Sch Board, June 1979. (Excellent description of the opposing points of view)

Parker B: Leadership: political battles offer you the challenge of a lifetime, Exec Educator **3**(8):24, 1980. (Describes ways special interest groups gain control of meetings and organizations and how to deal with them)

Parker B: National groups can light fires in your own backyard, Exec Educator, Aug 1980. (Excellent awareness article on the highly organized special interest groups; describes the networking capabilities)

Quackenbush M and Villarreal S: Does AIDS hurt? Educating young children about AIDS, Santa Cruz, 1988, Network Publications. (A book for teachers and parents of young children about AIDS. It includes an extensive section of children's questions and possible answers in terms understandable by children. Additionally, one chapter illustrates how AIDS education can be woven into early elementary school classroom activities.)

Scales P: Barriers to sex education, J Sch Health **50**(8):337, 1980. (Includes useful descriptions of strategies communities can use to overcome the barriers to sexuality education)

Sex education in the public schools, J Sch Health, April 1981. (A special issue containing 24 articles about sexuality education in the schools)

United States Department of Education: What works: schools without drugs, 1986. (A booklet, free of charge, that outlines the proposed methods for a complete community-wide effort to rid schools of drugs.)

CHAPTER 9

A Scope and Sequence Plan for Elementary School Health Instruction

When you finish this chapter, you should be able to:

- **Identify objectives appropriate for an elementary school level of interest in health education.**

- **Develop measurable objectives, the content of which is appropriate to the abilities of a given level of elementary health education.**

- **Explain objectives in a scope and sequence increase in complexity to address the developmental capacity of children ages 6 through 12.**

Planning the scope and sequence of health teaching is a critical step in curriculum development. A scope and sequence plan serves as the framework for structuring teaching and learning at every grade level. *Scope* here refers to what health content areas will be addressed and is presented as the vertical axis of Table 9-1. *Sequence* specifies *when* each content area will be studied and even *how* it is to be addressed as implicit in the objectives. The plan for sequence is explicit in the progression provided in the headings of Table 9-1.

Scope and sequence development is more critical in elementary school than in high school, since it must address about 9 years of a child's school life. Decisions governing scope

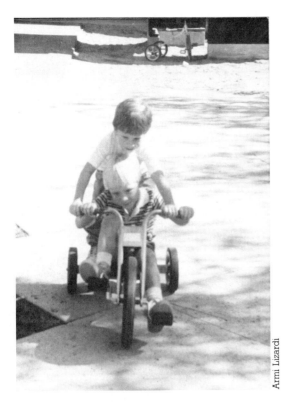

Armi Luzardi

and sequence ordinarily are made by administrators, once the sources of curriculum have been studied. Ideally, however, these decisions are made with the advice and participation of teachers, students, parents, and other significant community members. This involvement is essential to identify the needs and interests of the youngsters for whom the program is intended; it ensures the support of the community and builds bridges of communication between the school and community.

This chapter presents an example of a scope and sequence plan appropriate for health education from kindergarten to grade 8. The sequence of these objectives follows that of the plan explained in Chapter 4. Each objective provides a clue to the intended content and is appropriate for the abilities that can be expected of children of that age. These are curriculum-level objectives, which are broadly designed to afford teachers flexibility in lesson planning while serving as a stabilizing frame of reference and means of maintaining consistency among approaches used. Objectives in each area move from simple to complex and from concrete to abstract. However, the most abstract content to be mastered and behaviors expected from students are at the high school and college levels.

Although this scope and sequence plan is but one of many possible arrangements, it is consistent with current recommendations relative to comprehensive school health education at the elementary and middle school levels.

The content areas used in this scope and sequence plan and brief descriptions are as follows. More specific content indications for kindergarten to grade 3, grades 4 to 6, and grades 7 and 8 are presented in chapters 10, 12, and 14 respectively.

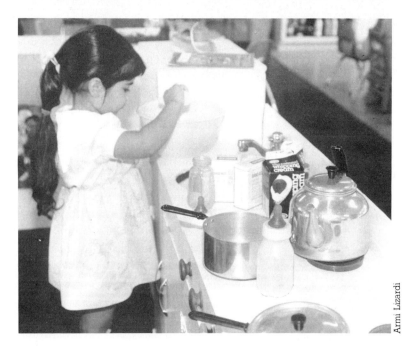

Armi Lizardi

1. *Personal health and fitness:* the development of positive health care habits, including grooming, cleanliness, physical fitness, and other habits that maintain the structure and function of the body and promote overall wellness.
2. *Mental and emotional health:* the individual's achievement of a positive self-concept and social awareness; understanding and managing emotions; the ability to apply problem-solving skills; respecting the rights of others to be different; and acceptance of responsibility for one's own health.
3. *Family life:* the roles and interactions of individuals within the family; the responsibilities and privileges of various family members; the physical, mental, and social progression through the life cycle from birth to death; and the communication necessary in families.
4. *Nutrition:* sources and characteristics of food; the importance of eating a variety of foods from each food group; the components of a balanced diet; the potential influence of food fads on nutrition; and the differences in nutritional requirements of individuals of varying ages, body types, and activity levels; and the difference in nutritional qualities of foods within a food group.
5. *Disease prevention and control:* differences between illness and wellness; factors that lead to the development of diseases and disorders; ways to control and prevent the spread of diseases; and appropriate courses of action when disease is suspected.
6. *Accident prevention and safety:* the identification and elimination of hazards; reasons for safety rules in the home, school, and community; basic first-aid procedures; obtaining help in emergencies; and the hazards of risk-taking behavior.
7. *Consumer health:* the identification of various health services and health-related products; the forces that influence the selection of a health product or service; the criteria used when making these selections; and evaluation of commercial appeals motivating the purchase of health-related products and services.

8. *Use and abuse of drugs:* the beneficial and appropriate uses of drugs and medications, as well as the harmful and inappropriate uses; reasons why people abuse drugs; laws regulating the sale of drugs; and the impact of peer pressure on the decision to abuse drugs.

9. *Environmental health:* ways to conserve natural resources and prevent environmental pollution; ways people can work together to improve the environment; and ways the environment enhances mental, physical, and social health.

10. *Community health:* the characteristics of a healthy community; the services of various health agencies; the role of various health workers; and community health career opportunities.

The scope and sequence plan in Table 9-1 is included to provide examples of objectives. Although the plan is not exhaustive, it does demonstrate the range of possible objectives appropriate at the various grade levels. Additionally, because objectives form the cornerstone for the development of teaching plans, several have been selected from the scope and sequence at every level to illustrate learning opportunities (Chapters 11, 13, and 15). Each plan includes learning opportunities that describe one possible way to achieve the selected objective. The objectives selected are identified by an asterisk in Table 9-1. Learning opportunities and fully developed lessons for the primary level (kindergarten to grade 3) are found in Chapter 11, those for the intermediate level (grades 4 to 6) in Chapter 13, and those for the middle school level (grades 6 to 8) in Chapter 15. You will notice an overlap with regard to grade 6, which is found in both the intermediate grouping and the middle school grouping. This occurs because grade 6 can be found in either setting depending on the district's preference.

As evidenced by the scope and sequence plan in Table 9-1, the depth and breadth of health information covered in the elementary school is vast. To complicate matters, "facts" change rapidly as research continues in health science. What is believed to be true one day may be proved wrong the next. Therefore it is impossible for one text to include all the pertinent health facts an elementary school teacher might need. The kinds of health topics and content that would be appropriate for the elementary school teacher to address in each of the 10 content areas are described in following chapters. Most likely further research is necessary for the teacher to feel comfortable with the subject matter when teaching health, so readings in each of the 10 areas are given in the bibliography at the end of the book. Since specific factual information is constantly changing, a school or college librarian could be of help in locating the most current information on a specific topic before preparing lesson plans.

TABLE 9-1. A scope and sequence plan

Content area		Student objectives by grade levels		
	K and 1	2 and 3	4 to 6	7 and 8
Personal health and fitness	The student 1. Names health habits that protect self and others* 2. Explains the importance of regular visits to health advisers 3. Explains why daily dental care is essential for the growth and development of teeth	The student 1. Describes how decision making affects personal health practices 2. Interprets the relationship of personal health care habits to optimum growth and development 3. Identifies physical, mental, and social benefits of good health 4. Explains the importance of health screening procedures	The student 1. Explains how personal health behavior is influenced by friends and family members* 2. Describes the relationship of personal health behavior to the optimum structure and functioning of the body 3. Explains the relationship of physical fitness to sound body function	The student 1. Analyzes the relationship between food choices and fitness 2. Proposes personal health care and fitness programs to meet individual needs and interests* 3. Compares immediate and long-range effects of personal health care choices and behaviors
Mental and emotional health	The student 1. Names positive personality characteristics 2. Describes experiences that elicit different emotions 3. Differentiates between pleasant and unpleasant emotions	The student 1. Classifies social behaviors as acceptable or unacceptable 2. Describes ways actions or words can make one feel different emotions 3. Illustrates ways to show friendship*	The student 1. Explains the relationship between physical well-being and mental and emotional health 2. Identifies positive and negative effects of stress 3. Synthesizes acceptable ways to deal with strong negative emotions*	The student 1. Identifies constructive ways to manage stress* 2. Analyzes the influence of peer pressure on health choices 3. Describes the importance of setting realistic goals 4. Explains the interrelationship among physical, mental and emotional, and social well-being

*These objectives are illustrated by sample learning opportunities in Chapters 11, 13, and 15.

Continued.

TABLE 9-1. A scope and sequence plan—cont'd

Content area		Student objectives by grade levels			
		K and 1	2 and 3	4 to 6	7 and 8
Family life		The student 1. Describes the meaning of family 2. Explains the role of various family members 3. Lists ways family members can work together as a unit 4. Explains that all living things come from other living things	The student 1. Identifies responsibilities and privileges of various family members 2. Explains ways family membership changes* 3. Describes the importance of consideration among family members	The student 1. Proposes ways to solve conflicts with friends and family members 2. Interprets changes in social activities as family members mature 3. Describes the progression of the individual through the life cycle from birth to death 4. Identifies growth and developmental characteristics common in puberty*	The student 1. Predicts physical, mental and emotional, and social changes that occur during adolescence 2. Explains why growth is individual, although in many ways predictable 3. Describes the reproductive processes* 4. Identifies social and cultural factors in the development of responsible health behavior
Nutrition		The student 1. Explains the importance of a nutritious breakfast 2. Identifies a variety of nutritious foods 3. Lists different characteristics of food*	The student 1. Explains the importance of eating a variety of foods 2. Identifies foods according to food groups. 3. Proposes food combinations that provide a balanced meal 4. Explains how foods with limited nutritional value are related to growth and development	The student 1. Identifies factors that influence personal food choices 2. Classifies foods according to their major nutrients 3. Analyzes the nutritional worth of food choices for meals and snacks* 4. Explains reasons for differences in nutritional requirements from person to person	The student 1. Evaluates diets appropriate for individual needs 2. Explains the relationship between calorie intake and level of activity to body weight* 3. Analyzes nutritional value of food in fad diets 4. Predicts long-range outcomes of poor food choices

Disease prevention and control	The student 1. Explains the difference between illness and wellness* 2. Identifies ways to prevent the spread of disease 3. Explains the importance of health checkups and screening procedures	The student 1. Differentiates between communicable diseases and other diseases 2. Illustrates ways the body fights disease 3. Explains the role of immunizations in the control of disease 4. Describes health actions that can hasten recovery from disease	The student 1. Identifies factors that may cause diseases and disorders 2. Differentiates between control of communicable diseases and of noncommunicable diseases* 3. Explains the contribution of science to the detection, prevention, and control of disease	The student 1. Analyzes the relationship of personal life-style choices to disease prevention* 2. Identifies the symptoms of diseases common among youth 3. Explains the effects of disease on individuals, families, and communities 4. Describes appropriate courses of action when a disease is suspected
Accident prevention and safety	The student 1. Defines the meaning of a hazard 2. Explains the importance of safety rules 3. Describes safe behavior when going to and coming home from school	The student 1. Explains how to obtain help in an emergency 2. Illustrates basic first aid for minor injuries* 3. Identifies potential hazards at home, school, and community	The student 1. Differentiates between hazards and accidents 2. Evaluates actions of bicycle riders 3. Concludes personal responsibilities for reducing hazards and preventing accidents 4. Illustrates basic first aid for stopped breathing*	The student 1. Proposes a home safety program* 2. Illustrates standard first-aid procedures in life-threatening situations 3. Compares risk-taking behavior to the causation of accidents

Continued.

*These objectives are illustrated by sample learning opportunites in Chapters 11, 13, and 15.

TABLE 9-1. A scope and sequence plan—cont'd

	Student objectives by grade levels			
Content area	**K and 1**	**2 and 3**	**4 to 6**	**7 and 8**
Consumer health	The student 1. Names people who help promote and protect health* 2. Lists products commonly purchased for health-related purposes 3. Explains the function of advertising in promoting sale of health products	The student 1. Differentiates between health products and services 2. Explains the relationship between health consumers and health providers 3. Identifies reasons that people choose health products commonly found in the home	The student 1. Analyzes information provided on health product labels 2. Names sources of reliable health information and services 3. Describes appeals that promote the sale of foods and medications used by children* 4. Differentiates between health quackery and licensed health care	The student 1. Analyzes methods used to promote health products and services 2. Compares scientific and faddish bases for choices among health products 3. Describes the function of consumer-protection agencies 4. Identifies criteria for the selection of an appropriate health adviser*
Use and abuse of drugs	The student 1. Defines the meaning of drug use and abuse 2. Names hazardous substances people use or abuse 3. Explains reasons for consulting adults before using an unknown substance	The student 1. Interprets methods for identifying potentially hazardous substances* 2. Describes the difference between the use and abuse of drugs 3. Explains why some people avoid certain mood modifiers such as tobacco and alcohol	The student 1. Identifies the effects and hazards associated with the use of any drug 2. Explains reasons for laws regulating the use of drugs* 3. Analyzes reasons that some people abuse drugs	The student 1. Predicts the effects of certain drugs on physical, mental and social functioning 2. Analyzes the factors motivating individuals to use or abuse drugs 3. Evaluates the significance of peer pressure on the decision to abuse drugs*

Environmental health	The student 1. Identifies environmental (air, land, and water) pollution* 2. Lists ways individuals can help keep their surroundings clean	The student 1. Identifies ways to conserve natural resources 2. Describes ways to work with others to help provide a healthful environment	The student 1. Describes ways that improving the environment can enhance physical, social, and mental health 2. Identifies causes of and ways to prevent environmental pollution*	The student 1. Analyzes ways individuals and communities can promote a healthful and safe environment 2. Evaluates the efforts of community groups and agencies in improving and protecting the environment*
Community health	The student 1. Identifies familiar community health workers (health helpers) 2. Explains the role of various health workers in the community	The student 1. Describes characteristics of a healthy community 2. Lists services provided by community health agencies and organizations	The student 1. Illustrates ways community members work together to solve problems 2. Lists ways to help agencies in the promotion of health 3. Identifies career opportunities in the health field*	The student 1. Describes community efforts to prevent and control disease 2. Concludes that individual participation is essential if community health activities are to be successful* 3. Contrasts the functions of various health concerned specialists

*These objectives are illustrated by sample learning opportunities in Chapters 11, 13, and 15.

TABLE 9-2. Where to introduce AIDS information

Content area	Student objectives by grade levels			
	K and 1	**2 and 3**	**4 to 6**	**7 and 8**
Disease prevention and control	The student †1. Explains the difference between illness and wellness †2. Identifies ways to prevent the spread of disease †3. Explains the importance of health checkups and screening procedures	The student †1. Differentiates between communicable diseases and other diseases 2. Illustrates ways the body fights disease 3. Explains the role of immunizations in the control of disease 4. Describes health actions that can hasten recovery from disease	The student *1. Identifies factors that may cause diseases and disorders *2. Differentiates between control of communicable diseases and noncommunicable diseases *3. Explains the contribution of science to the detection, prevention, and control of disease	The student *1. Analyzes the relationship of personal life-style choices to disease prevention 2. Identifies the symptoms of diseases common among youth *3. Explains the effects of disease on individuals, families, and communities *4. Describes appropriate courses of action when a disease is suspected

†Indicates foundational learning opportunities for understanding AIDS.
*Indicates where specific information about AIDS can be presented.

HOW DO WE DEAL WITH INFORMATION ABOUT AIDS?

Certainly the AIDS crisis demonstrates that health information changes quickly. A well-planned curriculum is flexible enough to integrate new information as it appears. In the case of AIDS, basic health instruction does not deal specially with the disease or with specific methods to prevent HIV infection. In the lower grades, instruction deals with all diseases, and prevention techniques are generic to disease in general. Students in later grades are able to deal with more specific information about AIDS and its prevention; however, this assumes that basic foundational lessons have already been experienced by students. The objectives in Table 9-2, taken from Table 9-1, illustrate places in the curriculum where AIDS information can be addressed. The early grades help to provide a conceptual foundation for study in later grades where more specific information about AIDS, HIV infection, and prevention techniques can be introduced.

EXERCISES

1. Contact your state department of education or a school district office to find out if a scope and sequence chart for health education is currently being used. (These charts often are called *state frameworks*.) Find out how these charts are distributed in your state and how the chart was developed. If it was done by committee, who was on the committee? Was that committee representative of teachers, administrators, and community members? Draw some conclusions regarding the development and use of the scope and sequence plan that you have examined.

2. Using the learning opportunities in Chapters 11, 13, and 15 as a model, develop accompanying teaching plans for selected objectives not fully developed in this text. (Those which have accompanying learning opportunities are identified by an asterisk in Table 9-1.)

3. Develop expanded content for an objective. Use library references for the most current factual information.

CHAPTER 10

Content Appropriate for Primary Level Students

When you finish this chapter you should be able to:

- **Describe appropriate content in ten areas of health education for students in grades K through 3.**

- **Select content appropriate for health instruction relative to the needs and interests of selected primary school age children.**

- **Match information in chapter corresponding to content component of an instructional objective designed for a given primary school grade.**

This chapter presents content appropriate for children in grades K through 3 in ten health areas. Since the audience for the information in this chapter is young children, the concepts addressed are basic, providing a necessary foundation of health knowledge. The complexity and depth of information will increase as children move from kindergarten to grade three. And, since children's needs, interests and base level knowledge differ from area to area (even from district to district within the same city), teachers will need to modify the health content addressed as directed by district guidelines. Particular attention to developmental levels and interests can also serve as a guide in planning classroom activities.

PERSONAL HEALTH

Recognizing, valuing and adopting good health practices at an early age help children establish the foundation for a healthful life style as adults. Personal health goes beyond cleanliness and hygiene to the affective dimensions of feeling good about practices that promote health and fitness. Good health is a personal responsibility. It is the individual who makes the daily decisions in life that promote or adversely affect health. A child's health status is in a state of constant change, the desired goal being that children adopt habits that promote general health throughout their lifetimes. Certainly it is not possible to be in a state of "excellent" health at all times in one's life, but it is possible to be working consistently toward the highest possible level of wellness as determined by hereditary and environmental factors.

Cleanliness

Clean hands, clothes, and eating utensils help to prevent the spread of disease. Washing with soap and water helps to kill the germs that cause disease. Simple rinsing with water is not adequate. Thorough washing will kill most germs that may have been picked up on the hands. It is particularly important to wash hands before eating or preparing foods. Additionally, being clean is a pleasant feeling for many people. Good grooming, including maintaining clean, neat hair and trimmed fingernails, wearing clean clothes and bathing regularly not only promotes health but is socially desirable.

It is also important to avoid sharing items that can carry germs. Combs, brushes, toothbrushes, towels, tissues, cups, glasses, and other eating utensils can be the means of transmitting disease from one person to another. Before using any of these items, children should be sure that such items have been properly cleaned, particularly those borrowed from others.

What to Wear?

Dressing appropriately for the weather is an important practice for primary level children. While the body does a good job of regulating temperature, it is necessary to help by wearing the correct clothing for different weather situations.

- Warm or hot weather—Lightweight clothes made of materials that "breathe" such as cotton are best. This type of clothing allows perspiration to dry on the skin and cool the body.
- Rainy, cool weather—Clothes that repel water and keep the feet and underclothing dry are important. When clothing next to the body gets wet, its effectiveness in maintaining body heat is diminished.
- Cold weather—Wearing several layers of clothes causes warm air to be trapped between the layers for added protection against heat loss. Some kinds of clothing

are specially designed for cold weather, such as jackets with insulating materials like feathers or wool. In cold weather, gloves or mittens should be worn and the head covered with a warm hat. A hat is especially needful because the body loses heat rapidly from the head. Gloves or mittens should not be allowed to get wet, for then they will not protect against the cold.

Sleep and Rest

Children in elementary school need anywhere from eight to eleven hours of sleep per night. The actual amount of sleep needed is different for each individual and usually decreases with age. Lack of adequate sleep will interfere with a child's ability to learn and achieve.

Fatigue can be physical or mental. Knowing how to relax after play or stressful events is an important skill and should be related to personal interests. Engaging in "quiet time" activities that are enjoyable and restful can be healthful for children. These could include:

- reading
- daydreaming
- playing with puzzles
- watching TV
- drawing
- creative writing
- listening to music
- going to the movies

Exercise

Physical fitness is an important component of health. Physical exercise can become an integral part of everyone's life. In order for exercise to be incorporated into an individual's lifestyle, it should be fun and interesting. Anyone, regardless of physical ability, can establish a regular exercise regime that will be beneficial. Exercises for children should be age-appropri-

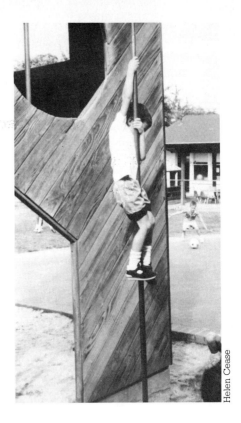

Helen Cease

ate, building upon coordination skills and including a variety of activities that involve all parts of the body.

Dental Health

Dental health is a major topic at the primary level. Establishing correct and consistent toothbrushing and flossing habits can help prevent dental caries, which in previous years was a frequent health problem in children. Flossing and toothbrushing help to prevent the build up of plaque on the teeth. Plaque is a film of bacteria that grows and is enhanced by the presence of sugar in the mouth. If allowed to build up on the teeth, plaque will break through the tough enamel layer and attack the softer tissue underneath, forming a cavity.

BASIC PARTS OF A GOOD EXERCISE ROUTINE

A good exercise workout should include:

Warm-Up Activities—These are the "get ready" activities. They help get muscles stretched and ready for more vigorous movement. Some possible warm-up activities you might provide your students include:

- Toe reaches—Sit on the floor with the legs stretched apart and straight. Slowly bend and reach for the right ankle. Stretch as far as possible without straining and count to ten. DO NOT BOUNCE. Alternate to the other ankle. Do several sets of toe reaches up to ten.
- Side stretches—Stand in a comfortable stance. Stretch arms up and bend at the side slowly. Count to ten as you stretch. DO NOT BOUNCE. Straighten up and bend to the other side. Do several sets of the side stretches up to ten.

Aerobic Activities—These are activities that exercise not only the skeletal muscles, but major body organs, the heart and lungs. Aerobic activities get the heart pumping blood (and therefore oxygen) to all parts of the body. To be effective, an aerobic activity should be sustained. Some examples of aerobic activities for children include:

- running
- jumping and hopping
- bike riding
- jumping rope
- skating
- swimming
- climbing

Cool Down Activities—Similar to warm-up activities, these are the "slow down" activities. Instead of stopping vigorous aerobic activity abruptly, stretching and balance activities are recommended.

- Knee pull—Lie on the floor on your back and pull one knee up to your chest as you bend your leg. Hold your knee close to the chest and count to ten. Alternate with the other knee. Repeat several times with each leg.
- One-foot balance—Stand in a comfortable position. Stretch your arms out straight to the sides. Slowly lift one leg and balance for a count of ten. Repeat with alternate legs up to five times.

FLOSSING TECHNIQUES

- Floss the teeth before you brush them
- To floss the teeth, break off about a foot and a half of dental floss and wind most of it around one of your middle fingers.
- Wind the remaining floss around the middle finger of the other hand.
- Steady the floss between your hands with your thumbs and forefingers.
- Leave about 1¼ inches of floss between your thumbs to go between your teeth.
- Move the floss between your teeth and gently guide it into the space between your tooth and gum.
- Bend the floss toward each tooth as you scrape the floss up and down against the sides.
- Do the same thing for *each pair* of teeth, *using a new piece of floss as needed.*

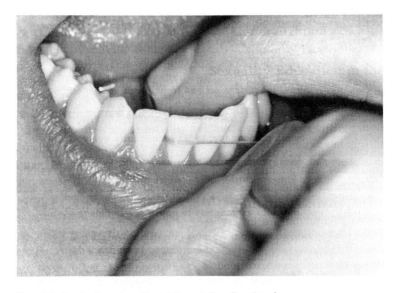

Copyright by the American Dental Association. Reprinted by permission.

BRUSHING TEETH

- Starting with the brush near the gum line, use the top surface of the brush in a back and forth motion.
  a. Brush the outside surfaces of the upper teeth.
  b. Brush the outside surfaces of the lower teeth.
  c. Brush the tops of the upper and lower teeth.
  d. Brush the inside surfaces of the upper and lower teeth.
- Using the tip of the brush and brushing gently with an up and down motion, brush the inside surface of the top front teeth and the bottom front teeth.
- Then rinse the mouth with water.

While there are several different methods suggested for brushing teeth, one good way is described below. Always use a flat, soft-bristled toothbrush.

Flossing and brushing are desired after every meal, but it is not always possible. At least once a day is recommended. Special care should be taken to brush after eating foods containing sugar. While it is obvious that cakes, candies and cookies are high in sugar, other foods such as apples, raisins, and oranges also contain sugar.

Young children need practice in the techniques for effective brushing and flossing. Using oversized models of teeth and toothbrushes to demonstrate the techniques is both fun and informative for children. If invited, dentists and dental hygienists will often be willing to come to primary level classrooms to provide such instruction.

Children in the primary grades will be losing primary teeth and cutting permanent teeth. This is a normal process of the body that proceeds on a child's individual timetable. Comparisons between and among children should be discouraged with the explanation that each child will lose primary teeth whenever the body is ready for this to occur.

The Body and Its Care

At the primary level, children explore the five senses and the functions of taste, touch, sight, hearing, and smell. The senses enhance the quality of life and help keep one safe. Keeping the body parts associated with the senses healthy is important in helping a person to stay in touch with the environment. At the primary level, care of the eyes and ears is of *particular importance* because the individual can take concrete steps to ensure the health of these two sensory areas. Most school districts across the country arrange for screening of sight and hearing as a part of the primary grade experience. This screening provides a unique opportunity for the students to receive instruction related to experiences they will have.

The function and importance of other body parts are addressed at the primary level. The human organism is an amazing and efficient machine. Although certain characteristics such as our height and body type are determined by genetic factors, the student needs to learn ways to make the most of his or her physical potential.

- The skeleton—The bones in the skeleton provide a framework for the body and protect the internal organs. Over 200 bones

---

CARE OF THE EYES

- Protect eyes from chemicals and foreign objects.
- Keep dirty hands, materials, or objects away from the eyes.
- Inform an adult of any discomfort of the eyes.

CARE OF THE EARS

- Protect ears from loud noises.
- Never put anything into the ears.
- Report any discomfort or drainage to an adult.

---

make up the human skeleton. The skeleton has joints that allow the "framework" to move. Bones are made of an inner layer of spongy tissue surrounded by hard bony material. The maturation process, exercise, and what we eat influence the quality of a person's bone tissue.

- The muscles—Some muscles attach to bones and as they contract, move the bones in different ways. These muscles are called "voluntary" because they work as an outcome of conscious commands sent by the brain. Other muscles like those of the heart are called "involuntary" because they work without our having to think about them. The heart is a powerful organ and contracts to send blood throughout the body to deliver oxygen and nutrients (food) to the cells and to pick up waste materials. The heart muscle pumps the body's blood throughout the body, during the process of which waste materials are absorbed so they can later be excreted.

MENTAL HEALTH

It is as essential to establish mental health practices at an early age as it is to practice good physical health habits. The difficulty in teach-

ing in this area arises from the fact that good mental health habits are more difficult to define and, to a large degree, are more dependent upon the individual. Mental health learning tasks issues for the primary grades center around the development of a positive self-concept and the ability to express emotions comfortably and appropriately.

Self-Concept

One's major emotional need is to feel good about oneself. Everyone needs to have a positive feeling about who he or she is, as well as a strong sense of self-worth. A positive sense of self gives one the necessary confidence to try new things and to reach out to other people. Primary school children should be given the opportunity to experience a sense of accomplishment in a nonthreatening atmosphere. Even though the earliest links to self-concept develop in the home, you can do much to encourage your students to appreciate their individual strengths.

Feelings

Everyone has emotions, or feelings. Some of these feelings are pleasant, while others are uncomfortable. It is normal to experience a wide variety of emotions daily. Common emotions include happiness, sadness, anger, fear, love, frustration, and embarrassment. Feelings are often linked to circumstances that occur in life. Let your students explore the situations that cause certain emotions in them. For example, a hug from a mother may induce feelings of happiness and love, whereas not being allowed outside to play with friends may induce anger or frustration. Feelings are not "good" or "bad" but are reactions to what is happening to one.

Feelings can cause physical changes as well. Being aware of these changes can help a person to recognize emotions. When anger is experienced, an upset stomach or a headache may be the body's response. Being called on in class may make hearts speed up and palms perspire.

Behavior

An important step in the socialization process of children is learning what is acceptable and unacceptable behavior in response to feelings. They need opportunities to practice expression of emotions in a positive way. For example, if I am angry with my brother, rather than fight with him I may hit my pillow or run around the block. Children can understand that everyone loses control of his or her emotions to some degree now and then. This is normal and acceptable as long as losing control does not become the pattern of one's life style.

Students should understand that breaking rules usually is considered unacceptable behavior in our society. Help them to explore the reasons for rules (regarding behavior) in our society. In particular arrange for them to study school rules and share information on the kinds of rules that may be enforced at home.

Friendship

Friendship is an important concept for primary level children to understand. Many different kinds of friendship can be studied, such as friendship with classmates, family members, neighbors, and pets. Students should learn how to be a good friend and to become aware of some of the characteristics that encourage friendship. Friends share toys, treat each other courteously, can be trusted with a secret, and help each other out when necessary.

We Are Alike

All people are alike in certain ways. We all have a body made up of the same organs and parts. We all feel happy sometimes, and other times sad. Sometimes we want to be with our friends and sometimes we want to be alone. We all need to feel accepted and like to be kissed and hugged by the people we love. When children realize the similarities of people's experiences and needs, they can begin to enjoy the feeling of being a part of the "human community."

We Are Different

One of the nicest things about our world is that everyone is different in some ways. Children vary in their abilities, skills, appearance, and talents. Climbing a tree may be easy for Lauren and difficult for Brad. Brad may be better at drawing pictures. Children need opportunities to explore these kinds of individual differences and to appreciate the uniqueness of self and others. When their special differences are accepted, children feel better about themselves and are better able to appreciate those of others.

FAMILY LIFE

During early elementary school years family life focuses on the development of an appreciation of self and the family unit. Be careful to avoid stereotyping roles according to gender. Most school districts have standards for educational materials that require a nonsexist presentation of characters in stories. For example physicians should not be shown only as male or nurses only as female. A word of caution, however: Before other aspects of any family life curriculum are taught, parental, administrative, and school board approval must be considered and obtained.

Families

The membership and makeup of families are constantly changing. Families typically consist of parents, siblings, grandparents, aunts, uncles, and cousins. Pets often are considered family members as well. However, everyone's family is unique. It is common for children to be in a family having only one parent. Various factors affect membership in a family: divorce, the birth of a child, death, and remarriage are common events in our society. In any case, when there is a change in the makeup of the family, adjustment is required of family members. It is necessary in such cases for families to try to work out any problems and to be considerate of each other.

Role of the Family

All families fulfill a most important role in society; they provide stability and emotional support for the family members. In a family, no matter how large or small, the acceptance of individual responsibilities is necessary. Often these responsibilities are related to the age of the family member. For example, a parent or both parents may be responsible for working to support the family. Children often are assigned tasks around the home to help keep it neat and clean. Sometimes they help out with cooking and cleaning up after meals. Young children have fewer responsibilities; however, older children often have more privileges. Staying up later,

going places with friends, and having a private bedroom are common privileges earned as children grow in the ability to take on responsibility.

All Living Things Reproduce

All living things reproduce the same type of living organisms. Dogs have puppies, cats have kittens, and humans have infants. All human infants change as they grow into adults. They get bigger, stronger, and abler as they grow up. A boy will grow up to be a man and a girl to be a woman. It is always the mother who has a baby; however, once a baby has been born, both mother and father are responsible for its care. After the baby has grown to be a child and then an adult, he or she can be a parent too. And, when these children have children, he or she will become a grandparent. Some people live long enough to have great-grandchildren.

Abuse Prevention

Sexual abuse of children is a disturbing actuality. Children who are abused feel guilty and often feel that there is no one who can help. Children must realize that they have the right to accept or reject affection, and that strangers or even people they know can be harmful. If a child is approached by a stranger offering a gift, a promise, a ride, or a threat, they should say "no" or run to tell someone they trust. As a part of primary grade instruction, children can be helped to identify people who can be trusted in dealing with personal or family difficulties.

NUTRITION

One of the most important principles for the maintenance of good health is that the body needs a variety of foods daily to promote growth, repair, and optimum functioning. Because eating is an everyday activity, most people don't stop to think about what they use to fuel their bodies. The eating habits of children are often poor. Habits of their families, lack of knowledge, hurried family life styles, and peer-influenced attitudes about eating are contributing factors. Even primary grade children can learn to think of wise "food choices" rather than thoughtless consumption of fad foods or sugar-laden snacks.

Food Choices

The foods we eat often have too little to do with the nutritional needs of the body. The food choices of parents and siblings usually become the food choices of younger children. These eating patterns, once established, are not easy to change. For example, having potato chips and pop as an after school snack is not easily changed instead to eating a banana and drinking a glass of milk. Food customs are also influenced by ethnic beliefs and traditions. Jews may refrain from eating pork or may eat only kosher foods. Mexican-Americans may prefer tortillas to sliced bread, Young children enjoy learning about different cultures and trying new foods. Primary grade students can learn to identify the various characteristics of foods by tasting them. Foods are sweet, salty, crunchy, watery, greasy, smooth, sour, or chewy. Often, school dietitians will cooperate with teachers in offering new foods or featuring "special" foods for taste tests to complement nutrition information presented in the classroom.

The Food Groups

Foods are often grouped according to their major nutrient content. A balanced daily diet includes something from each food group.

- The *Milk group* contains all milk products (except butter and sour cream), such as cheeses and yogurt. These foods are good sources of protein, calcium, riboflavin, vitamin A, and phosphorus. Children need three servings per day from the milk group.
- The *Meat or Protein group* contains red meat, fish, poultry, dried beans and peas, and nuts. Protein, iron, and minerals come from this group. Elementary children need two servings from this group daily.
- The *Vegetable and Fruit group* contains all vegetables and fruits, including the juices. Potatoes are in the vegetable and fruit group, as are apples, oranges, green beans, peas, carrots, lettuce, tomatoes, corn, and squash. Foods from this group are most nutritious when eaten fresh or only lightly cooked. Overcooking removes much of the vitamins from foods. The fruit and vegetable group provides vitamins A and C as well as fiber. Four servings from this group are recommended daily for children.
- The *Bread and Cereal* group (sometimes called the *Cereal and Grain group*) contains all breads, cereals (hot and cold), muffins, tortillas, corn bread, rice, noodles, pasta, grits, and pizza crust. These foods provide thiamin, iron, niacin, and carbohydrates. Whole grain breads and cereals also provide fiber. Children need four servings daily from this group.
- There are many other foods that are not in one of these four food groups and sometimes are called *Extra* or *Other* foods. These include candies, cakes, pies, cookies, chips, soft drinks, mustard, mayonnaise, relishes, and almost all sauces. Extra foods contain many calories but few nutrients. For this reason, they should not be eaten in place of a food in a food group and

should be minimized in diets of people who are overweight.

Breakfast

It is particularly important to eat a nutritious and balanced breakfast because it has been so long since the evening meal, and breakfast (meaning "break the fast") is the first meal of every day. It helps get the body going and provides energy for the day's work and play. Sometimes the foods thought of as "breakfast foods" are not appealing in the morning. But there are no "right" or "wrong" foods for breakfast. The important thing to remember is to eat foods from at least three of the food groups. For example, if a menu of toast, scrambled egg, and orange juice is not appealing, a peanut butter and jelly sandwich with a glass of milk may be more tempting while fulfilling the same nutritional needs.

Snacks

Elementary school children often have more control over snack foods than foods that are served as part of a meal. Snacks can provide needed nutrients if wise choices are made. Children enjoy sharing ideas about healthful snacks and can be taught to apply the same basic principles of nutrition to choosing snacks as when planning meals.

DISEASE PREVENTION AND CONTROL

The nature, spread, and prevention of diseases are topics that can be too sophisticated for young children. However, it is important for them to learn the difference between illness and wellness, ways to avoid certain illnesses, and what steps should be taken if an illness occurs. Although all people are exposed to disease-producing organisms from time to time, persons who take care to get proper sleep, eat balanced diets, engage in regular exercise programs, and manage the stress in their lives are less susceptible to illness. If these persons do become ill, they recuperate more quickly. Even persons with chronic diseases can enhance their health by adhering to sound personal health practices.

Categories of Disease

There are two basic categories of disease: communicable, which can be spread from one person to another directly or indirectly; and noncommunicable, which cannot be spread to others. Communicable diseases are caused by pathogens that invade the body and disrupt the body functions. Pathogens, commonly called "germs", are very small organisms that live almost anywhere but are usually invisible to the naked eye. Although the term "germ" is not scientifically correct, it is much easier for the primary level child to learn. More specific and correct terminology can be introduced at the intermediate level.

Prevention of Communicable Disease

The purpose of many recommended health habits is to prevent the spread of disease. Cleanliness habits are important because soap and water deter the growth of potentially harmful germs.

Noncommunicable Disease

Noncommunicable diseases result from life style patterns, the social and physical environment, and any genetic weaknesses that we inherit. For example, people who smoke or chew tobacco are more likely to develop lung and oral cancer. Other noncommunicable diseases like cyctic fibrosis can be inherited from one's parents. People can not be immunized against noncommunicable diseases and they cannot change their heredity; however, in some

---

CLEANLINESS HABITS

- Hands should be washed after using the bathroom and before eating.
- Fresh fruits and vegetables should be washed before eating them.
- Cooking and eating utensils should be washed with hot, soapy water after each use.
- Hairbrushes, combs, towels, and toothbrushes should be used by only one person and should be washed regularly to help prevent the spread of disease or harmful organisms (e.g., lice).
- Covering one's nose and mouth when coughing or sneezing helps to prevent germs from spraying into the air where they can infect someone else.
- Used tissues should be disposed of immediately after use.
- Staying at home in bed when feeling ill prevents contact with others who can "catch" the disease and helps speed recovery and prevents transmission of the illness to others.

---

cases they can develop life styles that reduce their chances of developing certain noncommunicable diseases. An example of a life style change is beginning an exercise program to reduce the risk of heart attack. In other cases, like epilepsy and diabetes, there are medical treatments that can help minimize or control the effects or severity of the disease.

When a Person is Ill

The human body has a wonderful ability to fight off disease when it is attacked by pathogens. Certain substances in the body, called antibodies, can prevent disease by killing pathogens and prevent or hasten recovery from a disease. However, whenever a person feels ill, it is important to take certain steps to help existing antibodies do their job. Getting extra rest, which often means staying out of school and not playing with friends, and drinking plenty of liquids are both helpful practices. Sometimes a doctor's advice and help are needed as well. Medicines may be prescribed to help the body fight a disease.

ACCIDENT PREVENTION AND SAFETY

Accidents are the primary cause of death among children. Many people mistakenly believe that accidents are merely bad luck. Most accidents, however, are the result of risk-taking behaviors or the failure to follow safety precautions. Knowing and following safety rules helps children avoid hazardous situations and prevent accidents. Rules are made to help reduce the chance of getting into hazardous situations, not to curtail fun.

It is essential that children know what to do if an emergency situation arises. Even primary grade children can learn to apply simple first aid procedures in the case of minor injuries.

Lessons learned in class can be reinforced by distributing safety checklists for students to take home and share with parents. To help correct potential hazards and to help *ensure* a safe environment, these things can be done at home:

- Store knives in a special knife holder or a separate compartment away from the other utensils.

- Keep matches out of the reach of small children.
- Use matches only in the presence of an adult.
- Keep pot handles turned so they don't protrude past the stove top.
- Do not run electrical cords under carpets or rugs.
- Promptly wipe up any spills on the floor.
- Keep toys and other items off stairways and floors.
- Avoid the use of slippery throw rugs.
- Install smoke detectors.
- Practice evacuation routes in case of fire.
- Store dangerous chemicals and medicines out of the reach of children.

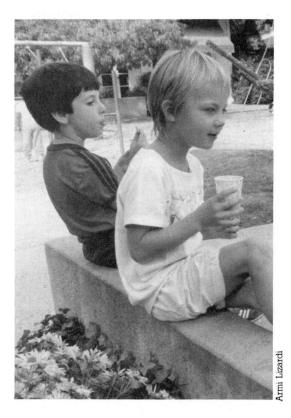

Armi Lizardi

Injuries that occur during recreational activities can be avoided by following these rules for play:

Around Water:
- Never swim alone or without adult supervision.
- Don't play in or around flooded drainage ditches or other bodies of water.
- Wear life preservers when riding in a boat.

On Land:
- Be cautious when walking or climbing in unfamiliar terrain.
- Be alert around all moving vehicles.
- Wear the proper protective equipment for sports.

When Riding a Bike:
- Ride bicycles on the right side of the road, with the traffic.
- Obey all traffic signs when bike riding.
- When bicycle riding, look both ways before crossing an intersection.
- Use hand signals to indicate turns when riding a bicycle.
- Wear white if riding a bike at night.

Even when rules are followed, accidents still occur, and it is important for students to know what to do in such an emergency. The first step is to call for help. An adult always should be summoned to the scene. It may be necessary to call for help loudly, to run to the house next door, or to telephone for help. Children should know how to use the telephone in case of an emergency. The front of the phone book contains the procedure for the local area. Necessary information to give when calling for help includes:

- your exact location
- type of injuries
- the telephone number from which the call is being made.

It is always a good idea to ask the person to

repeat the above information to be sure it has been correctly recorded.

Young children can learn to apply simple first aid measures for minor injuries. For cuts and scratches they can wash the wound with soap and water and cover it with a dressing if necessary. For minor burns they can learn to apply cold water until the burning sensation ceases and never to put butter or oil on a burn. For bleeding, children can be instructed to hold some clean material firmly on the wound and ask someone to seek help. Classroom practice of simulated emergencies gives primary children experience in dealing with common emergencies and reinforces ability to perform simple first-aid procedures.

CONSUMER HEALTH

Everyone is a consumer, including children in primary grades. Consumers can select from a variety of services and products that may directly or indirectly affect health. The goal of consumer health instruction is to help children make informed choices about the worth of products and services that may positively or negatively affect their health.

Products

Examples of health-related products are medicines, toothpaste, shampoo, foods, vitamins, and first-aid products. Youngsters are constantly barraged with advertising that seeks to promote purchase of a particular health product. This persuasion begins to be encountered at a very young age, usually through Saturday morning television commercials. Products related to health whose advertisements are often specifically directed toward children include vitamins, cereals, candies, and soft drinks. The purpose of advertising is to convince the consumer that a particular product is needed or desirable, as well as the best choice. Often advertising sells people on the idea that they need a certain product they have never before thought about. Even at this age, children can learn that the goal of advertising is sales, not health. They can also recognize the fact that advertised products are not necessarily worthwhile, useful, or even harmless. Yet advertising directed toward children is very effective, even though they themselves do not do the actual purchasing. Early health instruction can make a difference in their children's acceptance of advertising claims.

Services

Services include the advice and help of physicians, nurses, druggists, and dentists. These people are often called "health care providers." Primary grade children can become acquainted with the work of professionals who provide health services as well as with the kinds of equipment and procedures these persons employ. Appropriate instructions about "trips to the doctor and dentist" can help to allay fears that children may have and help primary students view health professionals as "helpers."

USE AND ABUSE OF DRUGS

In the early years content in this area should focus on safe behavior around unknown substances. Students in primary grades need to learn that drugs are medicines which should be used only under the direction of a medical advisor or parent. Some people choose to use certain mood modifiers such as tobacco and alcohol. These substances should not be used by children. Since these kinds of mood modifiers can be harmful to health, many adults also choose to avoid these substances.

Unknown Substances

Harmful substances may have special markings or special containers to help children identify them as dangerous. A skull and crossbones or "Mr. Yuk" stickers, showing a face with a sour expression, indicate that the contents are poisonous. Stickers of this sort often are available from local poison control centers. Some students may have them in their home already on products such as cleaners, medicines, and insecticides. Young children can learn the reasons for consulting adults before tasting or using an unknown substance and the importance of keeping harmful products locked out of reach of younger sisters and brothers.

Medicines

Medicines are drugs that are used to help sick people get well. Some medicines can be bought freely off the drugstore or market shelf (over-the-counter). Other medicines can be purchased only with a prescription from a doctor or dentist. If the medicine is a prescription drug, it will include special information on the label:

- prescription number
- name of the medication and the dosage
- directions for taking the medicine (how much, how often)
- name of the doctor
- patient's name
- date of its issue

Over-the-counter medicines will also have certain information on the label or package:

- indications (reasons for taking the medication)
- directions for taking the medicine
- warnings
- ingredients (chemicals that are in the medicine)

Whether the medicine is over-the-counter or prescription, it is very important to read and follow the directions and to pay attention to any warnings that appear on the label. Primary grade students should only take drugs from parents or medical care providers and should never medicate themselves. Medicines can help when used correctly but can be harmful when used incorrectly.

Mood Modifiers

Drugs are not always used to help sick people get well. Some drugs like alcohol and tobacco are used as mood modifiers (they cause a change in the way people think and feel). Mood modifiers can be harmful to health and certain ones should not be used at all by children. Primary grade students can learn how mood modifiers of this kind affect the body and the reasons why people choose to avoid some such substances.

ENVIRONMENTAL HEALTH

Students at this level can grasp the notion that the environment is everything around them. Air, land, and water are the three basic aspects of the environment. It is possible for the environment to get "dirty." This is called environmental pollution. A healthful, enjoyable environment is a clean one. As persons who live on Earth, children must become aware that they have certain responsibilities as well as rights. For example, it is important to try to conserve natural resources, such as water.

The Air

The air can be polluted by automobile and airplane exhaust, industrial *smoke,* forest fires, and even cigarette smoke. When the air becomes polluted, a variety of health problems can result. Some people sneeze and cough or develop breathing difficulties. Others who are more sensitive may have more serious health problems. People should always try to follow laws requiring that cars and industrial smokestacks have special devices to help filter out the pollutants. It is also helpful to walk, ride a bicycle, or use car pools and public transportation whenever possible.

The Land

The land is increasingly polluted by litter and graffiti (writing on walls in public places). As more and more people inhabit the earth, more and more trash is produced. Disposing of all of this waste is an increasing problem. Also, we are using more convenience products like paper plates, cups, and disposable diapers. These products add to the problem. Some of our waste can be recycled, other wastes cannot. Children easily learn to accept personal responsibility for the proper disposal of trash and deposit of aluminum and glass containers in recycling bins. These actions help keep schools, homes, and communities free of litter.

The Water

Water can become polluted by dumping trash and chemicals into lakes, streams, and other waterways. This pollution can make the water unsafe to drink and can also kill plants and animals that live in the water. Certain laws have been enacted to help prevent further pollution of our water resources. Efforts are underway to clean up waterways that have already been polluted; however, it is much better to prevent such pollution before it occurs. Clean-up efforts are expensive, time-consuming, and in some cases can never return a body of water to its natural state. Children must become aware that it is people who are destroying the Earth's water environment. People can protect the environment if they will, and "people" is you, and me.

COMMUNITY HEALTH

Health resources exist within each community to deal with the solution of community-wide health problems. Students in the primary grades *can learn the names and roles of persons* who promote and protect the health of others as well as the places that provide health services in the community.

Health Helpers

People who help promote and protect the health of others are often called "health helpers" by primary level teachers. Health helpers are all members of the community who contribute to the health of others, including physicians, nurses, dentists, hygienists, fire fighters, police officers, crossing guards, pharmacists, parents, and teachers. Each person plays a different role in the protection and promotion of the health of community members. Physicians, nurses, and pharmacists help people who are sick become well. Fire fighters, police officers, and crossing guards help people stay safe or help them if they are hurt. Parents and teachers teach children how to stay healthy and safe.

Health Facilities

In most communities there are various *places* that provide health services, including the local hospital, pharmacy, clinic, dental office, doctor's office, and public health department. Schools, fire departments, and police departments, also may provide certain health services like emergency care and health and safety education. People who work in these places help keep others safe and healthy.

REFERENCES

American National Red Cross: Standard first aid and personal safety, Garden City, NY, 1979, Doubleday & Company, Inc.

Branden N: The psychology of self-esteem, New York, 1983, Bantam Books.

Cooper K: Fitness: the facts, Milwaukee, 1981, Ideals Publishing, (615) 885-8270.

Food, Washington, DC, US Department of Agriculture.

Growing Healthy, New York, 1986, National Center for Health Education.

Hales D and Williams B: An invitation to health, Menlo Park, Calif, 1986, The Benjamin/Cummings Publishing Co, Inc.

Maslow A: Motivation and personality, ed 3, New York, 1987, Harper & Row.

Pipes P: Nutrition in infancy and childhood, St Louis, 1989, The CV Mosby Co.

Richmond J and Pounds E: You and your health, Glenview, Ill, 1981, Scott Foresman and Co.

US Public Health Service: Healthy people: the surgeon general's report on health promotion and disease prevention, Washington, DC, 1979, US Department of Health and Human Services.

Van Amerongen C: The way things work book of the body, New York, 1979, Simon and Schuster.

CHAPTER 11

Primary Level Teaching Activity Ideas

When you finish this chapter, you should be able to:

■ **Develop learning opportunities in elementary health education for grades K through 3 which appropriately provide practice of the behavior and content specified in an objective.**

This chapter presents several fully developed health education learning opportunities for kindergarten and grade 1 and grades 2 and 3. They are designed to meet objectives selected from the scope and sequence plan in Chapter 9. Each learning opportunity described here is an example of *one way* to meet a stated objective. Ten different teaching plans are presented, one in each of the ten content areas identified in the scope and sequence plan in Chapter 9. Although the teaching plans in this chapter do not represent a comprehensive health education program, they do provide examples for the creation of plans when developing one.

The teaching plans are divided into those for kindergarten and grade 1 or grades 2 and 3 because the capabilities of the kindergarten child are so different from those of the third-grade child. These learning opportunities are based on the assumption that the second- and third-grade students have some reading and writing abilities. The teaching techniques have been chosen carefully for their appropriateness for the primary-level child. The components of the teaching plan, as well as the teaching technique used, are consistent with those described in Part I. Plans include an objective, content

generalizations, ("big ideas"), initiation activity, sample learning activities, and an evaluation activity that relates directly back to the objective. The last activity in each lesson serves as the culminating activity. Other helpful components included are vocabulary words, integration possibilities, lists of specific materials and resources needed, and actual worksheets, patterns, and bulletin board examples for the activities described.

In developing these learning opportunities the teachability was of primary concern. Although each has a beginning, a logical sequence, and an ending that evaluates the stated objectives, the activities are only *samples* of those that can be used. Teachers must add, delete, and modify activities to meet specific student needs. The actual time needed to teach the activities will vary for every classroom situation, and teachers will need to plan accordingly. It can be assumed, however, that several days will be required to complete all the activities included in each plan.

The activities described here show the interrelationships among health content areas. For instance, activities for disease prevention and control are also appropriate for personal health and fitness. Community health workers could be discussed in relation to community health, consumer health, accident prevention and safety, disease prevention and control, and so forth. This overlapping demonstrates the dynamic nature of health education content. A skilled teacher will recognize these interrelationships and use them to enhance classroom activities.

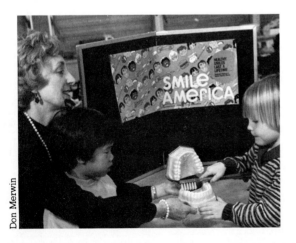

Don Merwin

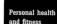

PERSONAL HEALTH AND FITNESS

Objective. The student names health habits that protect self and others.

Level. Kindergarten and grade 1

Integration. Art, writing, coming to conclusions

Content generalizations. The adoption of habits such as washing hands before eating, covering sneezes, using clean eating utensils, limiting or avoiding contact with sick people, and staying home from school when sick helps to keep diseases from spreading.

Vocabulary. Habits, health, protect

Initiation. ''Mystery Health Bag''
Fill a bag with items that often are used when practicing good health habits. Identify the bag as the ''Mystery Health Bag.'' Use a bag that will allow the students to feel the items when they handle the bag (such as a pillowcase, opaque plastic bag, or cloth bag). Place the bag in a prominent spot in the classroom, or set up a table display using the bag in the center and placing items around the bag as they are discussed. Printed name signs for the items can be made for the table display.

    Allow a student to feel the outside of the bag and guess what might be in it. Then pull out one item. Ask the students to identify the item and tell about its use. Supplement their answers as necessary. Repeat this for two or three items a day. Ask the students to bring items that might go into the ''Mystery Health Bag.''

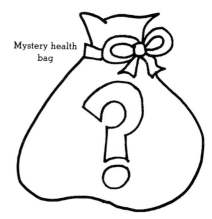

Mystery health bag

Materials
''Mystery Health Bag'' (pillowcase, plastic bag, or cloth bag)
Items for bag: brush, soap, toothbrush, shampoo, tissue, etc., raincoat
Optional: name signs for each item for table display

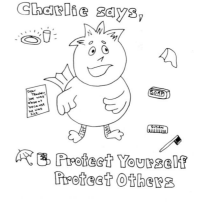

Charlie says, Protect Yourself Protect Others

Activities

1. Protect Yourself, Protect Others
Put up a bulletin board display, *Protect Yourself, Protect Others,* with Charlie Chicken in the center. Point out to the students that there are many things we can do to help stop the spread of disease, and these habits all help protect us and others.

Materials
Bulletin board display: *Protect Yourself, Protect Others* (p. 254)

2. "Dirty and Clean" Demonstrations

Rotate small groups of students into a demonstration on washing hands, preferably near the sink. Explain to them that proper handwashing is an important health habit to learn.

a. Have students rub a few drops of salad oil on their hands.

b. Then they should sprinkle some cinnamon on their hands.

c. Have them wash their hands with water *only,* and observe. Ask, "Are your hands clean?" (No.) "How can you tell?" (The cinnamon is still sticking.) "Does washing hands with just water get hands clean?" (No.)

d. Now have the children wash their hands with *soap* and water, and observe. Ask, "Are your hands clean now?" (Yes.) "How can you tell?" (The cinnamon is gone; they smell clean.) Ask the students to draw some conclusions on proper hand washing. Ask, "What is needed to get hands clean?" (Soap and water.)

e. Ask the students if they know when to wash their hands. Explain that sometimes we cannot see the dirt, so it is important to wash hands even if they do not look dirty, particularly before we handle or eat food and after we go to the bathroom.

f. Ask the students if they can think of other items that should be washed before use. (Dishes, utensils, combs, brushes, clothes.) Ask, "What is the best way to get these objects clean?" (Wash them with soap and water.)

3. Covering Sneezes Experiment

In another small group conduct an experiment about covering sneezes. Fill a spray bottle with water with several drops of red food coloring added, and set it on the table. Hand students the worksheet, *Look What Happens When I Don't Cover My Sneeze!,* and have them draw pictures of their family members or friends on the worksheet. Then have the students take turns using the spray bottle to squirt their picture. Suggest that they say "ah choo" when they squirt. Then the students should try it again using a tissue to "catch" the spray. (More than one tissue may be needed if the spray is strong.) This activity could be done outside.

Materials

Sink or bucket of water
Salad oil (not in glass container)
Cinnamon
Paper towels

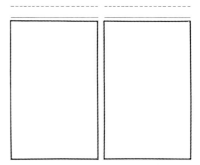

LOOK WHAT HAPPENS WHEN
I DON'T COVER MY SNEEZE!

Directions:

1. Draw a member of your family.
2. Draw a friend.
3. Write their names above their pictures.

Materials

Spray bottle with colored water (use several drops of *red* food coloring)
Tissues
Worksheet: *Look What Happens When I Don't Cover My Sneeze!* (p. 255)

4. Well Child, Sick Child
   a. Use a flannel board and figures to create a story about a child who went to school while sick, exposing the other children to the germs that caused their illness.
   b. Ask the children to remember what Charlie says (protect yourself, protect others). Ask them how staying home when you are sick "protects." (It protects others from catching the sickness you have and protects you from getting sicker.) Ask how they can protect themselves from someone who is sick. (Stay away; do not play with a sick friend.)

Materials

Flannel board figures: *Charlie Chicken* (p. 254); *Well child* (p. 256); *Sick child* (p. 257)

Flannel board

Personal health and fitness

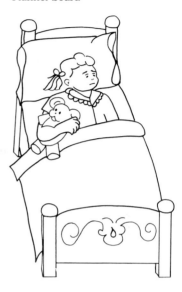

Evaluation. "Charlie Chicken Says"

Have the students form a circle. Start out saying, "Charlie Chicken says . . .," and then all the students say "Protect yourself, protect others." Then spin a bottle in the middle of the circle, and the student to whom the bottle is pointing must name a protective habit studied. Then that student spins the bottle, and the next student replies. They may name a habit mentioned before but not the one named the turn before. Continue until all students have participated.

NOTE: You may wish to use a name other than Charlie if there is a student with that name in the class. (The same applies to other worksheets.)

Materials

Bottle

Bulletin board display

PROTECT YOURSELF, PROTECT OTHERS

Directions: Make a large Charlie Chicken for the center of the board. Fill the board with good health habits and pictures that represent each habit. Leave enough room to mount student work.

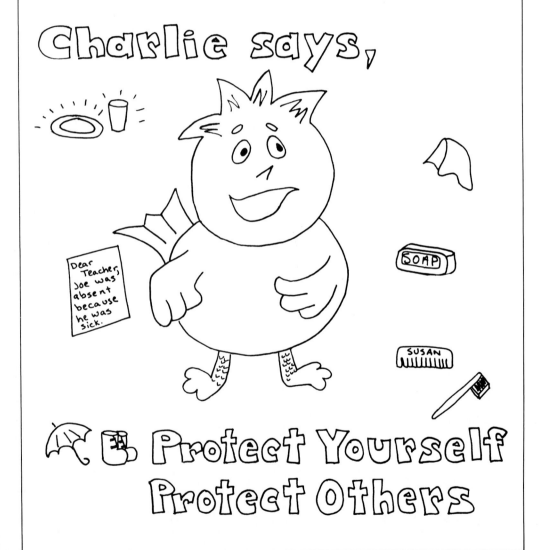

Worksheet   Name _____

LOOK WHAT HAPPENS WHEN
I DON'T COVER MY SNEEZE!

Directions:

1. Draw a member of your family.
2. Draw a friend.
3. Write their names above their pictures.

_____   _____

_ _ _ _ _ _ _ _ _ _ _ _ _   _ _ _ _ _ _ _ _ _ _ _ _ _

_____   _____

Flannel board figures

WELL CHILD

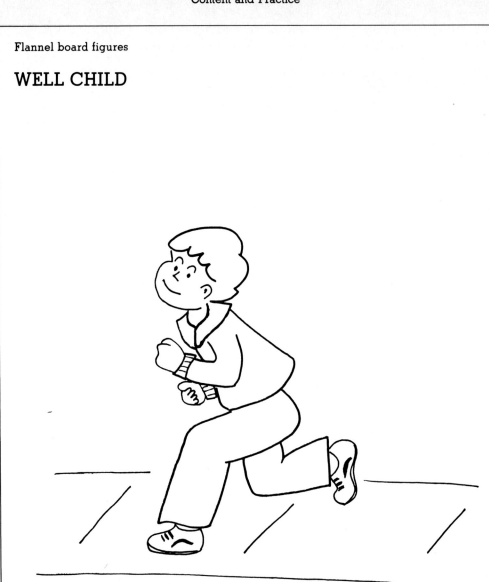

Flannel board figures

SICK CHILD

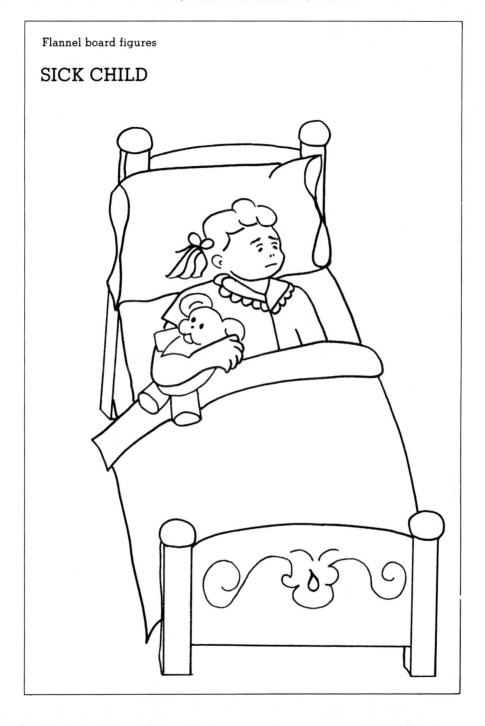

MENTAL AND EMOTIONAL HEALTH

Objective. The student illustrates ways to show friendship.

Level. Grades 2 and 3

Integration. Reading, problem solving, drawing conclusions

Content generalizations. Friendship is an important aspect of life, but it has a different meaning for different people. A friend is usually someone you like to be with. Often friends enjoy the same activities, like playing baseball, roller skating, going shopping, or dancing. A friend is also someone who cares and helps out when needed. A friend is someone who shares possessions (such as toys, books, and cookies) and feelings (such as happiness, sadness, frustration, and anger).

Vocabulary. Friendship, feelings, sharing, enjoyment

Initiation. Reporting on ''Friendship''
Ask for a volunteer to play the part of a television reporter. This student is to go around the room surveying other students in the class about friendship. The question should be something like, ''What are some ways that you show you are a friend?''

Activities. Ask the students if anyone in their survey said that sharing was a part of friendship. If no one did, explain that many people believe it is a very important part of being a friend. Tell them that the next activity will give them an opportunity to practice sharing.

1. A Crayon for my Friend
   a. Allow the students to form groups of five or six. A working space is needed for each group, ideally a table with six chairs or a table the children can stand around. Each working space should have six crayons of different colors: red, green, blue, yellow, orange, and purple.

Materials
Optional: prop microphone

A CRAYON FOR MY FRIEND
Directions: Color the crayons the correct color. Share crayons.

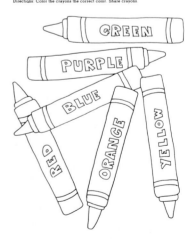

Materials
Crayons: red, green, blue, yellow, orange, and purple (1 set per group)
Worksheet: *A Crayon for My Friend* (p. 260)

b. Explain the task to the students before handing them the worksheets. The task is to color each crayon pictured on the worksheet the correct color. Since there are six children in a group and only six crayons, the members of the group will have to share the crayons for all to finish the worksheet.

c. Hand out the worksheet, *A Crayon for My Friend,* and circulate around the room, observing the sharing in each group. Stop at each group and ask how they are doing.

d. When everyone has finished, ask a person from each group to tell about his or her experiences with the activity. Ask the students, "What are some other ways that you share and show friendship?"

2. Showing Friendship

Tell the students they are going to practice some more ways to show friendship. Use the worksheet, *Showing Friendship,* which portrays a situation where friendship can be demonstrated. Students are to read about the picture and draw or write a way that the character in the picture could be a friend. Post the finished worksheets on the bulletin board.

Materials

Worksheet: *Showing Friendship*
   (p. 261)
Crayons

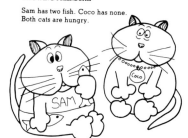

SHOWING FRIENDSHIP

Sam has two fish. Coco has none.
Both cats are hungry.

How can Sam be a friend? Draw or write below.

Evaluation. Friendship Mural

Have the students cooperatively make a large mural on friendship. Each student in the class must participate by painting one way to show friendship on the mural. Mount the mural in the classroom or hallway of the school.

Materials

Large piece of butcher paper
Poster paints

Worksheet   Name _____

A CRAYON FOR MY FRIEND

Directions: Color the crayons the correct color. Share crayons.

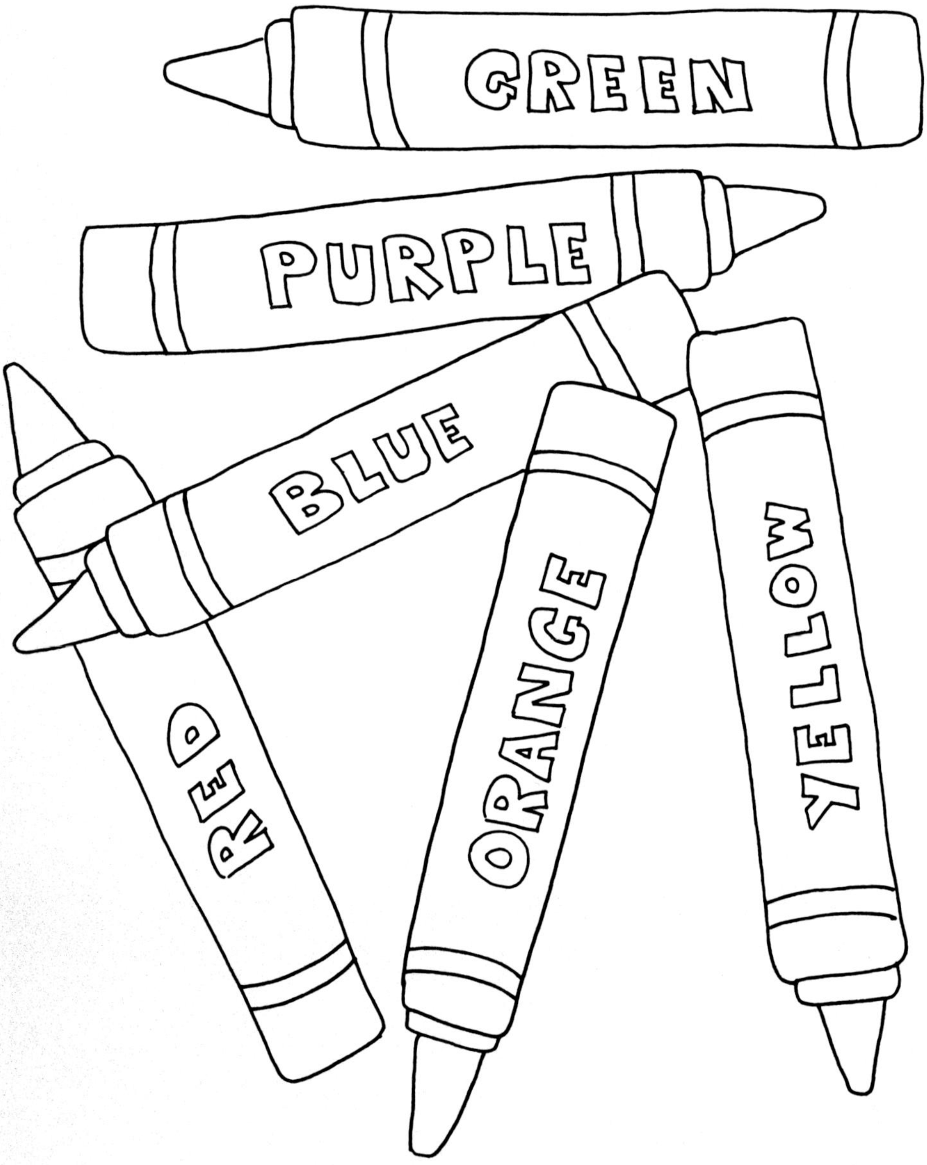

GREEN

PURPLE

BLUE

RED

ORANGE

YELLOW

Worksheet   Name _____

SHOWING FRIENDSHIP

Sam has two fish. Coco has none.
Both cats are hungry.

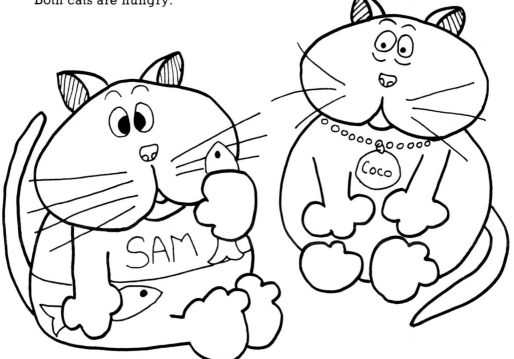

How can Sam be a friend? Draw or write below.

FAMILY LIFE

Objective. The student explains ways family membership changes.

Level. Grades 2 and 3

Integration. Mathematics, social studies, creative writing, art

Content generalizations. The membership of different families is varied, and the composition of an individual family is dynamic. Family membership can involve many combinations of people, such as mother, father, siblings, uncles, aunts, grandparents, and cousins. Many people consider pets to be family members too. The membership in any one family can grow from one to many members. The changes in the family are usually a result of marriage, birth, death, and divorce. Moving from one location to another also can affect family membership.

Materials
Worksheet: *Family Portrait* (p. 265)
Crayons

FAMILY PORTRAIT

MY FAMILY

Vocabulary. Family, increase, decrease

Initiation. Family Portrait

Ask the students, "What is a family?" After they have given their responses, explain that we are all part of a family, and everyone's family is different. Hand out the worksheet, *Family Portrait,* and ask the students to draw their family. (Some children will include pets.) Tell them to count the number of persons (and pets) in their family.

Ask the students if this number was always the same for their family, and if not, why it was different. (My little sister was born. My grandfather died. My parents got divorced. My mother remarried, and now I have a father and a stepfather.)

Activities

1. Our Families
   a. Construct a bulletin board display, *Our Families.*
      (1) Mount a class picture, individual school pictures, or both on a bulletin board.
      (2) Have the students mount their completed worksheets, *Family Portrait,* randomly around the class picture.

Materials
Class picture or individual school pictures
Worksheet: *Family Portrait* (completed) (p. 265) and/or actual family photographs brought from home
Scissors
Crayons
String

(3) Instruct them to draw, color, and cut out the same number as there are family members in their picture. When finished, they should mount their number next to the family portraits.

(4) Help the students connect a string from their picture in the class picture to their family portrait.

b. When finished with the bulletin board, ask the students to count and record on a piece of paper the number of families with two members, three members, four members, and so forth. Then ask which number was the most common and which was the least common. Finally, explain to the students that all families are unique and that there is no "right" number of members in a family.

2. The Story of Two Families

a. Tell the students they are going to meet two families: the Red Family and Blue Family. Prepare a flannel board with the two families side by side as follows.

Red Family	Blue Family
(mount pictures here)	(mount pictures here)

b. Read or present a story such as the following to the students. Have a student put pictures of the characters and their names on the flannel board as they are introduced and remove them as they leave.

TWO FAMILIES

I'd like you to meet two families: the Red Family and the Blue Family.

The Red Family is composed of Grandma Red and Rick, who lives with his Grandma. The Blue Family is composed of Father Blue, Mother Blue, and their daughter Beverly. How many people are in each family? [Place each number on the board.] Which family has more members? Which has less members?

One day Grandma Red received a telephone call from her daughter Dorothy and son-in-law Samuel. Dorothy and Samuel were moving to Grandma's town, where they have jobs. Grandma says, "Come live with Rick and me in our house. Join our family. We have plenty of room." So Samuel and Dorothy moved in with Grandma and Rick.

The Blue Family changed too. Mother Blue was pregnant—she was going to have a baby. One day Mother and Father Blue went to the hospital. When they returned home, they introduced Beverly to her new baby brother.

Materials

Flannel board

Pictures of family members (cut from magazines or group pictures)

Name signs for family members to mount on flannel board:

Grandma Red

Rick Red

Daughter Dorothy

Son-in-law Samuel

Mrs. Yellow

Mother Blue

Father Blue

Beverly Blue

Baby Blue

Various numbers to mount on flannel board

Now how many are in each family? Which family has more members? Which has fewer members? [Change the numbers on the board.]

Grandma Red got another telephone call. One of her oldest friends, Mrs. Lettie Yellow, said that her husband Mr. Yellow had died. Lettie Yellow said she did not like living by herself. Grandma Red said, "Come over and live with us. We have plenty of room." So her friend Lettie Yellow moved in too. How many are now in the Red Family? Which family has more members? Which has fewer? [Change the numbers on the board.]

c. Discussion questions
(1) Did the membership of the two families remain the same, increase, or decrease? (Both increased.)
(2) In what ways did family membership increase? (Birth, friends moved in, and relatives moved in.)
(3) How could family membership decrease? (Someone moves out when grown, to get a job, to go to school, or after getting married; or death.)

3. How the Green Family Changes
Then have the students write their own illustrated story about the Green Family. The Green Family changes from *three* members, to *two* members, and then to *four* members. Have the students draw a picture and write about the members of the Green Family in each stage—3, 2, and 4 members—and how the membership changed. (NOTE: Students may do each third of this assignment on three separate days.) Allow them time to tell the class or each other in small groups about their stories.

Materials
Paper
Pencils or crayons

FAMILIES CHANGE

Two people are new to this family. List two ways this *increase* might have happened.

1. _____
   _____
2. _____
   _____

List two ways this family might *decrease*.

1. _____
   _____
2. _____
   _____

Evaluation. Families Change
Each student should complete the worksheet, *Families Change,* and explain two ways family membership can increase and two ways it can decrease.

Materials
Worksheet: *Families Change* (p. 266)
Pencils

Name _____

Worksheet

FAMILY PORTRAIT

MY FAMILY

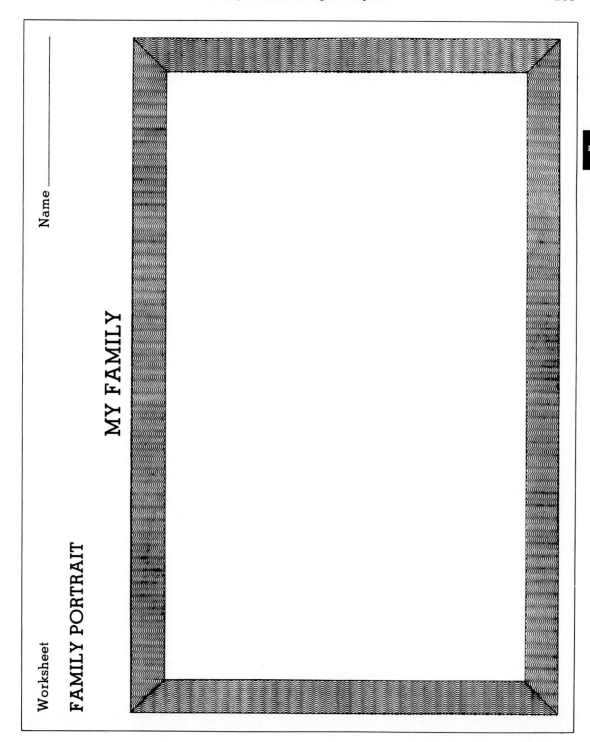

Family life

Worksheet   Name _____

FAMILIES CHANGE

Two people are new to this family. List two ways this *increase* might have happened.

1. _____

_____

2. _____

_____

List two ways this family might *decrease*.

1. _____

_____

2. _____

_____

NUTRITION

Objective. The student lists different characteristics of food.

Level. Kindergarten and grade 1

Integration. Color discrimination, reading readiness, art

Content generalizations. The characteristics that foods exhibit can be related to a person's likes and dislikes of different kinds of food. Taste, texture, smell, shape, and color often play a role in the selection of food.

Vocabulary. Salty, sweet, sour, rough, smooth, crunchy, slippery

Initiation. What Foods Can You Feel?

Pass a bag around to the students. Have them try to identify the food items within, without looking at the food. Instruct them to keep their ideas to themselves until everyone has had a chance to think about their guess. Then ask the students to identify different characteristics of the food item they observed. Ask questions like, ''Was the food rough or smooth?'' ''Did the food smell sweet or sour?'' ''Was the food long and narrow or round?'' and ''What is the food?''

NOTE: In this activity use a food that is easily identifiable by most students in shape, smell, or texture. Bananas, grapes, apples, pickles, or orange slices are good examples.

Materials
Paper bag
Food items: banana, grapes, pickle, apple,

Activities

1. Characteristics of Food
   a. Show pictures of different foods (from magazines or food models) or actual foods to demonstrate taste (salty, sweet, sour), texture (rough, smooth, crunchy, slippery), smell (sweet, sour), and color.
   b. Hold up three pictures of foods or food models of the same color (such as an apple, red jello, and a tomato). Ask ''How are these foods the same?'' (They are all red. ''How are they different?'' (They taste different: two are sweet, and one is not; one is crunchy; one is juicy.)

Materials
Pictures of foods from magazines or food models

c. Ask the students to draw a picture of another food that is red (e.g., strawberries, pizza, cherries, watermelon, beets, or spaghetti sauce). Then have each student show the picture to the class and tell about the food. (It is crunchy; it is sweet; it is juicy; it smells sour.)

Materials
Paper
Crayons

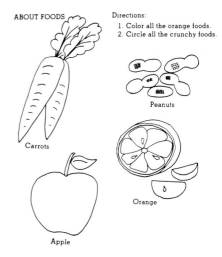

ABOUT FOODS

Directions:
1. Color all the orange foods.
2. Circle all the crunchy foods.

Peanuts

Carrots

Orange

Apple

2. About Foods
Hand out the worksheet, *About Foods*. Using crayons, students are to color the foods that are orange and circle the foods that are crunchy.

Materials
Orange crayons
Worksheet: *About Foods* (p. 270)

3. Three Dimensional Food Models
   a. Have the students make three-dimensional food models from butcher paper stapled together and stuffed with newspaper. Make the food larger than life, perhaps as large as the students. An alternative is to have them make clay models of food. It may be helpful to put the students into groups for this activity. Have parents, older students, or teacher aides help out in each group.
   b. Display the stuffed food models around the room. Ask students who worked on the model to tell about their food.

Materials
Butcher paper
Paints
Pencils
Staples
Scissors
Newspaper
Alternative: clay and paint

Evaluation. Name That Food
Play a simple game called "Name That Food." Begin by listing several characteristics of a food without naming the food. Continue describing the food until a student correctly guesses it. For example. "I am thinking of a food . . . it is red on the outside . . . it is crunchy . . . it is sweet . . . it is a fruit. . . . What is it?" (Apple.) Continue the game as time and the students' attention span permit.

Nutrition

Worksheet   Name_____

ABOUT FOODS

Directions:
1. Color all the orange foods.
2. Circle all the crunchy foods.

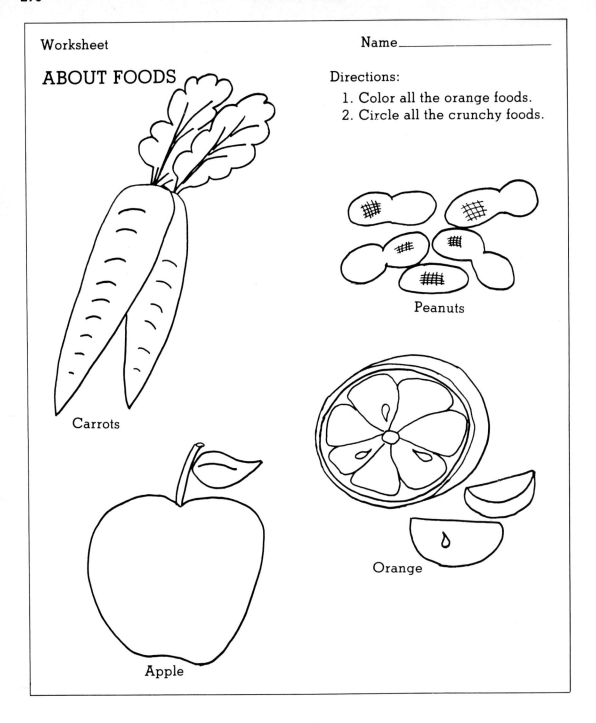

Peanuts

Carrots

Orange

Apple

DISEASE PREVENTION AND CONTROL

Objective. The student explains the difference between illness and wellness.

Level. Kindergarten and grade 1

Integration. Reading, writing, language arts

Content generalizations. Our degree of health may vary from day to day. Generally, when a person is ill, a disease, (severe or mild) is involved. The degree of illness or wellness usually affects the way we feel and the type of activities in which we can (or should) be involved. Most illnesses are accompanied by symptoms. If someone is ill, usually rest is recommended.

Vocabulary. Sick, ill, well, thermometer, fever, absent

Initiation. Being Absent
Read the following story, and follow up with the discussion questions.

BEING ABSENT

It was a beautiful Monday morning at school. When the school bell rang, Mrs. Owen opened the classroom door, and all the children in her first-grade class filed in. Mary noticed that the place where her friend Judy sat was empty. When Mrs. Owen called the roll, Judy did not answer. Mrs. Owen said Judy was absent. Mary wondered where she was.

Ask the following discussion questions:
1. Why do you think Judy was absent? (She was ill.)
2. Have any of you been absent? Why?
3. What kind of illness did you have?
4. How did you feel when you were ill?

Activities

1. Why Was Judy Absent?

   a. Continue the story started in the initiation.

WHY WAS JUDY ABSENT?

On Sunday Judy felt fine. She went to the park with her dog Tippi and played fetch. She and Tippi ran all the way home. Later Sunday night Judy started to cough; she felt tired and did not want to play with Tippi. Her dad felt her forehead with his hand and said. "You feel warm; maybe you have a fever. I'll take your temperature."

Sure enough, Judy's temperature was 101 degrees Fahrenheit. She had a fever. So her dad put her to bed and said, "You are sick, and you need to rest to get well." [NOTE: Decide if the use of a Fahrenheit or centigrade thermometer is more appropriate for the students in your class.]

The last time she had been sick, she had had to go to the doctor. She wondered if she would have to go again.

On Monday morning Judy's fever was down to 99 degrees Fahrenheit. Her mother said she should stay home from school until she was completely well again.

On Tuesday Judy's dad took her temperature again, and it was normal, so he said, "You may now go to school." Mary and Judy played as usual at school that day.

   b. Discussion questions
      (1) Why was Judy at school Tuesday and not Monday? (She was ill on Monday.)
      (2) Was it a good idea for Judy to stay home from school on Monday? (She still had a fever.)

2. Who Should Stay Home?

   Hand out and explain the worksheet *Who Should Stay Home?* (Maria is sneezing, feels tired, and has a fever; Donald feels good and full of energy and is happy.) Ask the children if they think either of the children should stay home from school. Have the students cut out the picture of the child who should stay home and paste that picture inside the house on the worksheet. Students then can take the worksheets home and explain them to their parents.

Materials

Worksheet: *Who Should Stay Home?*
  (p. 276)
Scissors
Paste or glue

WHO SHOULD STAY HOME?

Maria is sneezing.   Donald is smiling.
She feels tired.   He feels good.

Cut out the picture of the
child who should stay home.

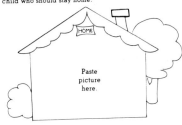

Paste
picture
here.

3. Reading a Giant Thermometer
   a. Show the children the *Giant Thermometer* (previously made from pattern.) Explain its purpose. Ask the children if anyone has ever had their temperature taken. Ask, "Has anyone ever had a fever? How did you know you had a fever?"
   b. Place the *Giant Thermometer* on the bulletin board. Tell the children that this thermometer reads "normal." Then show various pictures of well children and explain that they probably have normal temperatures and are not sick. Ask the children to try to think of activities they like to do when they are well. Ask, "Is it possible to do the things you like to do when you are sick? Why or why not?"

Materials

Pattern: *Giant Thermometer* (teacher made) (p. 277)

Pictures of well children having fun (skating, riding bicycles, playing games, etc.) from magazines or children's books

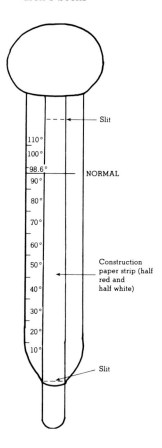

4. When We Are Well

   Send a note home to parents explaining that their child is learning about illness and wellness. Ask the parents if they could send a photograph of their child to school. The photograph should be of the child when he or she was well and preferably doing something enjoyable. When the photographs are brought from home, have the children mount them on a piece of construction paper. Then put all the photographs on the bulletin board next to the *Giant Thermometer* with the title, "When We Are Well." This activity could be done with pictures cut from magazines or drawn by students if the teacher determines that photographs from home will be difficult to obtain.

Evaluation. Who Is Well? Who Is Ill?

Hand out the worksheet, *Who Is Well? Who Is Ill?* Ask the students to identify the child who looks ill and to explain how they can tell. Help them complete the words *ill* and *well* on the worksheets. They should color the well child and circle the ill child.

Materials

Letter to parents
Construction paper
Photographs of students from home, if
  possible

Materials

Worksheet: *Who is Well? Who Is Ill?*
  (p. 278)
Crayons

Disease prevention and control

WHO IS WELL? WHO IS ILL?   Directions:
                                  1. Circle the ill child.
                                  2. Finish the words.
                                  3. Color the well child.

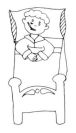 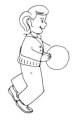

I_ _   We_ _

Worksheet   Name _____

WHO SHOULD STAY HOME?

Maria is sneezing.   Donald is smiling.
She feels tired.   He feels good.

sniff

Cut out the picture of the
child who should stay home.

HOME

Paste
picture
here.

Pattern

GIANT THERMOMETER

Directions:

1. Make a large thermometer out of white construction paper.

2. Mark the degrees in black.

3. Make a very large black line for 98.6° F (normal).

4. Make a long strip of construction paper, half red and half white.

5. Move it through the slits to demonstrate the way the thermometer works.

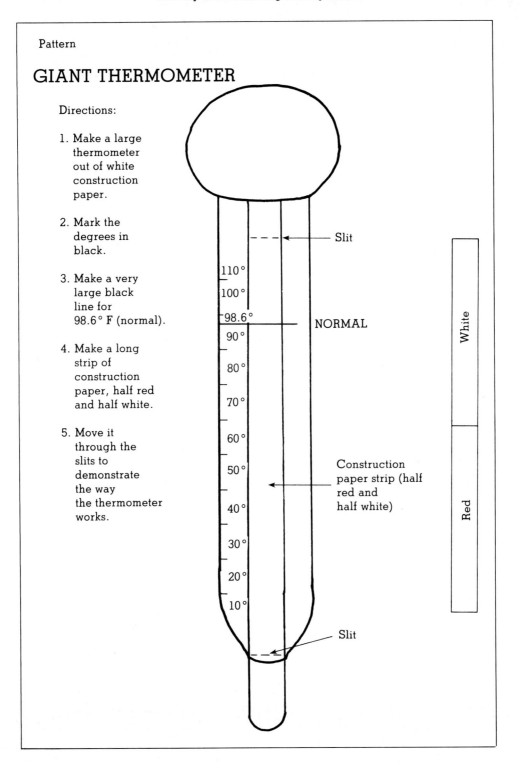

Slit

110°
100°
98.6°   NORMAL
90°
80°
70°
60°
50°   Construction paper strip (half red and half white)
40°
30°
20°
10°

Slit

White

Red

Worksheet   Name _____

WHO IS WELL? WHO IS ILL?

Directions:

1. Circle the ill child.
2. Finish the words.
3. Color the well child.

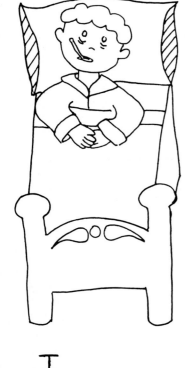

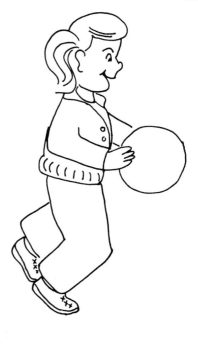

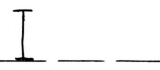

I __ __

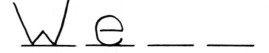

We __ __

ACCIDENT PREVENTION AND SAFETY

Objective. The student illustrates basic first aid for minor injuries.

Level. Grades 2 and 3

Integration. Writing, language arts, art

Content generalizations. First aid is the immediate care given to an injured or suddenly ill person. Those who give first aid must be trained specifically to know what to do, as well as what not to do. Basic first aid procedures include (1) wash wounds with soap and water; (2) apply direct pressure to stop bleeding; (3) treat minor burns with cool water; (4) always get help from an adult in an emergency situation or when an accident occurs; and (5) if a tooth is knocked out, save the tooth, and call the dentist immediately.

Vocabulary. First aid, pressure, adhesive tape, adhesive bandage, wound, sterile pad

Initiation. First-aid Box

Show the students a box covered with white paper with a red cross on the sides and top. Ask the students what they think might be inside a box like this. (Probably students will recognize the first-aid symbol and guess items such as bandages, first-aid cream, and adhesive tape.) Take out the items as they are guessed by students. Explain that the symbol on the box is recognized around the world. It means first aid to most people. First aid is the *first* help given to a person who is injured (hurt) or ill. It can be given to yourself or to another person, but help always should be asked of an adult as quickly as possible.

Materials

First-aid box (teacher-made)
Items to put in box: adhesive bandages, triangular bandages, sterile gauze pads, adhesive tape, first-aid cream

Activities

1. Four Accidents
   a. Following are four accident situations (stories). Use the same procedures for each story, and preferably do only one story a day.
   b. An option is to ask for student volunteers to dramatize the story, demonstrating the correct first-aid procedures.

Accident prevention and safety

BRANDON AND THE COOKIE SHEET

Brandon could smell cookies baking in the oven. His mother was making his favorite kind, oatmeal with raisins! He ran into the kitchen and saw them in the oven. They looked done to him, and his mother was on the telephone. He got the pot holder out of the drawer and opened the oven. He did not realize how heavy the cookie sheet was. He dropped the cookie sheet and burned his arm.

Ask students, ''What should be done?''

Brandon's mother ran into the kitchen. She saw that he had a minor burn on his arm. Immediately she lifted him up to the sink and ran *cool* water over the arm for a long time. That made Brandon's arm feel better. She looked at the arm very carefully and said, ''Brandon, you are very lucky. There are no blisters. We don't have to go to the doctor.''

Discussion questions
  (1) How did Brandon burn his arm? (He dropped a hot cookie sheet on his arm.)
  (2) What did Brandon's mother do? (She ran cool water from the faucet over his arm.)
  (3) What should Brandon do next time so he does not burn his arm? (Ask his mother or father for help when working in the kitchen.)

Hand out the worksheet, *Brandon and the Cookie Sheet,* and explain the directions. When the students are finished, allow them to tell about their pictures.

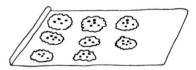

Materials
Worksheet: *Brandon and the Cookie Sheet* (p. 284)

JENNIFER AND THE ROLLER SKATES

Jennifer was at home alone while her Grandma, with whom she lives, went to buy groceries for lunch. Grandma said she would be back in about 10 minutes. Jennifer slipped on her roller skates and took a spin on the sidewalk. She tripped over some gravel, fell, and scraped her knee. Her knee did not bleed, but it was scraped and had gravel and dirt on the surface. The scrape was about the size of a quarter.

Ask students, "What should be done?"

Jennifer took off her skates and went into the house. She washed the scrape and the surrounding skin with soap and warm water. She dried the scrape with a clean cloth, and checked to make certain all the dirt and gravel was removed. Then she taped a sterile pad on the wound. When Grandma came home, Jennifer told her what had happened and how the wound had been cared for. Grandma said, "Why Jennifer, you could not have done any better!"

Discussion questions

(1) How did Jennifer care for her scraped knee? (Cleaned it with soap and warm water, dried it, and applied a sterile pad.)
(2) If the scrape had been smaller, about the size of a dime, what could Jennifer have used instead of a sterile pad and adhesive tape? (Adhesive bandage.)
(3) Ask students to identify the items Jennifer used from the display.

Materials

First-aid items to display: sterile pad, adhesive tape, adhesive bandage

Accident prevention
and safety

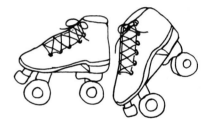

Hand out the worksheet, *Jennifer and the Roller Skates,* and explain the directions. When the students are finished, allow them to tell about their pictures.

Materials

Worksheet: *Jennifer and the Roller Skates* (p. 285)

TIMMY AND THE SWING SET

Shirley saw Timmy, the little boy who lived next door, playing on the swing set in his front yard. The swing accidently hit Timmy in the face, and his nose began to bleed. Frightened, Timmy yelled, "Help! My nose is bleeding!" and ran in circles while waving his arms.

Ask students, "What should be done?"

Shirley knew how to give Timmy immediate first aid for a nosebleed and went to help him. First she told him to sit down quietly. Then she gently applied pressure to the nostril that was bleeding. When Timmy was quietly sitting, she showed him how to apply the pressure to his nose himself. Then she knocked on the front door to tell his dad what had just happened. Timmy's dad sat with Timmy and told him to continue applying pressure while leaning slightly forward.

Timmy's Dad told Shirley, "Thank you for helping my son. You're a great neighbor who knew exactly what to do in this emergency." Timmy's nose stopped bleeding.

Discussion questions

  (1) What actions stopped Timmy's nose from bleeding? (Sitting down quietly, leaning slightly forward, and pinching the bleeding nostril.)

  (2) How can you stop your nose from bleeding? (Same actions, and tell a parent or teacher.)

Hand out the worksheet, *Timmy and the Swing Set,* and explain the directions. When the students are finished, allow them to tell about the pictures.

Materials

Worksheet: *Timmy and the Swing Set* (p. 286)

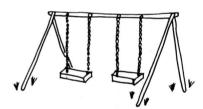

MEI LING AND THE SOFTBALL

When Mei Ling was playing softball one Saturday, the ball hit her in the mouth and knocked out one of her new front teeth. It was *not* a loose "baby" tooth, but a tight permanent tooth.

Ask students, "What should be done?"

Although Mei Ling was hurt, she knew exactly what to do. First, she found the tooth. She then wet a *clean* handkerchief at the drinking fountain and carefully wrapped the tooth in it. Mei Ling went home and told her mother, "My permanent tooth was knocked out. I wrapped it in this clean wet cloth."

Mei Ling's mother replied, "You knew exactly what to do. I'll call our dentist right away. I hope Dr. Palmer will be able to put your tooth back."

When Mei Ling and her mother arrived, Dr. Palmer said, "Yes! You have taken good care of this tooth and come to see me right away. I will be able to put Mei Ling's tooth back. You have helped save Mei Ling's tooth through good first aid."

Discussion questions

(1) How did Mei Ling and her mother help save Mei Ling's tooth? (Mei Ling found the tooth, placed it in a clean damp handkerchief, and told her mother right away; her mother brought Mei Ling and the tooth to the dentist right away.)

(2) It is best to wrap the tooth in a clean damp cloth. Mei Ling used her clean handkerchief. What else could have been used? (Clean damp paper towel, etc.)

(3) If no water, cloth, handkerchief, or paper towel had been available, what should Mei Ling have done? (She should have picked up the tooth with her hand and taken it home right away.)

Hand students the worksheet, *Mei Ling and the Softball,* and explain the directions. When they are finished, allow them to tell about their pictures.

2. Minor injuries bulletin board

Help students make a class bulletin board chart of minor injuries that happen in and out of school over the period of 1 week. For each injury record the type of first aid administered. Discuss with the students the appropriateness of the first-aid procedures administered for each injury. Then allow a child who has a minor injury to administer his or her own first aid with teacher supervision.

Accident prevention and safety

Materials

Worksheet: *Mei Ling and the Softball* (p. 287)

Evaluation

RANDY AND HIS BICYCLE

Randy was riding his bicycle home from school. He made the turn into his driveway too sharply and skidded and fell. When he looked at his elbow, it was bleeding and dirty. What should he do?

Have the students draw, demonstrate (act out), or write the proper first aid for Randy's injury. (He should wash the wound with soap and water, cover the wound with a bandage, and tell an adult what happened.)

Worksheet   Name_____

BRANDON AND THE COOKIE SHEET

1. What happened to Brandon in the kitchen?

_____

_____

_____

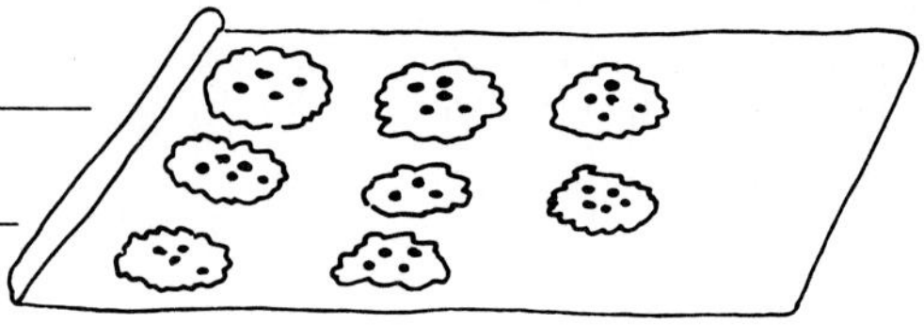

_____

_____

_____

2. Draw or write what Brandon's mother did
   in the space below.

The correct first aid is . . .

Worksheet   Name _____

JENNIFER AND THE ROLLER SKATES

1. What happened to Jennifer when her
   grandmother went to the store?

   _____

   _____

   _____

   _____

   _____

   _____

2. Draw or write what Jennifer did in the space below.

The correct first aid is . . .

Worksheet   Name _____

TIMMY AND THE SWING SET

1. What happened to Timmy in his backyard?

_____

_____

_____

_____

_____

_____

2. Draw or write what Shirley did in the space below.

The correct first aid is . . .

Worksheet   Name _____

MEI LING AND THE SOFTBALL

1. What happened to Mei Ling when she was
   playing softball?

   _____

   _____

   _____

   _____

   _____

2. Draw or write what Mei Ling did in the space below.

The correct first aid is . . .

CONSUMER HEALTH

Objective. The student names people who help promote and protect health.

Level. Kindergarten and grade 1

Integration. Art

Content generalizations. Many people promote *and* protect health. Some are health care workers, such as doctors, nurses, dentists, and hospital workers. Others in the community and school include fire fighters, police officers, crossing guards, custodians, school nurses, principals, and teachers. Family members also help protect and promote the health of others.

Vocabulary. MD, medical doctor, nurse, police officer

Initiation. Health Helpers

Read a story or book to the class about a health care worker, school worker, community worker, or family member who helps protect and promote the health of others.

Materials

Book or story

Activities

1. "Who Am I"—Puppet Game

   Use health puppets to play a game, "Who Am I?" Modify the patterns to make the puppets needed for your own version of the game.

   a. Hide the puppets behind a curtain while providing information regarding the role of each health helper, such as the following.

      (1) "I have a big light and a mirror so I can look inside your mouth at your teeth. I clean your teeth and tell you how to help your teeth stay healthy. Who am I?" (Dentist or dental hygienist.)

      (2) "I keep the school clean, and I watch out for things around the school that might be unsafe. Who am I?" (Custodian.)

   b. Have the students guess who each health helper is before bringing the puppet out from behind the curtain.

   c. Have the students use the puppets to put on a puppet show naming the health helpers in the show.

Materials

Health helper puppets (teacher-made paper bag puppets using patterns *Health Helpers* (pp. 290-292)
Puppet stage

HEALTH HELPERS

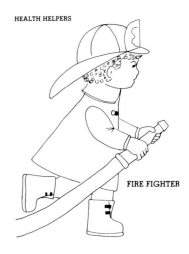

FIRE FIGHTER

2. Health helper pictures

   Have the students color pictures of health helpers. When the pictures are done, have them show the pictures to the class, naming the helper displayed.

   Materials

   Patterns: *Health Helpers* (pp. 290-292)
   Crayons

3. Health helpers we see every day

   Ask school health helpers such as the custodian, cafeteria worker, crossing guard, or nurse to visit the class and tell about their job. Speakers may suggest ways students can help keep the school healthful.

   Resources

   Guest speaker(s)

Evaluation. Health Helper Collage

   Have the students help make a collage of health helpers from pictures in magazines, or have the class paint a mural of health helpers.

   Materials

   Magazines, glue, and poster paper or butcher paper and poster paint

Consumer health

Pattern

HEALTH HELPERS

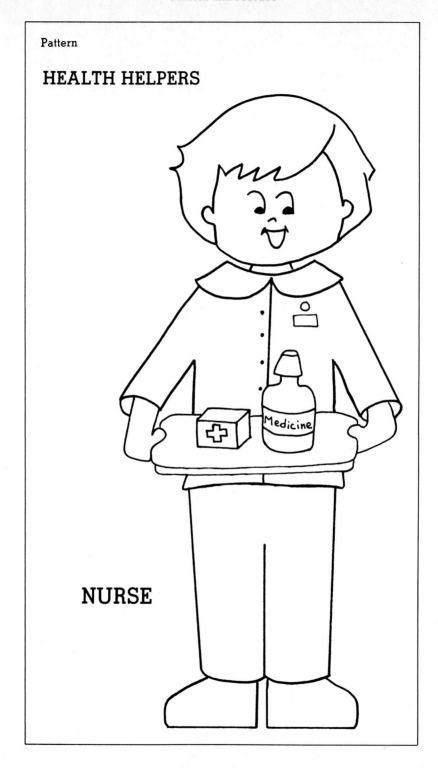

NURSE

Pattern

HEALTH HELPERS

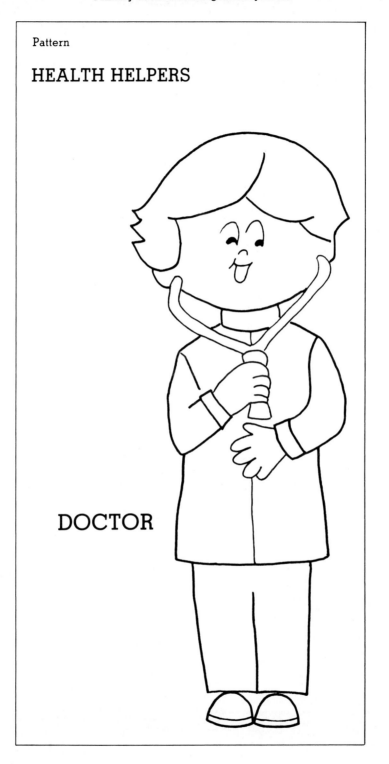

DOCTOR

Pattern

HEALTH HELPERS

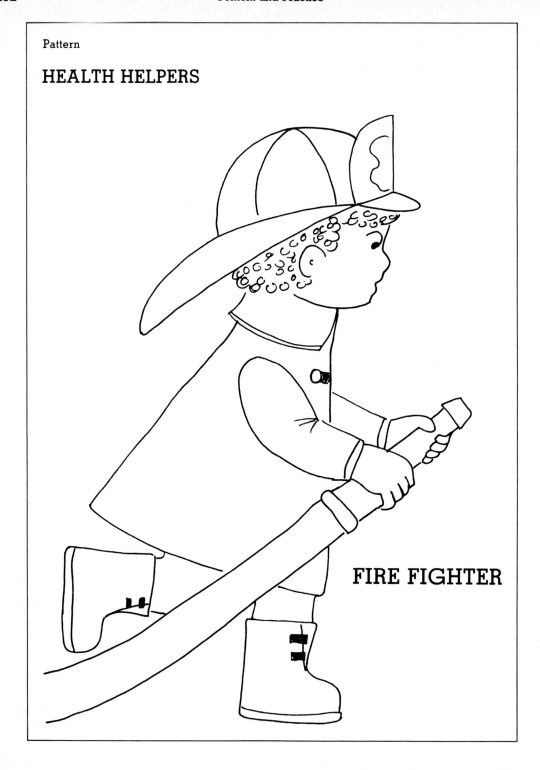

FIRE FIGHTER

USE AND ABUSE OF DRUGS

Objective. The student interprets methods for identifying potentially hazardous substances.

Level. Grades 2 and 3

Integration. Reading readiness, shape discrimination

Content generalizations. With the aid of specially designed warning labels, such as *Mr. Yuk* and the *skull and crossbones,* we can identify substances that potentially can damage our health. The senses, especially smell and sight, can be used to identify characteristics of many potentially harmful substances or spoiled foods that could be dangerous.

Vocabulary. Poison, label, warning, danger, mold

Initiation. "Safe" to Taste

Bring out one or several grocery bags filled with containers of various sizes, colors, shapes, and materials, such as soda bottles, milk cartons, gasoline cans, oil cans, detergent bottles, paint thinner cans, canning jars, and plastic bowls. Ask the students to indicate which normally contain substances that are safe to eat by placing the "safe" containers on a table labeled with a smiling face and the unsafe containers on a table labeled with Mr. Yuk.

Materials

Grocery bag(s)

Various containers, including food containers and containers of harmful substances.

Smiling face sign

Mr. Yuk sign

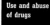

Use and abuse of drugs

Activities

1. What You See—Not Always What You Get

   a. Show the students two sealed identical soda bottles, each partially full of liquids that look the same. Explain that one bottle contains soda (which has been shaken so that the bubbles are gone), and one contains furniture polish. Invite the students to examine the sealed bottles to see if they can guess which is safe to drink.

   b. You may want to unseal the bottles and let the students use their sense of smell to discriminate further.

      NOTE: To avoid accidental ingestion of hazardous substances in the containers, you may wish to put the same nonhazardous substance in both jars and just *say* that they are two different substances. If you do this, do not open the containers for the students to smell.

   c. Repeat this several times with other look alikes (such as pills and candies or pancake mix and rat poison), stored in two baby food jars, two canning jars, two coffee cans, or other commonly used storage containers. They should look identical.

   d. Ask the students what could be done to warn others about containers that are used for storing hazardous materials.

2. Smart Sniffer

   a. Divide the class into small groups of four or five students. Display the worksheet, *Smart Sniffer*, and explain that each student will be given a worksheet to use to identify four mystery smells. Show a "mystery smell" jar to the class and demonstrate its use. (The top should not be removed. Students should sniff through holes punched in the lid.) Point out that each of the four jars is numbered. Show that each worksheet contains the names of the mystery smells. Tell the students that they are to smell one mystery jar, find the bottle on the worksheet that has the same number, and make a label by writing the name of the smell on the cut-out labels at the bottom of the worksheet. They should draw a smile face in the circle on the label if the smell is of something safe to eat or a Mr. Yuk face in the circle if it is hazardous. You should warn the students that smells can be deceiving. Not all things that smell good are safe and not all things that smell bad

Materials

Sets of identical see-through containers filled with look-alike substances

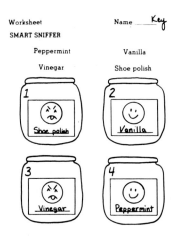

Materials

Worksheet: *Smart Sniffer* (p. 296)
Crayons
Scissors
Paste
"Mystery smell" jars (4 baby food jars containing cotton balls with drops of a different aromatic substance such as vinegar, shoe polish, vanilla, and orange or peppermint extract)

are hazardous. (For example, cyanide smells like almonds.) Then they should cut out the label and tape or paste it onto the picture of the jar with the correct number.

Give each group four baby food jars. The jars should be numbered 1 to 4 (with the jar labels removed, lids on, and holes punched in lids). Each should contain cotton balls that have several drops of an aromatic substance. The aromas should represent smells of safe substances, such as vinegar and vanilla and those that are hazardous such as shoe polish, and orange or peppermint extract.

Evaluation. Safety Labels

Show the students a copy of the worksheet, *Safety Labels,* and explain that they will color the Mr. Yuk labels yellow-green on the worksheet before taking it home to their parents. Then read aloud the letter to parents at the top of the worksheet, being certain that the students fully understand the intended use of the worksheet.

Distribute the worksheets, and have the students begin coloring as you circulate among them to complete the salutation on the letter and sign where "teacher" is indicated.

Materials

Worksheet: *Safety Labels* (p. 297)
  Crayons

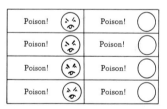

Use and abuse of drugs

Worksheet   Name _____

SMART SNIFFER

Peppermint   Vanilla

Vinegar   Shoe polish

1   2

3   4

Cut

Cut   Cut   Cut   Cut

Worksheet   Name _____

SAFETY LABELS

Dear _____

    Today's health lesson taught your child that some substances such as paint supplies, gasoline and oil, some medicines, garden chemicals and household cleansers can be extremely dangerous to their health if injested. We are concerned about the fact that each year young children suffer need- lessly because they consumed dangerous chemicals -- all too often the result of someone storing such materials in containers like canning jars and soda bottles that the youngsters associate with edible substances.

    In our effort to prevent needless accidents, your child has colored labels which can be attached to all hazardous materials that might attract a child. Many containers, of course, already bear such labels. I ask that you and your child work together to locate dangerous materials in your home and that you attach a label where no warning is present.

                           Sincerely,

                        _____

                        Teacher

Use and abuse of drugs

Poison!	😠	Poison!	◯
Poison!	😠	Poison!	◯
Poison!	😠	Poison!	◯
Poison!	😠	Poison!	◯

ENVIRONMENTAL HEALTH

Objective. The student identifies environmental (air, land, and water) pollution.

Level. Kindergarten and grade 1

Integration. Reading readiness, writing readiness

Content generalizations. The environment is the world around us, including land, water, and air. All living beings are dependent on a clean, usable, stable environment. When living quarters become dirty, contaminated, or unusable, they are polluted. Environmental pollution means the land, water, and air are dirty and unusable.

Vocabulary. Environment, pollution, land, water, air

Initiation. Defining "Environment"

Tell the students that they are going to learn a new long word today. It is a very important word. The new word is *environment*. Offer them the opportunity to say this new word individually and as a group. Applaud and praise their ability. Tell them that environment means *everything* in the world *around* us. This includes all the land, water, and air. Ask the students, "Are the land and all things on land a part of the environment?" "Are the air and all things in the air a part of the environment?" "Are the water and all things in the water a part of the environment?"

Activities

1. Air—Water—Land Learning Stations

   Show some environmental pictures to the class. Initially, show all pictures of one type, emphasizing what each is, for example, "This is a picture of land, which is a part of the environment." Mix up the pictures, show them, and ask the students to tell whether they are part of the land environment, water environment, or air environment.

   Rotate the students into learning stations in groups of four or five. They are to sort each picture into one of three appropriate boxes.

Materials

Land pictures: empty fields, playgrounds, city buildings, houses, freeways.

Air pictures: clear sky, clouded sky, stormy sky, sky with birds, sky with airplane.

Water pictures: drinking fountain, river, lake, stream

Three shoe boxes, one labeled *land* with a picture of land; the second *water* with a picture of water; the third *air* with a picture of sky

2. The Story of Diamond Lake
   a. Inform the students that we want to keep our environment clean and healthful so that all the people, plants, and animals can live well in the environment. When the environment becomes dirty and unusable, we say it is polluted. Ask the students to listen to the following story about an environment that became polluted. The flannel board figures, *Goldie, Water, Trash*, are used during the presentation.

Materials

Flannel board figures: *Goldie, Water, Trash* (p. 301)
Flannel board

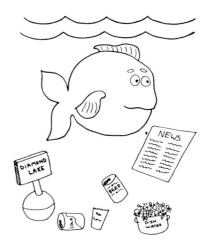

DIAMOND LAKE

Diamond Lake was so clean and beautiful that it sparkled. Many people and animals enjoyed Diamond Lake. Manuel and his family delighted in swimming at Diamond Lake each summer. Goldie Fish lived in the lake, which was clear and clean and filled with oxygen for her to breathe. Manuel and his family were careful not to throw trash in the lake so it would stay clean.

But some people who came to Diamond Lake dumped their garbage into the lake. Diamond Lake became filled with old newspapers, soda cans, and dirty dishwater.

Diamond Lake became a "polluted" lake. It no longer sparkled. Goldie Fish gasped for oxygen. Goldie's gills had to work very hard to get oxygen out of the polluted water. One summer Manuel and his family were very unhappy when they arrived at the lake. They could not go swimming because the water made their skin itch and hurt. Diamond Lake was dirty and polluted. Manuel said, "This is terrible! The lake is polluted, and we can no longer use it." Manuel was very sad. Goldie was very sad too.

   b. Discussion questions
   (1) Why were Manuel and Goldie sad? (The lake was polluted.)
   (2) What happened to make the lake polluted? (People dumped garbage into the lake.)
   (3) What does "polluted water" mean? (The water is dirty and unuseable.)
   (4) How can we keep lakes clean and unpolluted? (People must not throw garbage or other substances into lakes.)
   (5) Can Diamond Lake be saved? (Yes, with a great deal of work and help from many people, it is possible to restore Diamond Lake to its original beauty. It may take many years.)

Environmental
health

3. Air and Land Pollution

   Ask the students if they think that air and land can become polluted too. Ask them to speculate on what might cause the air to become polluted. Tell them to think about things that put smoke into the air. (Cars, airplanes, trucks, cigarettes, factories.) Use the same questioning for land pollution. Tell the students to think of things that might make the land and buildings messy and dirty. (Trash, litter, graffiti.)

   Using the worksheet, *Air and Land,* help the students trace around the words *air* and *land.* For each picture on the worksheet ask, "Does this pollute the air or land?" After each picture is discussed, students should draw a check mark by pictures of things that pollute the air and an *X* by those which pollute the land. Ask the students if they have any ideas on how they can help keep the air and land from becoming polluted. (Do not litter, do not write graffiti on walls, and walk or ride a bicycle instead of riding in a car when possible.)

Materials

Worksheet: *Air and Land* (p. 302)
Pencils or crayons

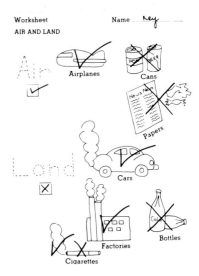

Evaluation. Stop Pollution

   Hand each child a picture of the land, air, or water. Ask them to identify the type of environment and tell what might make that environment polluted. Also have the students tell how we might keep the environment from becoming polluted.

Materials

Pictures of air, land, and water used
   earlier

Flannel board figures

GOLDIE, WATER, TRASH

Use the pictures below to make flannel board figures
for use with the Diamond Lake story.

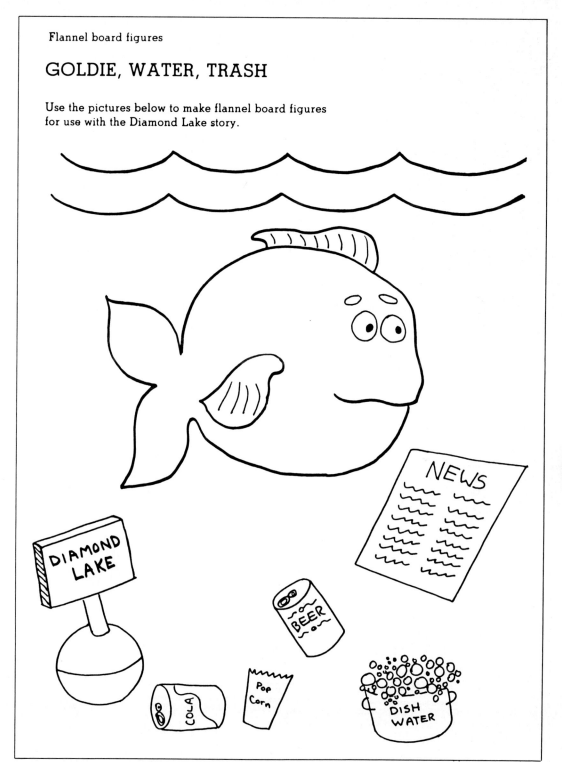

Worksheet   Name_____

AIR AND LAND

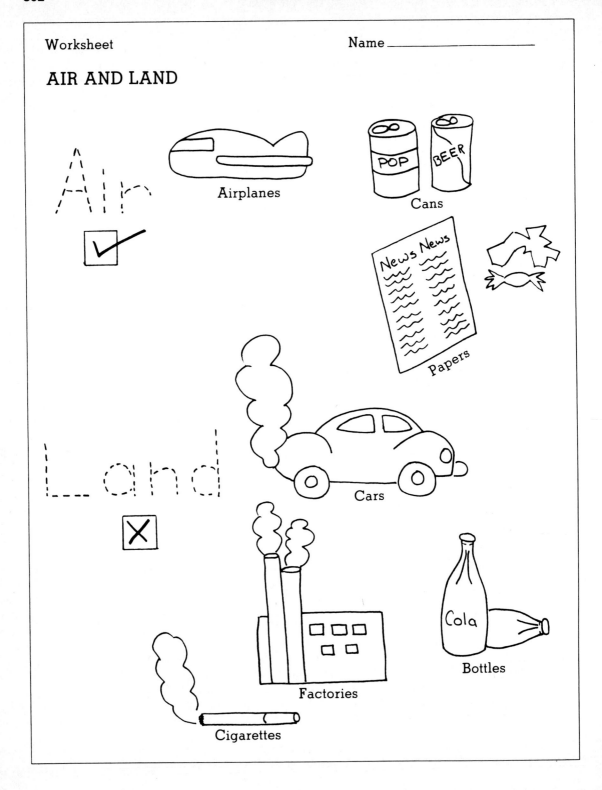

Air

Airplanes

Cans

Papers

Land

Cars

Factories

Bottles

Cigarettes

COMMUNITY HEALTH

Objective. The student lists the services provided by community health agencies and organizations.

Level. Grades 2 and 3

Integration. Map skills, social studies, writing

Content generalizations. A variety of health agencies and organizations exist in each community to safeguard the health of all people. There are many services needed and provided in communities. Agencies common in most communities include a hospital, health department, fire department, police department, sanitation department, and voluntary health agencies. Knowing where health services are available will enable citizens to take an active role in protecting the community's health.

Vocabulary. Community, hospital, health department, sanitation department

Initiation. "Health Worker" Play
Show picture or teacher-made posters of community health workers, and discuss a main function of each. Review the functions to be certain that each child is familiar with each health worker. Then divide the class into small groups, and secretly assign each group a different health worker. Have each group or a member from each group act out the functions of their assigned health worker, and have classmates guess the health worker being represented. As each is identified, place a name card for the health worker on the left side of the bulletin board.

Materials
Pictures of health workers or posters made from *Health Helpers* patterns (pp. 290-292)
Name card for each health worker

Community health

Activities

1. Be a Wise Willy!'' Bulletin Board Activity
   a. One at a time, display large photographs of your com-
      munity's health office building for each health worker
      you have studied. Use these pictures to complete the
      bulletin board display, *Be a Wise Willy!* For instance,
      show a picture of the local firehouse, doctors' building
      or hospital, police station, health department, and
      selected health agencies or organizations (such as the
      American Cancer Society and American Lung Associ-
      ation). For each photograph ask the following ques-
      tions.
      (1) How many of you have seen the building before?
      (2) What is the name of the building?
      (3) Which of the health workers works in this build-
          ing?
   b. If the students are unable to answer a question, pro-
      vide clues or the information for them.
   c. After the students identify a photograph and discuss
      it, mount it on the bulletin board display, *Be a Wise
      Willy!* Stretch pieces of large colorful yarn between the
      photographs and the names of the health workers in
      that building. There may be several strings attached to
      one card.
   d. After discussing the bulletin board and allowing stu-
      dents to match the names with the photographs,
      explain that the yarn will be disconnected from the
      name cards and that students can come to the bulletin
      board during their free time and try to reattach the
      yarn to the correct photographs. To check their
      answers as they work independently, students can lift
      the index card beside each photograph and read the
      correct answer (name of health worker) for that photo-
      graph.
   e. When a student has matched the items on the bulletin
      board correctly, he or she should write his or her name
      on the *Wise Willy* name card and detach the yarn
      pieces for the next student's use.

Materials

Photographs of local community
agencies (from the agencies' professional photographs or brochures
or taken by the teacher)
Bulletin board display: *Be a Wise Willy!*
(p. 306)

BE A WISE WILLY!

Know how to keep Toledo healthy!

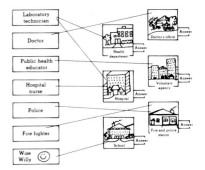

2. Health Workers in My Community
   a. Make a simple street map of your community similar to the sample worksheet provided here. If possible, it should include neighborhoods of all students in the class, school grounds, and downtown area. Using an overhead projector and a transparency of the handout, ask the students to point to the location of the school building, downtown area, their neighborhoods, and other familiar landmarks. Students should color significant points on the map (such as rivers, streets, and school).
   b. Ask volunteers to identify the location of the community health buildings that are posted on the bulletin board. As students show the correct location, have one student write it on the transparency so that others can write it on their worksheets properly.
   c. When all the worksheets are marked with the locations of the community health buildings, review the functions of each health worker.

Materials

Worksheet and transparency: *Health Workers in My Community* (p. 307)
Overhead projector
Transparency pen
Crayons

HEALTH WORKERS IN MY COMMUNITY

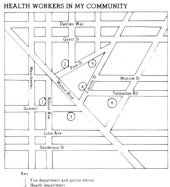

Key
1. Fire department and police station
2. Health department
3. Health agency
4. Doctor's office
5. Owen School
6. Custer Hospital

Evaluation. What Health Workers Do

Divide the class into two teams. Have the first student from team A draw a slip of paper with the name of a health worker from a hat or bowl containing the names of all of them. The student is to name the function of the health worker drawn and use the transparency to show the location of the corresponding community building. If the student does this correctly, the team gets 1 point. Team B now gets a turn, then team A, and so on.

Materials

Hat or bowl
Slips of paper with names of health workers
Transparency from worksheet: *Health Workers in My Community* (p. 307)
Overhead projector
Transparency pen

Community health

Bulletin board display

BE A WISE WILLY!

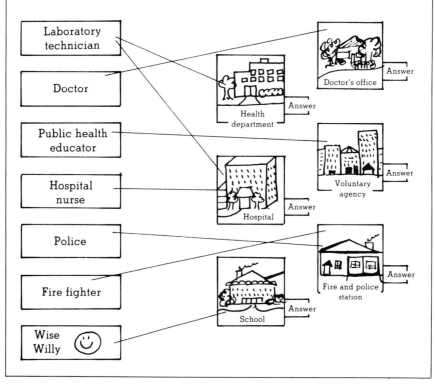

BE A WISE WILLY!

Know how to keep Toledo healthy!

Laboratory technician

Doctor

Public health educator

Hospital nurse

Police

Fire fighter

Wise Willy

Doctor's office — Answer

Health department — Answer

Voluntary agency — Answer

Hospital — Answer

Fire and police station — Answer

School — Answer

Worksheet   Name _____

HEALTH WORKERS IN MY COMMUNITY

Key:
1. Fire department and police station
2. Health department
3. Health agency
4. Doctor's office
5. Owen School
6. Custer Hospital

EXERCISES

1. Spend some time in the children's section of the library reading books that could be used in teaching health at the primary level. Write brief reviews of several books for your own use later. Indicate in which content areas each book could be used. You may wish to start by reviewing the books suggested in this chapter for mental and emotional health, family life, and consumer health.

2. Use some of the patterns in this chapter to make your own colorful flannel board figures or bulletin boards. Go into a primary classroom, and teach a lesson using your materials. Then evaluate their effectiveness in your particular situation.

3. Only a few patterns are included for "health helpers." Make other health helper patterns for use in the primary classroom. Share them with your classmates.

4. Using objectives in the scope and sequence plan in Chapter 9, develop at least one lesson for the primary level. Try to do one at the kindergarten and grade 1 level, assuming students will not be able to read or write. Any worksheets developed for this level must be very simple and visual. Then do another lesson for grades 2 and 3. Assume that these students have some reading and writing abilities. If possible, teach one of your lessons in a local school, or present it to your university classmates.

CHAPTER 12

Content Appropriate for Intermediate Level Students

When you finish this chapter, you should be able to:

■ Describe appropriate content in ten areas of health education for students in grades 4 through 6.

Students at the intermediate level, grades 4 through 6, are able to assume a greater degree of responsibility for themselves and others compared to previous years in the primary grades. Along with increased responsibility comes the opportunity for greater independence. Intermediate level children's bodies grow larger and stronger, enabling them to perform tasks requiring more physical strength and dexterity. Health instruction at the intermediate level provides the factual, affective and behavioral concepts that build upon previous experiences and address the increased physical, emotional, and social maturity of these children.

PERSONAL HEALTH

Students at the intermediate level have a great interest in the human body and its functions. Information about the body sets the stage for understanding the reasons for certain good health practices and the consequences of poor health choices. Students at this level learn that family and friends set examples for health practices that may influence their own health choices. Sometimes these influences can have positive results, such as wanting to keep clothes clean to make a good impression. Other results are negative, such as smoking cigarettes because others are "doing it."

The Skin

The skin is called "one of the body's most complicated structures" and is one of the most observable features of any individual. The skin:

- protects against foreign material
- regulates body temperature
- eliminates waste products
- converts ultraviolet light to vitamin D
- stores fat and water

A closer look at the skin reveals three layers of skin cells.

The outermost layer is called the "epidermis." The epidermis helps to keep germs out of the body. Folds and creases in the epidermis make it possible for the skin to stretch easily when the body moves. Tiny oil glands open onto the epidermis and supply oil that keeps the skin soft, smooth, and waterproof. The lower part of the epidermis makes millions of new cells each day which replace the old cells that die as they are pushed upward. These dead cells compose the upper layer of skin that is seen and felt.

The next layer of skin is known as the "dermis." Nerve endings, blood vessels and glands are located in this layer. The nerve endings are important for the sense of touch. Blood vessels, arteries, veins, and capillaries supply oxygen and food to keep the skin cells of the dermis alive. Two types of glands are located in the dermis, sweat glands and oil glands. The sweat glands take in liquid from the spaces around the skin cells and send the liquid up to the skin surface through the pores. Sweating cools the body and carries off small amounts of waste materials.

The fatty layer below the dermis is made up of threadlike structures with many spaces. Fat and fluid fills the spaces which cushion the body and help hold in body heat.

One of the most interesting features of the skin is the ridges that form fingerprints. No two people have the same fingerprint so fingerprints are a good method of identification. Fingerprints never change even if fingers get burned. When the skin heals the same fingerprint will appear. Each of the ten fingers show a different fingerprint.

Taking care of the skin is an important part of making sure that the skin stays healthy and able to perform all of its functions.

Keeping clean is one way to care for the skin. The face needs a thorough washing with soap and water at least once a day. The rest of the body can be cleaned by bathing or showering several times a week. Some people bathe once a day. Just how often a person bathes or showers depends upon how dirty a person gets, whether the skin is dry or oily, the temperature outdoors, and personal preference.

Avoiding sunburn is another way of caring for the skin. Wearing protective clothing like hats and long-sleeved shirts provides protection when one is exposed to sunshine for long periods of time. Sun screen preparations are also effective in preventing sunburn.

The Respiratory System

The body must have oxygen from the air to stay alive. The respiratory system uses the oxygen which enters the body in a process called **"inhalation."** During inhalation the diaphragm (a large tentlike muscle) contracts along with the rib muscles to make the chest expand or become larger. When the chest expands, air is sucked into the body through the nose.

The nose prepares the air for the lungs by filtering out some of the germs and large dust particles by means of the nose hairs. Mucus in the lining of the nose also helps to collect germs and dust as well as moistening the air that is breathed in.

The pharynx is a funnel-like structure that allows the air to pass from the nose into the trachea or windpipe.

The trachea extends down the neck and then divides into two large branches called bronchial tubes. One of these branches goes to the left lung, the other goes to the right lung.

The lungs are where the exchange of oxygen and waste products takes place. The bronchial tubes inside each lung branch into smaller and smaller tubes finally ending in balloon-like air sacs. The oxygen from the air goes through the thin walls of the air sacs into the capillaries that surround them. At the same time, wastes pass from the capillaries into the air sacs where they can be "exhaled" from the body.

In the process called **exhalation,** the diaphragm and rib muscles relax to make the chest become smaller. Air is forced out of the chest as the ribs and diaphragm push on the lungs. A person does not have to think about breathing most of the time because the nervous system controls the breathing movements.

The Nervous System

The nervous system allows us to receive, interpret, and react to the messages we receive from our senses. The brain, spinal cord, and nerves make up the nervous system.

The nerves are special "transmitter" cells that send messages to and from the spinal cord. The "sensory nerves" transmit the signals that come into the body from the sense organs (eyes, ears, nose, skin, and tongue). The "motor nerves" take messages to the muscles if action is needed.

The spinal cord extends from the base of the brain down the back. It is protected by a chain of bones called the backbone. The spinal cord carries messages to and from the brain.

The brain is a soft, spongy organ that is protected by a special fluid and three coverings or membranes. In addition, the brain is protected by the bones of the head or "skull." The brain interprets the messages that come into the body and decides what to do about them.

The nervous system is sometimes called the "master system" of the body because it controls many of the processes that are necessary for life. Besides making sure that our respiratory systems breathe in air and breathe out waste products, the nervous system controls the beating of our hearts.

The Circulatory System

The circulatory system moves blood around the body so that the cells can receive food and oxygen and get rid of waste products. The heart, blood vessels, and the blood are the parts of the circulatory system.

Your heart is about the size of your closed fist and is located behind the ribs in your chest. The heart is made of a special kind of muscle that constantly beats and rests. Each beat of the heart pumps the blood through the blood vessels.

The blood vessels carry the blood throughout the body. Blood vessels called "arteries" carry the blood away from the heart. Blood in arteries is rich in oxygen. Blood vessels called "veins" carry the blood back to the heart. The blood found in veins carries carbon dioxide and other waste products. Small blood vessels called "capillaries" connect the arteries and veins.

The Digestive System

The job of the digestive system is to convert the food that is eaten into substances that can enter the cells of the body by way of the bloodstream. When food is swallowed, it travels from the esophagus into the stomach, where digestive juices act upon it. Food is channeled from the stomach into the upper part of the small intestine where it is further metabolized by chemicals from the pancreas and liver. As the food moves into the lower part of the small intestine, the nutrients are absorbed through the walls into the bloodstream. Food substances that cannot be absorbed by the digestive tract pass into the large intestine, colon and rectum from which they are eliminated from the body.

Growth

Students at the intermediate level are approaching a period of very rapid growth. They are growing physically, emotionally, and socially.

Often students worry that they are too short, too tall, too heavy, too thin or are abnormal in some way. Not all parts of the body grow at the same time so for a while, hands and feet may seem out of proportion. It also takes time to get used to the changes in body size and shape. Everyone grows and develops on his or her own timetable. Girls generally start their growth spurts at an earlier age than boys. Even though no two individuals grow in exactly the same way or at the same time, everyone's growth depends on the same three factors.

1. Heredity is the passing of traits from parent to child. A person's looks, growth patterns, and special talents are traits that are influenced by heredity.
2. Environment refers to everything in a person's surroundings. The types of food that are eaten, where a person lives, and daily experiences influence physical, emotional, and social growth.
3. Behavior is a factor that each person can control. Maintaining a healthy diet, performing regular exercise, and making friends are examples of behaviors that can influence the growth of an individual.

Fitness

Since students at this level are learning about the functioning of the systems of the body, it is appropriate to introduce the concept of physical fitness. Regular exercise, including aerobic, endurance, strength, and flexibility exercises, contribute to a sound body. In particular, the respiratory, circulatory, musculoskeletal, and nervous systems benefit from exercise. And, since all systems must work together, the body as a whole benefits. It is also proven that regular exercise relieves tension and that physical fitness is usually accompanied by feelings of well-being.

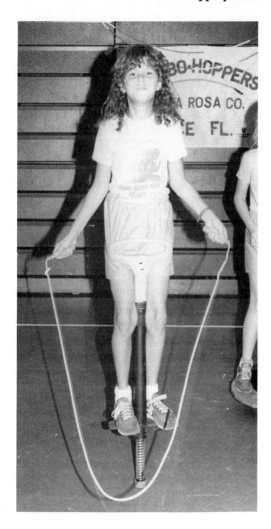

MENTAL HEALTH

The concept of a "sound mind in a sound body" can be introduced at this level. Health is more than physical well-being; it is a dynamic interaction among the physical, mental, emotional, and social aspects of the individual.

Stress

Stress is a normal part of life. There are general stressors in everyday life, such as having responsibilities at school and at home. Sleeping through an alarm and being late to school or being responsible for the dinner dishes can be stressful. Such a negative reaction to stressors is called "distress." However, stressors are positive as well. The anticipation of the school field day and trying for the best test score in the class are examples of stressors that may result in a positive reaction. When the body is under stress certain changes occur:

- the heart beats faster
- muscles tense
- palms feel sweaty
- breathing becomes faster

Even though stress is a normal part of life, sometimes we are under too much stress. Too many changes may occur at once or we may feel that we don't have control. There are steps a person can take to help combat the stress in life:

1. Do something physical. Ride a bike, go for a walk, or play a game of basketball.
2. Get plenty of sleep and rest. When a person doesn't get enough rest, dealing with everyday problems is more difficult.
3. Talk with someone who cares about you. It helps to talk about your worries. A friend, a parent, or a teacher can listen to your problems.
4. Take things one at a time. Complete one task before going on to the next one. Plan to do the most important things first.
5. Make time to work and time to play. Be sure to take the time to do things that you enjoy doing.

Emotions

Ways to deal with strong emotions, particularly anger, are important for students to learn. Positive ways to handle anger and other emotions include practices such as participating in a physical activity, talking it over with a friend or family member, and refocusing one's energy on

---

HOW TO MAKE A DECISION

1. Identify the exact decision to be made.
2. Think of all the possible outcomes.
3. Look at each outcome. Ask yourself what will happen if you choose that outcome. Think about how that decision will affect you and other people.
4. Make the decision that seems the best. Remember that you are responsible for your decisions.

---

something else such as cleaning out a closet, washing the car, or going for a walk. Negative ways to deal with strong emotions include drug use, physical violence, verbal abuse, and property damage.

Decision-making

Students in the latter part of the intermediate grades develop the ability to think abstractly and thus make decisions about the future. When decisions and actions reflect the attitudes and values of the individual, self-esteem remains intact. If decisions are contradictory to strongly held values, stress and emotional conflicts arise. Decision-making patterns and resulting actions give valuable clues about the individual's value system. Good mental health can be promoted by learning to make decisions through consideration of one's own beliefs and attitudes.

Emotional Needs

People are alike in that we all have basic emotional needs. Students in the intermediate grades can come to recognize human needs and to understand how these needs can be met in a healthy way.

All people have the need to love and receive love. There are many ways to show love that is felt; a hug, a smile, or doing something nice for the person you care about. Giving love also helps you to feel better about yourself.

Everyone has the need to feel that they belong. Your family is the first group to which you belong but as you grow older you enjoy having groups of friends. Friends are the people that accept you as you are and care about what you think and feel. Real friends do not pressure you into doing things that you don't want to do or that would make you feel bad about yourself. In other words, friends let you be yourself. The best way to make friends is to be a friend.

All people need to feel worthwhile. Individual talents and skills can make you feel more worthwhile. Trying new things and learning new skills can increase the feelings of self-worth. It is also important to recognize the achievements of others. Everyone thrives on personal abilities and the recognition of these abilities by others.

FAMILY LIFE

Family life education at the intermediate level focuses on the exploration of the roles and interactions of individuals within the life cycle. Students explore the responsibilities and privileges experienced by each family member and develop an awareness of the physical, mental, and social changes inherent in the life cycle as a person progresses from birth to death.

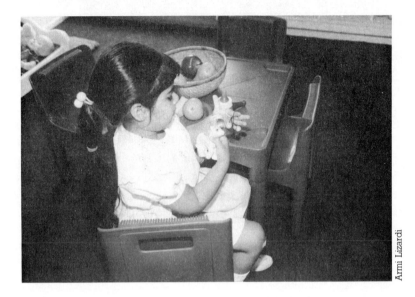

Armi Lizardi

Conflict Resolution

Conflicts with family members and friends are normal as children assume greater responsibility and independence. School and home experiences are particularly important in learning how to resolve conflicts. Looking at all possible options before making a decision, being willing to compromise, being able to see another point of view, and admitting mistakes are examples of positive conflict resolution.

Puberty

Puberty involves an important series of events in the growth and development of an individual. It is the period when girls and boys sexually mature into young women and men who are able to have children of their own. Stimulated by hormones, the secondary sexual characteristics for males and females emerge. Both sexes experience a growth spurt, thickening of the skin, a new interest in the opposite sex, and growth of pubic and other body hair. The amount of body hair that develops is largely inherited. Breast development, widening of the

hips, and menarche (the onset of menstruation) are significant physical changes that occur for girls. Boys grow more muscular, their voices get deeper, and they begin to experience nocturnal emissions. It is important that adolescents realize that they will develop and mature at their own rate. Some girls and boys mature early, and others mature late. There is no right time for puberty to begin because everybody is different.

The Reproductive Process

The physical changes of puberty prepare the body of a girl for future parenthood. Each month hormonal changes cause a mature ovum to be released from the *ovary* into the fallopian tube. Estrogen signals the *uterus* to prepare for a possible pregnancy by building up a nutritive lining. If the egg is not fertilized, the uterus sheds its blood-rich lining through the *vagina*. This process is called *menstruation*.

At puberty, boys begin to produce mature sperm in their *testes*. Sperm cells pass from the testes into the *vas deferens*, tubes that carry the sperm cells, along with nutritive fluids into the *urethra*. The urethra is a tube that runs the length of the *penis* and is the outlet for urine and sperm.

Adolescents become physically capable of having babies, even though parenthood also involves the emotional and social skills necessary for taking complete responsibility for a child. Adolescence is a time of transition, moving from childhood to adulthood. It takes several years to make all of the changes necessary to complete this exciting and important transition.

The Life Cycle

The life cycle extends from birth to death, and the stages are universal and predictable. It can be said that aging begins at conception and continues until death. The stages of the life cycle can be identified as:

- infancy—a time of total dependency
- toddler stage—a time of rapid physical and mental changes and growth in independence
- early childhood—a time to explore the world and test abilities
- middle childhood—a time when greater responsibility and independence are assumed and typically children develop a sense of accomplishment from being successful in tasks at home and at school
- adolescence—the transition from childhood to adulthood, when peers are highly significant and physical sexual maturity is reached
- early adulthood—a time to take total responsibility for oneself, to build intimate relationships with friends and perhaps a member of the opposite sex
- middle adulthood—typically a time to have a family, to develop a sense of accomplishment with work, and to become a contributing member of a community
- later adulthood—a time to relax, often to retire and pursue creative interests that time did not allow previously, such as returning to school, reflecting on one's life and enjoying grandchildren.

Dying and death are a part of the life cycle as well. It is common and normal to fear death and to avoid talking of such a depressing subject. However, most experts believe that the study of death and dying will enhance life and living. Kubler-Ross (1967), in her book *On Death And Dying,* observed five stages that terminally ill patients go through (although all persons do not experience all stages): *Denial* of imminent death, *Anger* about dying (often called the "why me?" stage), *Bargaining* to buy a little more time, *Depression* at the realization of losing all loved ones and mourning one's own loss of life, and *Acceptance* of the inevitable.

Death is when all life signs disappear. It has been increasingly difficult to define the exact time of death as medical science improves its abilities to forestall death. The most often agreed on determination of death is a flat electroencephalogram (EEG), which means that no brain waves can be measured. When death occurs or is imminent, it is essential for family members and friends to grieve. Grief is a human reaction to loss. We grieve not only for the sake of the person who has died, but also for the loss of that person in our life. Just as dying and death are a normal part of life, so are grief, mourning, and coping with the death of friends and family members.

NUTRITION

People eat for many reasons—because they are hungry, for enjoyment, and for the social interaction. Food provides the body with the fuel it needs to work, grow, and repair itself. As students get older, they become more responsible for food choices. By understanding the importance of nutrition in the functioning of the body, students can become more aware of how their personal eating habits affect their health.

Nutrients

Foods contain substances called nutrients. There are over 50 essential nutrients which are grouped into six main classes.

- Carbohydrates—provide energy
- Fats—provide energy and carry vitamins in the body
- Proteins—necessary for the growth and repair of tissue
- Minerals—regulate body functions and build strong bones and teeth
- Vitamins—regulate chemical reactions that convert food into energy
- Water—helps eliminate wastes, regulates body temperature, and carries nutrients

A well-balanced diet helps to ensure that a person gets all of the nutrients that the body needs to function optimally. The best and easiest way to be sure a diet is balanced is to choose foods from each of the four food groups every day.

- Milk Group—Children under the age of 12 should have three servings from this group. A serving is one cup of milk or a slice of cheese, for example. (Teenagers need four servings and adults two servings.)
- Meat Group—Children, teenagers, and adults all need two servings from this group. A serving could be one hamburger patty or two eggs.
- Bread & Cereal Group—Everyone needs four servings each day. A slice of bread is a serving.
- Fruit & Vegetable Group—Children, teens, and adults all need four servings daily from this group. A serving is one banana or apple or a half cup of corn or beans.

Sometimes people do not get enough of the essential nutrients in their diets. When this occurs, deficiency diseases may appear.

- Scurvy—A disease that causes bleeding gums, internal bleeding, and death. Scurvy is caused by a lack of vitamin C. Citrus fruits like oranges and grapefruit contain vitamin C.
- Beriberi—A disease that affects the nerves, causing paralysis. Lack of vitamin B_1 is the cause of beriberi. Meat and whole grain cereals are good sources of vitamin B_1.
- Rickets—A disease that causes crooked bones and crippling. A lack of vitamin D causes rickets. Milk contains vitamin D. Doctors have also discovered that people can manufacture their own vitamin D when they are exposed to sunlight.
- Pellagra—A disease that results in skin rashes, mouth sores, and memory loss. Pellagra is caused by a lack of the vitamin called niacin. Lean meat and bread contain niacin.
- Kwashiorkor—A disease that results in swelling of the abdomen, brain damage, and death. A lack of protein is the cause of kwashiorkor. Meats, fish, eggs, and nuts are good sources of protein.

Fad Diets

Advertisements for special diets are everywhere. Most of these diets are for losing weight. Some diets say to eat just one kind of food, like grapefruit or rice. Others advertise, "eat anything you want and still lose weight." These diets are examples of "fad diets." Usually, fad diets promise a quick way to lose weight or a way to lose weight without having to change eating habits. Most fad diets are unhealthy and can even be dangerous for children. When a person's body is growing it is especially important to take in all of the nutrients available through foods. The best way to stay healthy is to regularly eat a variety of foods from the four food groups. If a person needs to lose weight, he or she can achieve this by increasing exercise and reducing the amount of foods from the "extra" or "other" foods. "Extra" or "other" foods are those products that have calories but very few nutrients, like candy, cookies, and soda pop.

Food Choices

Various factors influence an individual's food choices. Many are related to family and cultural preferences. If the father does not like peas, they are not served often at the family table, and chances are good that other family members, especially the children, will dislike peas as well. Conversely, if the mother's favorite vegetable is broccoli, it is served often, and she comments on how much she likes it. Other family members may therefore learn to "love" broccoli as well. Adolescents are also influenced by peers in their food choices.

Other influences are related to taste and texture preferences. Some people eat certain foods because they are on special diets for health reasons. Diabetics need to watch sugar intake, people on weight-reduction diets need to watch calories, and people with high blood pressure should monitor salt intake if they are salt sensitive.

Cost and availability of foods are other factors affecting food choices. Usually the more abundant the food, the lower the cost. Therefore travelers are often surprised to find higher or lower prices for food than at home.

DISEASE PREVENTION AND CONTROL

There are many factors that contribute to disease. Some factors such as pathogens can be prevented or eliminated through antibiotics, vaccines, or improved sanitary conditions. Diseases that are caused by pathogens are said to be communicable diseases. Once these pathogens can be isolated, more specific research can be conducted regarding ways to prevent or cure the disease. Researchers and health care providers have developed methods that are effective against most of the communicable diseases. Other factors such as environment, habits, and heredity contribute to the conditions called noncommunicable diseases. Sometimes it is a combination of factors that leads to the development of disease. Research continues on significant diseases in our society such as cancer, heart disease, diabetes, arthritis, and many other diseases that still mystify scientists.

Pathogens

Pathogens (disease-causing organisms or other substances) come in many forms:

- Bacteria—One of the basic types of pathogens is bacteria—single celled plant-like organisms that live on or around human cells and flourish on or in every environment, including soil, water, air and all plants and animals. Major bacteria-caused diseases are typhoid fever, streptococcus and staphylococcus infections, tuberculosis, some sexually transmitted diseases, meningitis, and diphtheria.
- Viruses—Viruses are submicroscopic organisms that are hard to study because they are not visible by regular light microscopes. Consequently there is still a great deal to learn about viruses. Some disorders that can be traced to viruses are the common cold, polio, viral hepatitis, herpes,

smallpox, and AIDS. Researchers also believe that some cancers may be caused by viruses.

- Protozoa—This group of pathogens is made up of single celled organisms larger than bacteria but not visible to the naked eye. Malaria is the best known disease caused by protozoa.
- Fungi—Fungi are plants that can live on the skin and cause disease. Athlete's foot and ringworm are diseases that are caused by this pathogen.
- Parasitic worms—These pathogens are animals that live from the nutrients supplied by the ''host,'' the organism that is infected with the worm. Tapeworm and pinworm infections are examples of diseases that are caused by this type of pathogen.

The elimination of the pathogen will usually cure the disease. However, damage that the body suffered because of the disease usually will not be reversed.

Barriers to Disease

The body has many natural defenses that help to protect it from infection:

- The skin—Pathogens cannot enter the body through the skin unless a cut or opening is present. This is why it is important to keep sores and cuts clean.
- Mucous membranes—Mucous membranes are the tissues that line the openings of the body, the mouth, nose, and throat. Mucous is a sticky fluid that coats these body openings to trap dirt and pathogens.
- Tears—Tears are always washing the surface of the eyes to clean out dirt and germs. They also contain chemicals that kill pathogens.
- Saliva and stomach juices—These secretions of the body contain acid to help

digest food. Pathogens cannot live in this environment.

If the pathogens do get past all of these protective barriers, the body has additional weapons to use in fighting the infection.

- White blood cells—These special cells surround the pathogen and destroy it.
- Antibodies—Antibodies are substances that circulate in the bloodstream to help white blood cells destroy pathogens.

Noncommunicable Disease

Many noncommunicable diseases are ''chronic'' diseases, that is, the disease starts slowly and develops over a period of years. Not all of the causes of chronic disease are known; however, we do know that environmental and congenital factors are involved. Cigarette smoke damages the tissues of the lungs and can be related to lung cancer and emphysema. Air pollution similarly damages the lung tissues. Smokeless tobacco damages the delicate membranes of the mouth, increasing the risk of oral cancers. These are examples of environmental or behavioral factors that may cause diseases. Diseases or weaknesses that contribute to diseases can be congenital, such as congenital heart disease. Health habits and life style are other factors that are related to disease in that they influence the environment (as in smoking). In addition, hereditary and environmental factors may work together in causing a disease. For example, a person may be genetically more susceptible to emphysema, but unless that person smokes or lives in a polluted area, he or she may never develop the disease.

Preventing Disease

Even though many factors influence the disease process, there are some simple steps a person can take to help the body combat disease:

- Get adequate amounts of rest and sleep.
- Eat well-balanced meals each day.
- Exercise regularly.
- Keep the body and its environment clean.
- Wear clothing that is appropriate for the weather.
- Keep immunizations up to date.

ACCIDENT PREVENTION AND SAFETY

Many people believe that accidents are just bad luck, but accidents have causes that can often be prevented or controlled in some way. Being safety-conscious is one way intermediate students can help to prevent accidents. Being aware of and following rules can reduce the risks of becoming an accident victim. It is also important for students to master first-aid procedures for emergency situations.

Keeping Safe as Pedestrians

A pedestrian is someone who is walking. When walking from one place to another:
- Walk on the left side of the street when there is no sidewalk.
- Walk single file on a street with no sidewalks.
- Wear light colored clothing and carry a light when walking at night.
- Cross streets only at corners of crosswalks.
- Look both ways before crossing the street.
- Obey traffic lights.
- Wait on the curb, not on the street, before crossing.

Keeping Safe on Bicycles

When riding a bike a person must follow the same rules as someone driving a car. Adhering to all of the rules involves knowing what high-way signs mean and obeying them. When riding a bike:
- Use the correct hand signals.
- Stay close to the right side of the street.
- Drive in a straight line; don't zigzag.
- Carry packages and other objects in a basket or carrier.
- Walk your bike across busy intersections.

Keeping Safe in the Water

Swimming is an activity that is fun and provides good exercise for the body. In order to swim safely:
- Never swim alone.
- Avoid swimming when you are tired.
- Avoid pushing and shoving others.
- Know your own swimming abilities.
- Obey the rules and the lifeguard.
- Know where the shallow and deep water begin and end.

Keeping Safe at Play

Everyone has favorite activities and sports. Being safe while playing means knowing which of these activities are suitable for your age, size, and ability. Being safe while playing also means using the protective equipment for your sport. For example, tennis players wear special shoes to keep from slipping and skaters wears knee pads to prevent injury. Knowing safe places to play in your neighborhood, away from traffic or other hazards, also helps to keep you safe.

CONSUMER HEALTH

Intermediate students are health consumers anytime they buy or use a health product or use a health service. As a consumer, it is important that students receive practice in making informed health choices.

SEVEN STEPS FOR ARTIFICIAL RESUSCITATION

(1) **Tap and shout,** "Are you okay?" If no response, proceed to the next step.

(2) **Check for a pulse** by placing two fingers (not the thumb) on the neck, just to the side of the trachea.

(3) **Tilt the head,** with the chin pointing up. Place one hand under the head and gently lift. At the same time push with other hand on the victim's forehead. (This moves the tongue away from the back of the throat and opens the airway.)

(4) Immediately place your cheek and ear close to the victim's mouth and nose. **Look** for chest to rise and fall. **Listen** for air exchange. **Feel** for air blowing on your cheek.

(5) For an adult, pinch the nostrils, take a deep breath, and blow into mouth **two quick full breaths.** (For a baby, cover the nose and mouth with your mouth and give puffs of air.)

(6) **Look, listen, and feel for air;** if there is still no breathing, proceed to the next step.

(7) **Give 1 breath every 5 seconds** for an adult. To count each 5 seconds, blow, then say, "One thousand, two thousand, three thousand, four thousand." Blow, then continue the sequence. (You continue until help arrives or until the victim starts breathing.)

Sources of Consumer Information

The first step in making an informed choice is to have reliable information. Reliable sources for health information include certified medical advisers such as physicians, dentists, nurses and school nurses. Places to receive reliable health services include public health departments and clinics, physicians' offices, dental offices, and the school nurse's office. Television shows, radio shows, and magazines may or may not have reliable health information. Books can contain reliable health information if they are written by certified health advisers, but they may be out of date.

Labeling

When purchasing health-related products, it should be kept in mind that many products contain valuable health information on the label. Packaged foods must have the ingredients listed on the label in order from greatest to least, according to the amount present. An ingredient list for cranberry juice cocktail might be water, cranberry juice, sugar, vitamin C. This means that there is more water than cranberry juice in the product. It also shows that it has been fortified with extra vitamin C and that sugar was added. Understanding and using the information provided on food labels is one way to be a good consumer.

Advertising

Advertising also influences which health products are purchased. The purpose of advertising is to sell a product by convincing the consumer that she or he needs the product. Advertisers often use models or celebrities to help make the product seem more attractive. Consumers who buy only health products that they need can save money.

Quackery

Health quackery is health care performed by unlicensed practitioners or by licensed practitioners in an unethical manner. Health quacks often prey on people with incurable diseases. In particular, arthritis, cancer, diabetes, and multiple sclerosis patients are targets for quacks who promise quick, painless cures. These practitioners sometimes claim that medical science does not use their special method because they want the cure to be kept a "secret" so that physicians will make more money on ill patients. Quacks do not often hurt people directly, but when patients are in the care of a quack, they are not getting the proper medical help they may need. Whenever seeking medical services or other health advice, it is important to investigate the qualifications and limitations of the individual involved. Most states require licensing of health advisers. This usually involves successful graduation from a recognized professional school and a satisfactory score on a state examination. Continuing education to keep the health professional up to date is usually required for renewal of the license. Most health professionals display this license in a prominent place in an office, clinic, or pharmacy. If quackery is suspected, the Better Business Bureau or American Medical Association can be contacted.

DRUG USE AND ABUSE

Any drug or medication has the potential of being useful or hazardous to health. Drugs change the physical and mental workings of the body. When used correctly, drugs can save lives, cure illness, prevent disease, and relieve pain. However, inappropriate use of drugs can lead to physical or psychological drug dependence or both.

There are many laws that regulate the use of drugs. Federal, state, and local laws exist regarding drugs. Certain federal laws determine standards that drugs must pass to be legally sold in the United States. The Food and Drug Administration (FDA) sets these standards. The FDA also determines how drugs are sold legally. Some drugs are sold over the counter, which means that they can be purchased without a prescription. Others are prescription drugs and can be purchased only with a physician's orders. Certain drugs are not usually taken for medical reasons. Some of these drugs are legal (such as alcohol and tobacco), and others are not (such as marijuana, cocaine, LSD and PCP). There are often state and local laws that regulate the sale of legal drugs, alcohol and tobacco. Such laws regarding the age for purchasing these drugs, the penalty for drunk driving, hours when alcohol can be sold, and where a bar can be located, vary from state to state. Some counties do not allow the sale of alcohol at all. These are called *dry* counties.

Laws regulating the use of drugs are made for the sake of protection. In the case of prescription and over-the-counter drugs, the laws make drug companies prove that their drug is safe if used as directed. This means that drug companies must research their drugs carefully before they can sell them to the public or suggest that physicians prescribe the drugs. Thalidomide is an example of a drug that was thought safe and was used in other countries. It was taken by many pregnant women in England and by some in the United States who got it while travelling or stationed abroad, or were given it by physicians who received the drug as samples and assumed that it was safe to distribute. Later the drug was found to be the cause of severe birth defects in their babies. It had not been made legal to use in the United States because there was not enough research completed to meet the standards of the FDA.

Other drugs are thought to be unsafe and

unhealthful and are not legal to use at all. However, there is certainly controversy over whether some of these illegal drugs should be legalized. Marijuana has been shown to help cancer patients counteract the nausea of chemotherapy and is being prescribed for this purpose by physicians in some states. Some argue that marijuana is not as unsafe or unhealthful as the legal drugs alcohol and tobacco. Others argue that, even if marijuana is not as harmful, it is not wise to legalize it and add to the problems that are caused by the use and abuse of alcohol and tobacco.

Laws concerning driving an automobile while under the influence of alcohol are meant to protect the innocent people who are involved in traffic accidents. Drunk drivers are responsible for about half the fatal automobile accidents in the United States. Many states have strict laws about driving while drinking.

Age requirements to legally buy cigarettes and alcohol exist because it is known that these drugs can be physically harmful. It is generally believed by society that the legal use of these drugs should be limited to adults who are better able to understand the consequences of their actions.

Over-the-Counter Drugs

Over-the-counter (OTC) drugs can be bought without a prescription—at food stores, drug stores, and in many other places. There are OTC drugs for headaches, allergies, colds, coughs, and stomach aches. OTC drugs can be helpful if:
- taken only with parental guidance
- taken only according to directions

Prescription Drugs

Doctors often treat illnesses with special medicines that can only be bought with a prescription. These drugs are unsafe for self-medication and therefore must be filled by a *pharmacist*.

The pharmacist is specially trained to prepare the prescription and will provide directions for using the medicine safely. It is particularly important to have an adult administer the medication and to follow the directions carefully.

Drug Misuse and Abuse

Drug misuse occurs when a drug is used in ways that can harm the body. Taking more medicine than the directions indicate or taking someone else's medicine are examples of drug misuse. Drug abuse occurs when drugs are used for purposes other than those for which they are intended. A person who abuses a drug risks becoming dependent upon the drug, in addition to possibly suffering other ill effects.

Alcohol

Alcohol is a drug that is found in beer, wine, and liquor. It is a "depressant" drug that affects a person's body and mind and can cause dependency in certain individuals. Because alcohol is a depressant, it affects the way the brain works. Movement becomes slower, coordination is affected, and the heart and respiratory systems slow down.

Tobacco

Tobacco contains a powerful drug called *nicotine*. Nicotine is a "stimulant" drug and when taken into the body, causes the circulatory and respiratory systems to speed up. Nicotine also causes the blood vessels to narrow so that the heart has to work harder to pump the blood through the body. Tobacco can be smoked in the form of cigarettes, cigars, and pipes, or used in a smokeless form. Snuff and chewing tobacco are forms of smokeless tobacco.

Inhalants

Inhalants are substances that give off fumes that cause a feeling of drunkenness. Glue, gasoline, and aerosol sprays are examples of inhalants. There is no medical use for these chemicals; even small amounts of these poisons can cause permanent damage to the brain and other body systems.

ENVIRONMENTAL HEALTH

Four major types of environmental pollution that can be explored by intermediate level students are: air, water, land, and noise pollution. Maintaining a clean and safe environment can enhance the individual physically, mentally, and socially. A clean environment will decrease the spread of disease-causing microorganisms and lessen the chance of physical harm from unhealthy chemicals. A clean and safe environment is mentally restful; many people believe that the enjoyment of nature and a pleasant environment help reduce stress and stimulate the mind and emotions in a positive way. Finally, it is much easier to relate to others in an environment where the noise levels are tolerable.

Air Pollution

Pollution of the air is a major problem in modern society. Even though air pollution usually is a greater problem in metropolitan areas, pollutants are found in the air everywhere. Air pollutants are the actual substances found in the atmosphere that contaminate the air. The major pollutants are carbon monoxide, hydrocarbons, nitrogen oxides, mold, and dust. The sources of these pollutants include: smoke and noxious fumes from industry; smoke from forest fires, tobacco, and volcanos; and exhaust from incomplete combustion of petroleum products in automobiles, trucks, or airplanes. Recent technological advances include the development of engines that are less air polluting.

Water Pollution

Along with clean air, clean water is essential for sustaining life. In developing countries the most important health concern is the availability of clean and safe water. Many people in the United States have taken the abundance of good, clean water for granted; however, they are beginning to realize that the water resources must be protected to maintain the current standard of living. Waterways and resources can be polluted by sewer waste, solid debris, and chemicals. Contaminated water can breed disease, thereby posing a great danger to animal life as well as to humans.

The sources of water pollution are numerous and varied. Often pollution is related to the use of water in agriculture, industry, sewage drainage and treatment, and cooling nuclear power plants. In all cases the balance of nature is disrupted, causing a chain reaction that results in various problems. Many scientists believe that we have only scratched the surface in the detection of problems (many health-related) that result from water pollution.

Land Pollution

Pollution of the land often is related to its destruction, which takes many forms. Agriculturally, land can become unproductive or worn out if not used wisely. Cities and communities need to be planned carefully so that valuable watersheds, timber, lakes, and streams are protected and erosion is avoided. The land can be polluted aesthetically as well. Grafitti and litter are unsightly and even unhealthful. Industry can have a profound effect on the environment. The lumber industry, strip mining, oil drilling, waste disposal, and nuclear power production have caused destruction of the land. However, many of these industrial operations have now been modified so that the damage to the environment is lessened. In some situations steps are taken to restore the land to its original state. With the increased awareness of the importance of a clean and safe environment, industry probably will be required to examine the possible health and environmental hazards of their operations and, ideally, to take steps to correct any aspect that poses a threat to health or the environment.

Noise Pollution

Noise pollution has become a problem in societies which are becoming increasingly technological. With the recognition of the potential hazard to hearing, attempts have been made to reduce the level of noise in everyday life. Houses and offices can be shielded from highways with large berms of land planted with trees and shrubs. Airplanes can be built with quieter engines. Automobiles and trucks are required to have mufflers. People who work in noisy environments should be encouraged to wear protective devices to prevent hearing loss; this may even be required by law.

COMMUNITY HEALTH

In every community, members must work together to solve certain problems. Examples of this cooperation are the organization of a volunteer fire department in an area inaccessible to a staffed department, organization of a recycling center, provision of special classes informing community members of certain health problems, organization of a blood bank, and individual contributions of time or money to certain charities or health causes. Elected officials have a responsibility to work with health professionals and other community members to identify the health needs of the community and determine variable courses of action.

Many communities have local offices of voluntary health agencies. Individuals can volunteer time and money to these agencies to help fight certain problems both locally and nationally. Such agencies that may need volunteer help include the American Lung Association, American Cancer Society, American Heart Association, American Red Cross, National Foundation—March of Dimes, and Society for the Prevention of Blindness. Students can help by participating in various fund-raising and educational programs organized by these types of agencies. Common activities include raising money by hiking or bicycling competitions, working at camps, and teaching younger children about a particular health problem. Local hospitals usually need volunteer help as well. Students can join the hospital volunteer staff and often work directly with hospital patients.

Becoming involved in various health-related activities as an adolescent often stimulates interest in a health career. It is appropriate for teachers to encourage this interest in the intermediate years. More specific details about the actual duties of various health professionals can be explored by students in junior high and high school.

REFERENCES

American Automobile Association: Safest route to school, Falls Church, Vir, 1980, American Automobile Association.

Arena J and Bachar M: Child Safety is no accident, Durham No Car, 1978, Duke University Press.

Ashley R: Human anatomy, New York, 1976, John Wiley & Sons.

Barrett S: The health robbers, Philadelphia, 1980, George F Stickley.

Branden N: The psychology of self-esteem, New York, 1969, Bantam Books.

Cohen S: "The hallucinogens and the inhalants," The psychiatric clinics of north america, 7(4), 1984.

Eliot R and Breo D: Is it worth dying for? New York, 1984, Bantam Books.

Growing healthy, New York, 1986, National Center for Health Education.

Jenkins G and Schacter H: These are your children, Glenview, Ill, 1975, Scott Foresman and Company.

Kubler-Ross E: On death and dying, New York, 1967, Macmillan Inc.

Selye H: Stress without distress, New York, 1974, JB Lippincott.

Taylor K and Anthony L: Clinical nutrition, New York, 1983, McGraw-Hill.

CHAPTER 13

Intermediate Level Teaching Activity Ideas

When you finish this chapter, you should be able to:

■ **Develop learning opportunities in elementary health education for grades 4 through 6 which appropriately provide for practice with the behavior and content specified in an objective.**

Several fully developed health education learning opportunities for children in grades 4 to 6 are presented in this chapter. These plans contain activities designed to reach objectives selected from the proposed scope and sequence in Chapter 9. Ten plans are presented, one in each of the ten health education content areas. They demonstrate only one way to reach an objective and cannot be viewed as a total health education program for this level. They can serve as models for the further development of learning opportunities to round out a comprehensive health education plan.

The specific activities explained in these learning opportunities were chosen because they are particularly appropriate for these grades. Most should be successful in any of the three grade levels. Some are more appropriate for one grade level or another depending on the growth and development of the students in a specific grade, and these plans are identified as such. However, in all cases the final decision as to the appropriateness of the activities for a given group of students must be left up to the teacher. In addition, the teacher will have to plan the time needed for each learning opportunity, since it will vary from class to class.

The components of these plans are consistent with the learning opportunities described in Chapter 5. Each includes an objective, content generalizations (big ideas), initiation activity, learning activities using a variety of methods, culmination activity, and evaluation activity that calls for students to demonstrate the ability specified in the objective. Other helpful items are included, such as worksheets that are explained in the activities. If the worksheet has specific answers, a key is provided in a reduced form within the body of the teaching plan. Other materials that may have to be purchased, obtained from school supplies, or gathered from around the classroom are indicated in the margins.

In developing these plans the sequence from one activity to another is of prime concern. Often one can have a brilliant idea for the classroom but forget the essential lead-in and follow-up acitivities. Another common error in the development of learning opportunities is losing sight of the objective. This is often the result of fully developed activities that are tangential to the objective. Frequent checking of the objective during the development of learning opportunities is essential.

The interrelatedness of health education topics makes planning complex. Even though 10 content areas are identified here, health topics do not neatly fit within a specific area. For example, when dealing with alcohol use, it is just as appropriate to place it in the content area of drug use and abuse as in accident prevention and safety. The teacher who is aware of these relationships can skillfully weave content areas together into learning activities that reinforce and demonstrate these interrelationships to students. However, to be effective, these activities should be planned, not tangential material included by chance.

PERSONAL HEALTH AND FITNESS

Objective. The student explains how personal health behavior is influenced by friends and family members.

Level. Grades 4 to 6

Integration. Language arts

Content generalizations. The personal health behaviors chosen greatly influence the quality of life. The adoption of a healthful life style or an unhealthful life style is a personal choice that is influenced by a number of outside variables. Initially personal health behaviors are learned from parents and family members. When children enter school, they learn about other habits perhaps not practiced in their family. Particularly in the adolescent years, peer pressure has a strong influence on health behaviors. It is not unusual to see great changes in personal health behaviors of adolescents because of peer pressure. These changes can be positive, such as the adoption of better grooming habits or a personal fitness and sports program. The changes also can be negative, such as the adoption of drug habits or risk-taking behaviors. Whatever the final life style chosen, the health behaviors determining the choice have been greatly influenced by friends and family members.

Vocabulary. Life style, peer pressure, influence

Initiation. Habits—Word Puzzle

Hand out the worksheet for the students to solve. When they are finished, go over the solution to the puzzle. Then ask how many students got everything correct. (Most students will do *very* well on the puzzle.) Ask, "Why did you do so well filling in the missing words when we have not studied anything about health habits in class yet?" Students probably will have answers such as, "I learned it last year in Mr. Smith's class," or, "My mom always tells me to brush my teeth."

Explain to the students that we learn what good health behavior is from many places. This starts when we are very young. Ask the students if they can think of a health habit that a parent has been telling them about for as long as they can remember. Also ask them "Just because you know you should do something (such as wash your hands after using the restroom), do you always do it?"

Materials

Worksheet: *Habits—Word Puzzle* (p. 333)

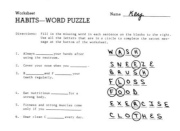

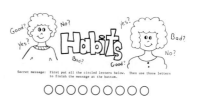

Have the students consider the following questions for
discussion.
(1) Can personal nutritional choices be influenced by
friends and family members?
(2) How can personal nutritional choices be influenced by
friends and family members?
(3) Can the influence of others be positive, as well as negative?
(4) How can you reinforce positive health behaviors in
your family or friends?
(5) How can you resist friends or family influencing you to
develop a negative health habit?

Activities

1. A Story About Maverick
   a. Tell the students they are going to hear a story about a
   10-year-old boy celebrating his straight-A report card.
   Ask them to think about what the boy, Maverick, does
   to celebrate his success.

MAVERICK CELEBRATES

Maverick flew into his house calling out, "Mom, Dad,
Grandpa, come look. I got all A's on my report card,
not even one A−. And the teacher's comments were
great. Mr. Adams said that I was exceptional in completing my assignments and a model student in class.
Listen to what he said about my health lessons:
'Maverick learned his health lessons and actually
applied them in class. He bought fruit and milk every
day during the nutrition break. Maverick successfully
led our "I don't smoke cigarettes" campaign in
school and received the highest grade in the class on
all his nutrition, science, and health examinations.' "

"Great!" exclaimed Maverick's dad. "You
weren't kidding when you said you could get straight
A's by studying after dinner every night."

"What a difference from last year when you
didn't study and got all C's," said Maverick's mom.
"You did better than get straight A's. It sounds as
though you're the star in school, particularly in
health."

Maverick could scarcely hold in his joy. He was
jumping up and down and shouting, "I did it!"

Grandpa said, "I'm proud of you too, Grandson.
I'm going to give you $5 to save or spend. A smart
boy like you will know the right thing to do with
$5."

Maverick thanked Grandpa, Mom, and Dad and ran upstairs to get ready for a party at his friend's house. Maverick brushed and flossed his teeth, put on a clean shirt, and stuffed the new $5 bill into his jeans pocket. He dashed out of the house, whistling as he walked to the party.

On the way Maverick ran into Albert, who was headed to the party also. Albert said, "Didn't you hear? The parents won't be home during the party. I'm bringing beer so that we can really celebrate. You especially have to celebrate your straight-A report card." "No thanks, I don't drink beer," said Maverick.

When they arrived at the party, Maverick noticed that the music was turned up loud, some people were drinking beer, and others were chewing or smoking tobacco. Maverick turned down several offers to chew or smoke tobacco or drink beer. But he did not turn down Albert's last offer.

Albert said, "Maverick, are you too good to celebrate with us just because you got all A's? You're not really one of us any more unless you have a couple of beers and a few cigarettes."

Maverick could not resist. He wanted to be one of the gang—their friend. They were all drinking and smoking, so why shouldn't he?

On the way home from the party Maverick had an upset stomach. He felt sick partly because he had had two beers and three cigarettes, but mostly because he had let himself down. As Maverick walked home alone, he was thinking, "Why did I have those beers and cigarettes? I really didn't want them, so why did I have them?"

b. Discussion questions
   (1) Why did Maverick drink two beers and smoke three cigarettes?
   (2) Why was Maverick able to turn down Albert the first time but not the second time?
   (3) Did Maverick's friends have anything to do with his decision to drink and smoke?
   (4) How could Maverick have avoided drinking beer or smoking cigarettes without jeopardizing his friendship with the others?

2. Lets Do It Together

   Identify a group health behavior that the class would like
   to collectively practice. It might be related to safety (not
   running in halls or putting away classroom materials that
   could cause someone to trip), environment (a litter clean-
   up campaign or a "be quieter in the lunchroom" campaign), nutrition (no junk food at school), or another area
   of health. Students should develop an approach to positively support and influence one another in practicing this
   positive health habit.

Evaluation. The Apple and the Candy Bar.

   Read the following story aloud to students.

> Marion has to make a snack choice. Her friend Kathy
> is going to have a SuperCocoCarmal Bar and thinks
> Marion should have one too. Marion has just gotten
> back from the dentist and has more cavities than she
> would like to admit. Marion's mother told her to eat
> apples instead of candy becaue they are naturally
> sweet and good for her. Besides, Marion likes
> apples.

   Ask the students to explain what influences Marion is
feeling before she makes her choice. The explanation can be
done as a paragraph or a cartoon.

Materials

Worksheet: *The Apple and the Candy Bar* (p. 334)

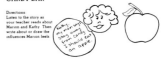

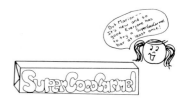

Worksheet   Name _____

HABITS—WORD PUZZLE

Directions: Fill in the missing word in each sentence on the blanks to the right.
Use all the letters that are in a circle to complete the secret message at the bottom of the worksheet.

1. Always _____ your hands after
using the restroom.

2. Cover your nose when you _____ .

3. B _____ and F _____ your
teeth regularly.

4. Eat nutritious _____ for a
strong body.

5. Fitness and strong muscles come
only if you _____ .

6. Wear clean C _____ every day.

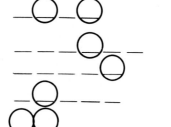
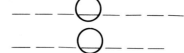

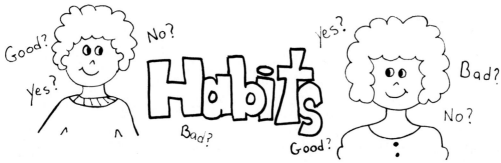

Secret message: First put all the circled letters below.   Then use those letters
to finish the message at the bottom.

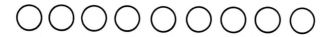

THESE ARE HABITS   __ __ __   __ __ __ __ __ __ __ !

Worksheet   Name _____

Worksheet   Name _____

THE APPLE AND THE CANDY BAR

Directions:
Listen to the story as your teacher reads about Marion and Kathy. Then write about or draw the influences Marion feels.

Kathy, my mom says stay away from candy. I should eat an apple.

But Marion — — It's new and so good. Everyone has to try a SuperCocoCarmel bar at least once!

SuperCocoCarmel

MENTAL AND EMOTIONAL HEALTH

Objective. The student synthesizes acceptable ways to deal with strong negative emotions.

Level. Grades 4 to 6

Integration. Art, language arts

Content generalizations. When our ideas or values are different from those of others or we do not get our own way, strong negative emotions, usually anger and frustration, arise, resulting in a stressful situation. Unacceptable ways that people deal with anger include fighting, swearing, breaking objects, and pouting. It is also unacceptable to "hold it in" and do nothing. Acceptable ways to deal with anger include exercise, "getting it off your chest" by talking it out, long walks, shouting into a pillow, and taking deep breaths. Some sort of physical exercise is probably the most effective. It is important to understand that anger is a normal emotion which everyone experiences. All these ways to deal with anger also can be used to deal with any stressful situation.

Vocabulary. Conflict, emotions, resolve, anger, appropriate, inappropriate

Initiation. It Really Makes Me Mad . . .
Ask the students to think about various things that make them mad using the worksheet, *It Really Makes Me Mad. . . .* Explain that they are to write down situations which make them angry. An example is, "I get mad when my little brother breaks the airplane model I spent 3 hours working on." Ask the students what they might do in this anger-causing situation. Ask for volunteers to tell what they really do when they get angry. Make no value judgment at this time regarding the appropriateness of their actions.

Explain that anger is normal. We need to learn how to deal with anger and other negative emotions because life is filled with both good and bad emotions. The good ones are easy to deal with; the negative ones are more difficult. Tell the students to hold on to their papers for use in later activities.

Materials
Worksheet: *It Really Makes Me Mad. . .* (p. 339)

IT REALLY MAKES
ME MAD...

1. When _____
   _____
   _____

2. When _____
   _____
   _____

3. When _____
   _____
   _____

GET YOUR HANDS OFF MY STUFF !!

Activities

1. Ways to Deal With Anger—Part I

   Write the words *acceptable* and *unacceptable* on the board. Explain to the students that anger can be dealt with in an acceptable or unacceptable way. Ask them to help you determine what is acceptable and what is unacceptable. Generally, unacceptable can be defined as any action that damages people, property, or feelings.

   Hand out the worksheet, *Ways to Deal With Anger*. Individually allow the students to read each situation in part I and determine if the action was acceptable or unacceptable. Tell them to leave part II blank for now.

2. Ways to Deal With Anger—Part II

   When students are done with the individual work on part I, put them in groups of four or five to discuss their choices. Part II is to be completed as a group. First, students should discuss and defend their choices in part I. Then, as a group, they should decide on an acceptable behavior for the situation described in part II. Everyone in the group must agree that the behavior chosen is acceptable. As a group, they should design a way to present their ideas to the class on a transparency. They can draw a cartoon, write a paragraph, or act it out as a skit.

   The groups should elect a representative to present their ideas orally to the class.

3. "Mad Feelings" Boxes

   a. A few days before this activity tell the students to bring to class an empty half-gallon milk carton. (Small milk cartons from the school cafeteria could be used if necessary.)

   b. Tell the students they will be making "Mad Feelings" boxes. First they are to decorate a milk carton as follows.

      (1) On one side print the word *acceptable*.

      (2) On another side print the word *unacceptable*.

      (3) On the two remaining sides draw two pictures of acceptable ways of dealing with anger.

Materials

Worksheet: *Ways to Deal With Anger* (p. 340)

Materials

Worksheet: *Ways to Deal With Anger* (with part I completed) (p. 340)
Transparency (1 sheet per group)
Transparency pens (at least one per group, but preferably several colors)

Materials

Overhead projector
Transparencies (completed by groups)

Materials

Half-gallon milk cartons (1 per student)
Construction paper (light colored)
Stapler
Felt pens, colored pencils, or crayons

c. Then every day for a week or so, at the beginning of class they are to write down the various situations that made them angry the day before. Each instance is written on a separate piece of paper, including the way that they handled their anger in that situation. Each piece of paper should be placed into the milk carton.

d. After about a week of collecting information about situations that make them angry, the students should draw out a slip of paper from the milk carton. The students should read each situation to themselves and consider whether the action taken was an acceptable or unacceptable way of dealing with anger. Students should paste a star on the "Mad Feelings" boxes either under *acceptable* or *unacceptable,* whichever applies for that particular situation. They continue the same process for each slip of paper in the box.

4. Dealing With My Mad Feelings

a. Ask the students to count the stars on their boxes. Ask, "Which side has the most stars? How well do you do at handling anger in an acceptable way?" Hand out the worksheet, *Dealing With My Mad Feelings.* Ask the students to use one of the situations where they behaved in an unacceptable way and to write a suggestion of a different way to behave in the same situation that would be acceptable. Allow them to work on this assignment in pairs if they desire. Review the written suggestions, and give them back to the students with comments.

Materials

"Mad Feelings" boxes (previously made by students)

Scratch paper

Mental and emotional health

Materials

"Mad Feelings" boxes filled with descriptions of anger-causing situations

Stars (all one color; at least 5 to 10 per student)

Materials

Worksheet: *Dealing With My Mad Feelings* (p. 341)

DEALING WITH MY MAD FEELINGS

Unacceptable
☆ ☆ ☆

★ ★ ★ ★ ★ ★
Acceptable

b. Have the students collect another week's worth of anger-causing situations and behaviors in their "Mad Feelings" boxes. At the end of the week they should analyze their behaviors again and give themselves a star on either the *acceptable* or *unacceptable* side. Ask if they improved during the second week. Explain that this is a very difficult behavior to learn and they should try not to be frustrated if they are having problems. Tell them it might be helpful to talk to someone they trust about further suggestions of appropriate ways to handle anger.

5. Take a Breather

Practice deep-breathing exercises with the students. Tell them this is often a very effective method of dealing with strong emotions, especially when it is difficult to do any physical exercise. Have the students sit up straight and inhale deeply from the abdomen. They should try to inhale slowly through their nose and bring their shoulders back slightly during inhalation.

A slow inhalation should take at least 5 seconds. Then have them exhale for 5 seconds *slowly* through the mouth. Have the students try this two or three times in class. Tell them to teach it to their parents if they like.

NOTE: For this activity you may want to consider playing soft music, darkening the room, and having the children close their eyes and lie down on a carpet. This will help the students relax. You could suggest that they try this type of relaxation at home if it is not possible at school.

Materials

"Mad Feelings" boxes (filled with anger-causing situations)

Stars (all one color but a *different* color than used previously; at least 5 to 10 per student)

Evaluation. What I Can Do When I'm Mad

Ask the students to look at the worksheet, *It Really Makes Me Mad . . .*, completed at the beginning of these activities. For each statement about what makes them mad, the students should write at least one acceptable way to deal with their negative emotions. Encourage them to use those behaviors when the anger-producing situations arise again.

Materials

Worksheet: *It Really Makes Me Mad . . .* (completed earlier) (p. 339)

Worksheet

Name _____

IT REALLY MAKES ME MAD...

1. When _____

_____

_____

_____

2. When _____

_____

_____

_____

3. When _____

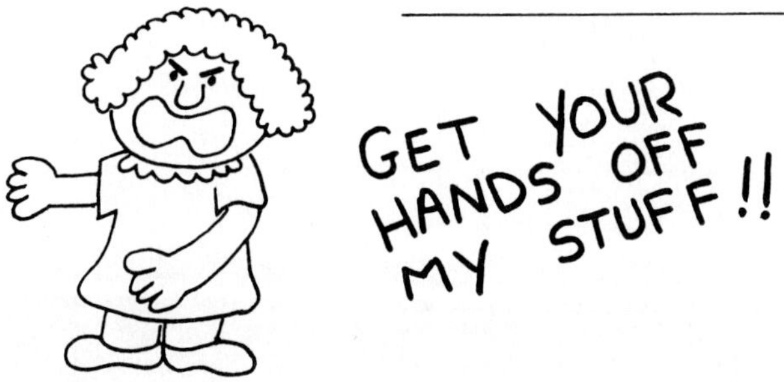

_____

_____

_____

GET YOUR HANDS OFF MY STUFF!!

Worksheet   Name _____

WAYS TO DEAL WITH ANGER

Part I

1. Susan has a new dress. She wore it to school for the first time on Monday.
    When she went to the cafeteria, one of the boys accidently squirted catsup
    on the dress. She grabbed the catsup bottle and squirted catsup all over
    his shirt.

               ACCEPTABLE   UNACCEPTABLE

2. Mary was working hard in her garden. She had just planted new seedlings.
    She had several neat rows of vegetables. Suddenly, Joe's large dog saw a
    cat and ran through the new garden. The seedlings were mashed but not too
    damaged. She shouted, "Oh, no!" and took a long walk around the block.
    When she came back from her walk, she asked Joe to help her replant the
    seedlings.

               ACCEPTABLE   UNACCEPTABLE

3. Rena was skating down the sidewalk. She hit a little pebble on the sidewalk
    and fell down. She got up and started to swear at the pebble. She picked
    up the pebble and threw it as hard as she could. She was so mad that she
    did not even look to see where the pebble landed.

               ACCEPTABLE   UNACCEPTABLE

4. Ken came home from school to find that his little brother Patrick had been
    looking through his closet again. He went downstairs and told Pat in a firm
    voice, "Please stay out of my closet." Then he went outside to play a hard
    game of touch football.

               ACCEPTABLE   UNACCEPTABLE

Part II

    Myrna studied hard for the mathematics test. She took her book home every
    day for 2 weeks. She had her brother quiz her on fractions. On the day of
    the test, Sam looked over her shoulder and copied her answers. The teacher
    graded the tests as the students finished them. Myrna did well, but Sam
    did the best in the class. Myrna was very angry. When she got out of class,
    she went over to Sam and gave him a good punch.

    Was Myrna's behavior acceptable? What other ways could Myrna have handled
    this situation and dealt with her anger?

Worksheet   Name _____

DEALING WITH MY MAD FEELINGS

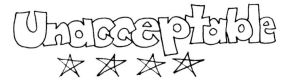

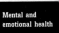

Mental and
emotional health

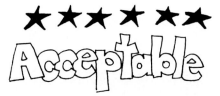

FAMILY LIFE

Objective. The student identifies growth and developmental characteristics common in puberty.

Level. Grades 4 to 6 (more appropriate for grade 5 or 6)

Integration. Science

Content generalizations. As boys and girls mature into men and women, many physical and psychological changes occur. Puberty is when these changes occur, and the result is the capability of sexual reproduction. Although puberty does not commence or end at the same time for each individual, the pattern of change is predictable. Puberty is a slow and gradual process that begins with a signal from the pituitary gland that stimulates the production of sexual hormones. These hormones in turn signal various parts of the male or female body to start growing and changing. Puberty is also a time when boys and girls begin to become more interested in each other. Generally, girls are about 2 years ahead of boys in both the physical and psychological changes of puberty.

NOTE: Before teaching any lessons regarding sexuality, state and local school district guidelines should be studied. It is highly recommended that parental consent forms be sent out with the help and advice of the school principal.

The teaching plan presented here deals primarily with puberty. Depending on the previous exposure of the students to information on reproductive processes, more or fewer activities may be required.

These activities are probably more appropriate for grade 5 or 6 and should be taught by a teacher who feels comfortable dealing with this material. It is also important to be sensitive to possible student anxiety and embarrassment.

Vocabulary. Puberty, hormones, menstruation

Initiation. My, Have You Changed!

A few days before starting these activities, ask the students to bring in a baby picture of themselves. It should be one that they don't mind others seeing (Fig. 13-1). (The best pictures are of students when they were toddlers rather than infants.)

Put up the bulletin board display, *My, Have You Changed!* Students should give you the picture *without* showing it to anyone else in the class. Allow the students to study the pictures on the bulletin board. Then have them number on their paper from 1 to whatever number of students there are in class. Ask the students to try to match each picture with a student's name. When they are finished listing names corresponding to the numbers next to the baby pictures, have all the students in the class go to the bulletin board and mount a slip of paper printed with their name under their baby picture. Have the students check their lists to see how many baby pictures they were able to identify correctly.

Materials

Bulletin board display: *My, Have You Changed!*

Slips of paper with each student's name

Student pictures as babies

MY, HAVE YOU CHANGED!

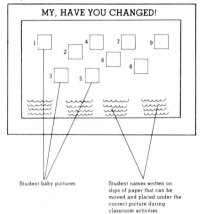

Student baby pictures   Student names written on slips of paper that can be moved and placed under the correct picture during classroom activities

Family life

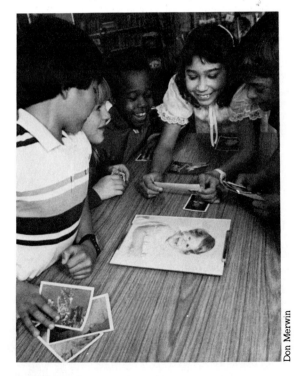

FIGURE 13-1

Don Merwin

Ask students the following discussion questions:
1. Were you able to identfy all the pictures correctly? Why or why not?
2. What are some of the ways that most students have changed since the picture was taken? (Taller, heavier, possibly more hair.)
3. Can you think of any changes that will occur in the next few years?

Activities

1. What Is Puberty?

   Conduct a short lecture on puberty. Bring out the following points in the lecture. As each of the words in italics is explained, write it on the board, and have the students write it on a piece of paper for use later.

   a. *Puberty* is triggered and regulated by the *endocrine system.*

   b. Chemical "messengers" called *hormones* regulate growth and development. They determine when and how you grow and change during puberty.

   c. The *pituitary gland* is a part of the endocrine system and is located at the base of the brain. This gland signals the body when puberty is to begin.

   d. The pituitary gland signals the female *ovaries* and the male *testes* to start producing hormones.

   e. One of the first signs of puberty is the *secondary sexual characteristics.*
      (1) For the boy:
         (a) Body hair (face, underarms, legs, pubic area, and possibly chest)
         (b) Deeper voice
         (c) Enlargement of penis and testes
         (d) Production of sperm
         (e) Broadening of shoulders
      (2) For the girl:
         (a) Development of breasts
         (b) Body hair (underarms, legs, pubic area)
         (c) Widening of hips

   f. Both boys and girls start producing mature sex cells: *sperm* in boys and *ova* in girls. (In girls all the eggs are present and begin to mature and be released at puberty.)

   g. An important part of puberty for girls is the onset of *menstruation.* This is a cyclical discharge of blood and *endometrial cells.*

Materials
Paper
Pencils

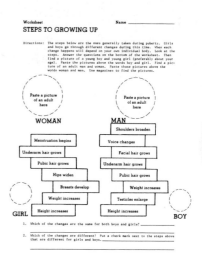

h. The changes that happen during puberty are natural and normal. Everyone will experience these changes at their own rate.

At the end of the lecture ask if there are any questions. It may be helpful to set up a question box so students can write questions anonymously on slips of paper.

2. Steps to Growing Up

Hand out the worksheet, and explain that these are the usual steps (sequence of events) in puberty. Have the students complete the questions at the bottom of the page. Orally review the answers to the questions on the worksheet, *Steps to Growing Up.* Tell the students to take the worksheet home and keep track of the changes as they occur in their own body.

Materials
Worksheet: *Steps to Growing Up*
(p. 346)

Evaluation. Changes, Changes

Students circle the growth and developmental characteristics occurring during puberty for boys and for girls on the worksheet *Changes, Changes.*

Materials
Worksheet: *Changes, Changes*
(p. 347)

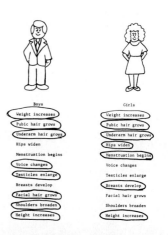

Worksheet   Name _____

STEPS TO GROWING UP

Directions: The steps below are the ones generally taken during puberty. Girls
and boys go through different changes during this time. When each
change happens will depend on your own individual body. Look at the
steps. Answer the questions on the bottom of the worksheet. Then
find a picture of a young boy and young girl (preferably about your
age). Paste the pictures above the words boy and girl. Find a picture of an adult man and woman. Paste those pictures above the
words woman and man. Use magazines to find the pictures.

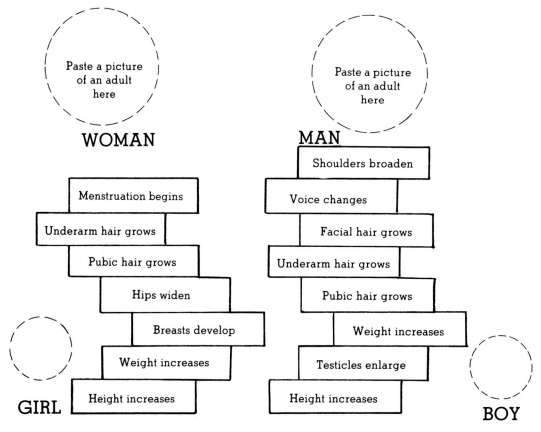

1. Which of the changes are the same for both boys and girls? _____

_____

2. Which of the changes are different? Put a check mark next to the steps above
that are different for girls and boys. _____

_____

Worksheet

Name _____

CHANGES, CHANGES

Directions: The two people below have both grown up. What changes did their
bodies experience during puberty? Circle the characteristics of
puberty for boys and girls.

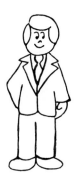
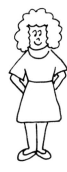

Boys   Girls

Weight increases   Weight increases

Pubic hair grows   Pubic hair grows

Underarm hair grows   Underarm hair grows

Hips widen   Hips widen

Menstruation begins   Menstruation begins

Voice changes   Voice changes

Testicles enlarge   Testicles enlarge

Breasts develop   Breasts develop

Facial hair grows   Facial hair grows

Shoulders broaden   Shoulders broaden

Height increases   Height increases

NUTRITION

Objective. The student analyzes the nutritional worth of food choices for meals and snacks.

Level. Grades 4 to 6

Integration. Science

Content generalizations. Fruits and vegetables, milk products, grain products, and protein products should be eaten daily to provide adequate nutrition. Each of these food groups provides specific nutrients that are required to promote growth and maintain health. Children in grades 4 to 6 should eat three servings from the milk group, two servings from the protein group (also called meat group), four servings from the fruit and vegetable group, and four servings from the bread and cereal group (also called grain group), daily for a nutritious diet. Certain foods are not placed in a food group because they are too low in nutrient content. These are called *other* or *extra* foods and are usually high in sugar, fat, or both. Foods in this category include cakes, candies, cookies, pies, salad dressings, mayonnaise, catsup, butter, margarine, jams, jellies, soda, and chips and should be consumed in moderation.

Vocabulary. Nutrients, protein, poultry, vitamins, minerals

Initiation. Three-Day Food Diary

Ask the students to keep a diary of all the foods they eat and drink, including meals and snacks. Begin the activity immediately by having the students write down everything they ate yesterday. That will be day 1 of the food diary. Today will be day 2, and tomorrow will be day 3. Tell the students they will be studying the foods they eat. Encourage them to eat normally. Allow a little class time each day to fill in the food diary from the previous day.

Materials

Worksheet: *Three-Day Food Diary* (3 copies per student) (p. 351)

Activities

1. Foods in the Four Food Groups

   Use food models to help discuss and identify various foods in each food group. Hold a picture of a food up, and have the children identify the group. Tell them that many foods we eat have more than one food group represented in the same dish. Beef stew has foods from the protein group and from the vegetable and fruit group. Ask the students what food groups are represented in a cheese sandwich. (Milk and bread and cereal.) Address the following questions in the discussion:

   a. What are the four food groups? (Milk, protein, vegetable and fruit, and bread and cereal.)

   b. What kinds of foods are in the milk group? (Milk, cheese, cottage cheese, and yogurt.)

   c. What kinds of foods are in the protein (or meat) group? (Meats, fish, poultry, dried beans and peas, and nuts.)

   d. What kinds of foods are in the vegetable and fruit group? (All vegetables and fruits, in all forms: juice, frozen, fresh, and canned.)

   e. What kinds of foods are in the bread and cereal (or grain) group? (Breads, cereals, rice, muffins, macaroni, pita bread, tortillas, and corn bread.)

   f. How many servings from each group are needed for children your age? (Three from milk, two from protein, four from vegetable and fruit, and four from bread and cereal.)

   Materials
   Food models or pictures of foods from magazines

2. Extra Foods

   Ask the students if they can think of any foods that have not been mentioned in any of the food groups. Explain that foods with a lot of sugar or fat do not have many of the nutrients needed for growth and health. Ask the children to help in making a list of extra foods. The following are examples.

Cakes	Cookies	Catsup
Candy	Jams	Jelly
Chips	Soft drinks	Mayonnaise
Butter	Margarine	Salad dressing

   Explain that these foods should be eaten in moderation and should not be substituted for a food in one of the food groups that is needed for a balanced diet. Have the students make collages of extra foods using pictures from magazines. They can work alone or in groups. When all have finished, put the collages on a bulletin board.

   Materials
   Construction paper
   Magazines
   Glue
   Scissors

Nutrition

3. How Well Did I Do?

Help students analyze their *Three-Day Food Diary* using the *Food Study Sheet.* Students should circle foods with a different-colored crayon to identify the group or to identify it as an extra food. Some foods should be circled with more than one color (for example, sandwiches, stews, pizza, and tacos). After the students have completed this, have them answer the following questions on a separate piece of paper.

a. How many days did you eat a balanced diet?

b. Which groups were you low in?

c. Did you eat extra foods all 3 days?

d. What kind of foods do you need to eat more of?

Evaluation How Well Does Pat Eat?

Have students analyze this worksheet in the same way that they analyzed their own diets by circling the various groups with crayons and answering the questions at the bottom of the page. Remind them that dishes which contain more than one food group should be circled with more than one color.

Materials

Worksheets: *Three-Day Food Diary* (completed earlier) (p. 351)

Student resource: *Food Study Sheet* (p. 352)

Crayons: red, green, black, blue, brown (1 of each color per student)

Materials

Paper

Pencils

Materials

Worksheet: *How Well Does Pat Eat?* (p. 353)

Crayons: red, green, black, blue, brown (1 of each color per student)

Worksheet   Name _Key_

HOW WELL DOES PAT EAT?

Directions: Read the diet that Pat ate one day. He is an 11-year-old boy who likes to play various sports. Did he get enough of the foods that he needs from each food group? Circle all the foods eaten from the various food groups with different colors to determine this. Then fill in the answers to the questions at the bottom.

BREAKFAST

     Bowl of cereal

     Glass of milk

     Glass of orange juice

SNACK BEFORE LUNCH

     1 Apple

LUNCH

     Hamburger on a bun

     Catsup

     Lettuce and tomato salad

     Salad dressing

     Glass of milk

     Chocolate brownie

SNACK BEFORE DINNER

     Bag of potato chips

DINNER

     Fried chicken

     Dish of carrots

     Lettuce and tomato salad

     Salad dressing

     Dinner roll

     Piece of cake

     Glass of milk

1. Did Pat have at least three servings in the milk group? _yes_

2. Did Pat have at least two servings in the protein group? _yes_

3. Did he have at least four servings in the vegetable and fruit group? _yes_

4. Did he have at least four servings in the grain group? _yes_

5. Did he eat any "extra" foods? _yes_

6. Did he substitute an "extra" food for a food needed in a food group? _no_

Worksheet   Name _____

THREE-DAY FOOD DIARY

Day   1   2   3
(Circle one)

BREAKFAST   Snacks between breakfast and lunch

_____   _____

_____   _____

_____   _____

_____   _____

_____   _____

_____   _____

_____   _____

LUNCH   Snacks between lunch and dinner
                                     (after-school snacks)

_____   _____

_____   _____

_____   _____

_____   _____

_____   _____

_____   _____

DINNER   Snacks after dinner

_____   _____

_____   _____

_____   _____

_____   _____

_____   _____

_____   _____

Nutrition

Student resource

FOOD STUDY SHEET

Grouping of food	Vitamins and nutrients	Purposes	Types of food
Fruits	Vitamin A Vitamin C Fiber	Healthy gums Healthy skin Growth and development	Apples Bananas Berries Strawberries Cantaloupe Grapefruit Oranges
Vegetables	Vitamin A Calcium Folic acid Iron Fiber	Healthy skin Growth and development Healthy bones Healthy teeth Healthy blood	Broccoli Carrots Celery Chinese pea pods Okra Greens Green beans
Milk	Calcium Phosphorus Riboflavin Protein Vitamin A Vitamin D (fortified)	Healthy bones Healthy teeth	Milk Nonfat milk Buttermilk Yogurt Cottage cheese Cheese

Grains	Carbohydrates
	B vitamins
	Iron
		Energy
		Digestive tract
		   (prevents constipation)
			Bread (whole wheat
			   or enriched)
			Cereal
			Pita
			Tortilla
			Matzo
			Rice
			Popcorn

Proteins	Protein Iron Calcium B vitamins	Build body tissues Repair body tissues	Eggs Cheese and beans (legumes) Cereal and milk Poultry Meat Fish

Worksheet   Name _____

HOW WELL DOES PAT EAT?

Directions: Read the diet that Pat ate one day. He is an 11-year-old boy who
likes to play various sports. Did he get enough of the foods that
he needs from each food group? Circle all the foods eaten from
the various food groups with different colors to determine this.
Then fill in the answers to the questions at the bottom.

Nutrition

BREAKFAST

   Bowl of cereal

   Glass of milk

   Glass of orange juice

SNACK BEFORE LUNCH

   1 Apple

LUNCH

   Hamburger on a bun

   Catsup

   Lettuce and tomato salad

   Salad dressing

   Glass of milk

   Chocolate brownie

SNACK BEFORE DINNER

   Bag of potato chips

DINNER

   Fried chicken

   Dish of carrots

   Lettuce and tomato salad

   Salad dressing

   Dinner roll

   Piece of cake

   Glass of milk

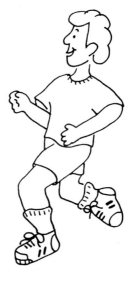

1. Did Pat have at least three servings
    in the milk group? _____

2. Did Pat have at least two servings in
    the protein group? _____

3. Did he have at least four servings in
    the vegetable and fruit group?_____

4. Did he have at least four servings in
    the grain group?_____

5. Did he eat any "extra" foods?_____

6. Did he substitute an "extra" food for
    a food needed in a food group?_____

DISEASE PREVENTION AND CONTROL

Objective. The student differentiates between control of communicable diseases and of noncommunicable diseases.

Level. Grades 4 to 6

Integration. Science, language arts, dictionary skills

Content generalizations. All women, men, and children are susceptible to both communicable diseases and noncommunicable diseases. Communicable diseases are infectious diseases in which a person serves as a host to an invading pathogenic agent. Communicable diseases are best controlled by prevention. Preventive measures include immunizations, minimizing exposure to pathogenic agents, and isolation during the contagious stage. Examples of communicable diseases are colds, measles, influenza, sexually transmitted diseases, and rabies.

Noncommunicable diseases are often diseases associated with life style, environment, and heredity. Examples of noncommunicable diseases are cardiovascular diseases, cancer, allergies, and arthritis.

Vocabulary. Life style, communicable, noncommunicable, pathogens, heredity, environment

Initiation. The Contagious "Handshake" Disease
Ask every student in the class to stand and shake hands with five students. Allow them to move around the room quickly to do this. Encourage them to shake hands with both good friends and those whom they do not know particularly well. When the handshaking is done, everyone should sit down again.

Have two students who are seated in different parts of the room stand. (Try to choose students who are not easily embarrassed.) Then ask all the students who shook hands with these two students to stand. Tell the rest of the seated students that they should stand if they see someone standing with whom they shook hands. Eventually the entire class should be standing.

When all the students are standing, ask, "What if Mary and Joe [the names of the first two students] had a disease that could be transferred by a handshake?" (The entire class would have been exposed.) Explain that a disease which can be "caught" is called a communicable disease. Reassure students that Mary and Joe do not have a disease that is transferred by a handshake, but if they did, all students in the class would have been exposed. Write the word *communicable* on the blackboard, and ask, "Who knows what this word means?" Through discussion with the students, reveal the meaning to be "catchable, transferable, and spreadable." Write descriptive words such as these under *communicable*. Similarly, write the word *noncommunicable* on the blackboard, and ask for the meaning of this antonym. Terms such as "not catchable, not spreadable, and not transferable" should be suggested. List these words under *noncommunicable*.

Inform the students that some diseases are communicable (transferable usually from person to person), whereas others are noncommunicable and cannot be transferred from person to person.

Disease prevention and control

Activities

1. What Kind of Disease?
   a. Divide students into six groups. Hand each group one *What Kind of Disease Card*. Instruct the groups to do the following.
      (1) Determine which of the diseases are communicable and which are noncommunicable.
      (2) Use health books, encyclopedias, or other references to find the information.
      (3) For the diseases that are communicable, identify the way each is spread and controlled.
   b. On the board or on two large pieces of butcher paper, start two lists. Label one *communicable* and the other *noncommunicable*. As the groups determine the category for the diseases on their card, they are to list them in the appropriate spot.
   c. Ask a representative from each group to briefly explain the spread and control of the communicable diseases they studied.

Materials

Teacher resource: What Kind of Disease Cards (a different card for each of the six groups) (p. 359)

Reference materials: encyclopedias, health books, pamphlets, charts

Teacher resource: Communicable Diseases (Chapter 2)

Optional: butcher paper (two large pieces), felt pens

Teacher resource   *Key*
WHAT KIND OF DISEASE CARDS   Communicable diseases are circled

1.	4.
(Hepatitis (viral))	Sickle cell anemia
Emphysema	(Rabies)
(Mumps)	High blood pressure
(Measles (rubella))	(Cholera)

2.	5.
(Chickenpox)	Rheumatic fever
Stroke	(Influenza)
(Tetanus)	(Mumps)
Heart attack	(Diphtheria)

3.	6.
(Diphtheria)	Skin cancer
Lung cancer	(Chickenpox)
(Ringworm)	(Ringworm)
(Influenza)	Emphysema

2. What are Communicable Diseases?
    a. In a full group discussion and lecture, present these concepts. Communicable diseases can be spread through disease-causing microorganisms (pathogens) that can be transferred from person to person or animal to person. Each type of pathogen causes a particular type of disease. The spread of communicable diseases can be prevented through *immunizations* (vaccines). We do not have vaccines for all communicable diseases. (An example of an immunization is a vaccine for some types of measles.) A second preventive measure is *isolation* during the contagious stage (an example would be staying home from school when you have the chickenpox). A third way is *minimizing your exposure* (an example would be not going to your cousin's house when you know that he or she has been exposed to mumps and probably will be getting mumps). And finally, *taking care of yourself* and staying healthy is important. People who get enough sleep, eat the right foods, etc., are more able to resist the pathogens and resist getting a cold for instance.

    b. Briefly review the four ways that communicable disease can be controlled, as discussed previously. Write them on the board if necessary. Have the students divide a piece of paper into four squares and draw a picture that represents each of the ways to prevent the spread of communicable disease. Post the finished pictures on the bulletin board near the list of communicable diseases.

3. What Are Noncommunicable Diseases?
    a. Review the concept of communicable diseases and the definition of pathogens. Referring to the two lists of diseases, explain that noncommunicable diseases cannot be transferred from person to person or animal to person. Through full group discussion, lecture, and use of the blackboard, present these concepts. Noncommunicable diseases are not caused by pathogens.

Materials
Paper
Rulers
Crayons or felt pens

Noncommunicable diseases result from how we live, the environment in which we live, and genetic weaknesses and resistances to disease that we inherit. An example of *heredity* is; a person might be born with an inherited disease such as sickle cell anemia or Tay-Sachs disease. Noncommunicable diseases can be caused by *lifestyle,* or how one lives. A person who is overweight, gets little exercise, and smokes is more likely to suffer a heart attack. People who smoke or chew tobacco are more likely to develop oral and lung cancer. People cannot be immunized against noncommunicable diseases. They cannot change their heredity; however, in some cases they can develop a healthful life style to prevent or lower the risk of noncommunicable diseases, and in other cases there are medical treatments available.

b. Discussion questions

(1) Why do immunizations not work against noncommunicable diseases such as heart disease or emphysema? (There is no pathogen to isolate and make a vaccine.)

NOTE: There is current research regarding the possibility that viruses are related to cancer. Research eventually may produce vaccines for what are now viewed as noncommunicable diseases as knowledge in medical science increases.

(2) How does lifestyle help prevent communicable, as well as noncommunicable, diseases?

NOTE: HIV infection is an excellent example of a communicable disease that is controlled by lifestyle choices. However, the example should only be used if students have had the opportunity to study this disease prior to this lesson.

4. What Do You Recommend?

Choose student volunteers to role play each of the following situations. Students may take turns being the patient with a disease and a physician who listens and discusses the problem. The student playing the patient should read the lines indicated, and the health educator should make up a response to the question.

SITUATION ONE

Patient: I need help. What do you recommend? I just had a slight heart attack and recovered after being in the hospital for a month. I do not want another heart attack. *Can you tell me where I can get an immunization against a heart attack?*

Physician:

SITUATION TWO

Patient: I am just about over my cold. I have had it for 3 days and feel much better. I cough and sneeze but only have a slight temperature. I am going back to work this afternoon. *Do you think this all right?*

Physician:

Evaluation. Preventing Disease

Have each student complete the worksheet, *Preventing Disease*. Grade the worksheets, and return them to the students. Suggest that the worksheets be taken home and shared with parents.

Materials

Worksheet: *Preventing Disease* (p. 360)

Worksheet   Name __Key__
PREVENTING DISEASE

1. Molly has the chickenpox, a communicable disease. She has itchy spots all over her stomach and her face. Tell Molly one way the chickenpox might have been prevented.

 She could have avoided exposure.

2. Harry had a heart attack, a noncommunicable disease. He is resting in bed, as recommended by the doctor. Tell Harry one way his heart attack might have been prevented.

 A more healthful life-style: good nutrition, exercise, not smoking.

3. How are communicable diseases and noncommunicable diseases different?

You catch a communicable disease by exposure to a pathogen. Noncommunicable diseases are not "catchable." They are diseases of life-style, environment, and heredity

Teacher resource

WHAT KIND OF DISEASE CARDS

1.
Hepatitis (viral)

Emphysema

Mumps

Measles (rubella)

4.
Sickle cell anemia

Rabies

High blood pressure

Cholera

2.
Chickenpox

Stroke

Tetanus

Heart attack

5.
Rheumatic fever

Influenza

Mumps

Diphtheria

3.
Diphtheria

Lung cancer

Ringworm

Influenza

6.
Skin cancer

Chickenpox

Ringworm

Emphysema

Disease prevention and control

Worksheet   Name _____

PREVENTING DISEASE

1. Molly has the chickenpox, a communicable disease. She has itchy spots all over her stomach and her face. Tell Molly one way the chickenpox might have been prevented.

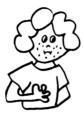

2. Harry had a heart attack, a noncommunicable disease. He is resting in bed, as recommended by the doctor. Tell Harry one way his heart attack might have been prevented.

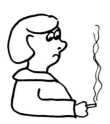

3. How are communicable diseases and noncommunicable diseases different?

AIDS AND THE IMMUNE SYSTEM—A Lesson for Young People*

Objective. The student will be able to demonstrate how HIV infection (AIDS) affects the functioning of the immune system.

Level. Grades 4 to 6

Content generalizations. For this lesson, examples are woven into the description of the activities as is the style for the entire *Growing Healthy* Program.

Vocabulary. AIDS, virus, germs, immune

Initiation. Germs, Germs, Germs
Review the fact that germs are often the cause of disease. Explain that germs are so small that they can only be seen with powerful microscopes. Ask students to brainstorm ways that germs can enter the body. Explain that a healthy immune system works to destroy all types of germs including bacteria and viruses. Ask a student to tell what is meant when someone is "immune" to something. Help students to conclude that it means "protected" or "safe."

Activities

1. Demonstration of the Immune System

   a. Hold the two ends of a 6′ hose in one hand so the hose forms a circle, illustrating the skin as a barrier to keep germs out. As long as the skin remains uninjured, it holds the body's insides in and keeps the rest of the world safely out.

   b. Reveal the break in the hose and explain that when there is a break in the skin, germs can enter. Have students name ways that breaks occur (cuts, scratches, punctures, etc.). Review proper care for breaks in the skin. (Wash with soap and water to kill germs.)

   c. Lay the hose on a flat surface where it can be seen by students and roll the tennis balls and golf balls into the circle through the break in the hose (skin). These balls represent bacteria. The bacteria are large germs and are plentiful. Roll in the marbles, explaining that these represent viruses, very small germs.

Materials
6′ hose
Tennis balls (3)
Golf balls (3)
Marbles (4)
Sock puppet (Teacher-made)
Foam cut in "T" shape (3)
Foam cut in "B" shape (3)

AIDS and the
immune system

---
*Adapted from *Growing Healthy, AIDS Integration*, 1988.

d. Explain that our blood contains white blood cells that fight germs. One kind of white blood cell (phagocytes) moves through the blood and tissues to surround and eat germs. Use the sock puppet to demonstrate the action of the phagocytes (the "eating" cells).

e. Another kind of white blood cell produces chemicals, called antibodies, that destroy viruses. Write "antibodies" on the chalkboard. These cells that produce antibodies are B-cells. Add B-cells to the circle.

f. T-cells are another type of white blood cells that help fight germs. Some T-cells attack and destroy viruses. Other T-cells direct the battle. Add T-cells to the circle. Stress that some T-cells serve as "command centers" for the body's battle against germs.

g. Explain that some of the antibodies stay in your blood and protect you in case you are exposed to the same disease again. That is immunity.

   Another way to get immunity is by having a vaccine. We do not have vaccines for all diseases.

h. Conclude the demonstration by pointing out that the immune system works 24 hours a day in every part of the body to ensure good health.

2. Discussion

a. Ask students what happens when the "command center" in a real battle is destroyed? Help students to conclude that when germs attack the white blood cells (in particular, the T-cells) that control the body's immune system, they cripple the body's ability to fight off disease and infection.

b. Ask students to name the new disease that destroys the immune system (AIDS). Explain that AIDS is caused by a virus called HIV (the AIDS virus). Once the AIDS virus destroys the "command centers" (T-cells) of the immune system, the body cannot defend itself against infections and diseases. The person with the AIDS virus does not die of AIDS but of other diseases that the body can no longer fight off. Most often, people with AIDS die of a type of cancer or pneumonia. Many people are infected with the AIDS virus and many people have died. It is a serious health problem.

Materials
Sock puppet (teacher-made)

c. How do you get AIDS? Explain that the AIDS virus is very fragile. It dies in air and light. The AIDS virus can be passed on through sexual contact with a person who has the virus. Some babies have been infected with the AIDS virus because their mother had the virus in her blood when she was pregnant. Since we now know more about AIDS women who want to have a baby can have a test to see if they have the AIDS virus before they get pregnant.

d. Ask students if they have heard of any other ways that people can become infected with the AIDS virus. Write the words "IV drug use" on the board and explain that people who abuse drugs using needles to put the drugs directly into their veins are at great risk. Sharing a needle with a person who has the AIDS virus risks exposure to the virus. Doctors and nurses are very careful when using hypodermic needles. Most of the time the needles used for giving shots or for giving blood are only used once and then disposed of. Students do not need to worry about needles used by doctors or nurses for medical reasons.

e. Ask students if they have any ideas how to prevent the spread of the AIDS virus. Help them to conclude that avoiding sexual contact (sexual abstinence) is a sure way and the appropriate way for young people to avoid the virus. Avoiding the use of IV drugs is another appropriate behavior. If they have any other specific questions about AIDS they should ask a trusted adult, a doctor, or call the local AIDS Hotline. Students can usually get the local Hotline number from the telephone directory or the directory operator.

Evaluation. The Immune System Demonstration Revisited. Using the materials for the demonstration of the action of the immune system, have students take turns rolling the tennis balls, golf balls and marbles and explaining what each represents. Students then should use the sock puppet to demonstrate the action of the white blood cells. Students should "throw" in the foam "T" shapes and "B" shapes and explain their role in the functioning of the immune system. In the demonstration, students should explain how the AIDS virus destroys the immune system. As each student demonstrates, other students in the class should critique the demonstration.

Materials
6' hose
Tennis balls (3)
Golf balls (3)
Marbles (4)
Sock puppet (Teacher-made)
Foam cut in "T" shape (3)
Foam cut in "B" shape (3)

AIDS and the immune system

ACCIDENT PREVENTION AND SAFETY

Objective. The student illustrates basic first aid for stopped breathing.

Level. Grades 4 to 6

Integration. Science

Content generalizations. When normal breathing stops and too little oxygen is being taken into the lungs, the victim is in danger. If breathing is not restored, the victim may die within minutes. Artificial respiration is the procedure for forcing air into the lungs of a person who has stopped breathing. Several specific steps should be followed. Mouth-to-mouth resuscitation should be continued until help arrives.

NOTE: This lesson is a presentation of the most basic principles of artificial respiration. Successful completion of these activities does not certify students in this procedure. The students should be aware that they should only administer this procedure in an emergency when no one else around can perform this life-saving technique. This procedure should not be confused with CPR, which involves chest compressions to start circulation, as well as mouth-to-mouth resuscitation. CPR should be taught only by a certified trainer. Contact the American Red Cross for guest speakers and other references.

Vocabulary. Lungs, inhale, exhale, artificial respiration, mouth-to-mouth resuscitation

Initiation. In and Out

Ask the students to place their hands on their chest and feel it rise as they inhale and fall as they exhale. Hand out the worksheet, *In and Out.* Explain to students that, when we inhale, the diaphragm muscle moves down to allow more space in the chest for the lungs to expand. The dotted lines on the worksheet represent the general position of the diaphragm and the expansion of the lungs. When we exhale, the diaphragm pushes up on the lungs, decreasing the chest capacity and pushing air out of the lungs, making them smaller. This is represented by the solid lines on the worksheet. Have the students take a few big breaths and observe the increased size of their chest on inhalation and the decreased size during exhalation. Then the students should color their worksheets, using different colors to represent the lungs and diaphragm during inhalation and during exhalation. The students also should label the basic parts of the respiratory system, including the trachea, bronchial tubes, lungs, alveoli (air sacks), and diaphragm. Put up a poster of the respiratory system, or have them consult an encyclopedia to correctly label these parts.

Materials

Worksheet and transparency: *In and Out* (p. 368)

Poster: *The Respiratory System*

Encyclopedias

IN AND OUT

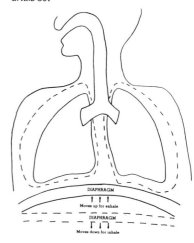

DIAPHRAGM
Moves up for exhale
DIAPHRAGM
Moves down for inhale

Accident prevention
and safety

Activities

1. Mouth-to-Mouth Resuscitation

Explain to students that breathing is called *respiration.* If a person is not breathing normally, another person can blow air into the nonbreathing person's lungs to try to keep him or her alive. This process is called *mouth-to-mouth resuscitation.* Tell students that they will be learning and practicing the specific steps in this process. If possible, have a guest speaker demonstrate the following steps. The speaker may have access to a mannequin. (If no mannequin is available, demonstrate the procedure on a student. Do *not* blow into the student's mouth; blow to the side of the student's head.) Tell the students that they will blow into Resusa Annie's plastic mouth and only to the side of their partner's head when practicing.

a. Write the following seven steps on the board.

(1) *Shout* and tap

(2) *Check* for pulse

(3) *Tilt* head to clear air passage

(4) *Look,* listen, and feel for air

Resources

Guest speaker: school nurse or Red Cross volunteer to demonstrate artificial respiration

Mannequin: Resusa Annie (American Red Cross)

       (5) *Give four* quick breaths

       (6) *Look,* listen, and feel for air

       (7) *Give 1* breath every 5 seconds for an adult

   b. Review the seven steps with the class, then demonstrate with a student volunteer. Blow air beside the head (not into the mouth) of the student.

   c. Have students pair up, one being the victim and the other the rescuer. Lead students through each of the seven steps. Have students trade roles and repeat the process.

   d. Inform students that, to be certified to actually give artificial respiration, young people and adults can take a class in basic first aid through the American Red Cross.

2. Practice Mouth-to-Mouth Resuscitation

   Organize the students into small groups of seven. In each group one student describes the first step in administering artificial respiration, then the person to the right states the following step and describes how it is done. The process continues until each student has identified one of the seven steps. Students may take turns being first so that the cycle is repeated and reviewed seven times. Optional: Have the students make flash cards with the seven steps for artificial respiration. They can quiz each other in pairs or in the groups.

Materials

Index cards (seven per student)

3. First Aid for Stopped Breathing
   Hand out the worksheet, *First Aid for Stopped Breathing,* and ask students to complete it individually. Go over the answers orally in class after everyone has finished.

Materials

Worksheet: *First Aid for Stopped Breathing* (p. 369)

FIRST AID FOR STOPPED BREATHING

Situation: You see a woman pull a man out of a lake. She says, "Can you help me? This man is not breathing. Do you know artificial respiration!"

Can you help? Write the steps below in the correct order. (Hint: The steps are at the bottom of the worksheet, but they are not in order.)

STEPS FOR ARTIFICIAL RESPIRATION

1. _____
2. _____
3. _____
4. _____
5. _____
6. _____
7. _____

Use these steps for help in remembering, if needed. If you do not need to look at these steps, all the better!

LOOK, LISTEN, AND FEEL FOR AIR
TILT HEAD
GIVE 1 BREATH EVERY 5 SECONDS
SHOUT AND TAP
GIVE FOUR QUICK BREATHS
LOOK, LISTEN, AND FEEL FOR AIR
CHECK FOR PULSE

Accident prevention and safety

Evaluation. Parent Letter

Give the students a letter to take home to their parents. Explain that the letter informs parents of their learning the steps of artificial respiration. Tell students to demonstrate these steps to their parents. Explain that the bottom half of the Parent Letter is to be returned after students have demonstrated the steps of artificial respiration.

Materials

Sample Parent Letter (p.370)

SAMPLE PARENT LETTER

Dear Parent:

Your child _____ has been learning how to perform artificial respiration during health class. To help him or her become more proficient, I have asked students to practice with their parents. These activities are limited to learning the steps of mouth-to-mouth resuscitation. We did not learn how to perform CPR (cardiopulmonary resuscitation). If you or your child is interested in becoming certified in first-aid procedures, I suggest you contact the American Red Cross.

As your child demonstrates the following steps, please check them off. Then return the bottom half of this sheet to me. Thank you for your cooperation.

Sincerely,

_____
(Teacher)

I have watched my son or daughter _____ demonstrate the following steps of artificial respiration.

1. Shout and tap ____
2. Check for pulse ____
3. Tilt the head to clear the airway ____
4. Look, listen, and feel for air ____
5. Give four quick breaths ____
6. Look, listen, and feel for air again ____
7. Give 1 breath every 5 seconds ____

_____
Signed (parent)

Worksheet
IN AND OUT

Name _____

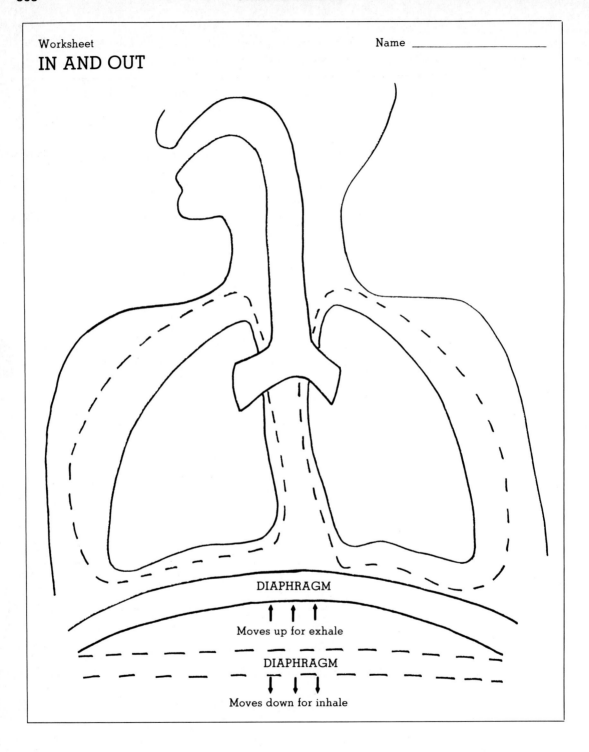

DIAPHRAGM

Moves up for exhale

DIAPHRAGM

Moves down for inhale

Worksheet   Name _____

FIRST AID FOR STOPPED BREATHING

Situation: You see a woman pull a man out of a lake. She says, "Can you help me? This man is not breathing. Do you know artificial respiration?"

Can you help? Write the steps below in the correct order.
(Hint: The steps are at the bottom of the worksheet, but they are not in order.)

STEPS FOR ARTIFICIAL RESPIRATION

1. _____

2. _____

3. _____

4. _____

5. _____

6. _____

7. _____

Use these steps for help in remembering, if needed. If you do not need to look at these steps, all the better!

LOOK, LISTEN, AND FEEL FOR AIR

TILT HEAD

GIVE 1 BREATH EVERY 5 SECONDS

SHOUT AND TAP

GIVE FOUR QUICK BREATHS

LOOK, LISTEN, AND FEEL FOR AIR

CHECK FOR PULSE

Teacher resource

SAMPLE PARENT LETTER

Dear Parent:

    Your child _____ has been learning how to perform artificial

respiration during health class. To help him or her become more proficient, I

have asked students to practice with their parents. These activities are limited

to learning the steps of mouth-to-mouth resuscitation. We did not learn how to

perform CPR (cardiopulmonary resuscitation). If you or your child is interested

in becoming certified in first-aid procedures, I suggest you contact the American

Red Cross.

    As your child demonstrates the following steps, please check them off. Then

return the bottom half of this sheet to me. Thank you for your cooperation.

                        Sincerely,

                        _____
                        (Teacher)

I have watched my son or daughter _____ demonstrate the following steps

of artificial respiration.

        1. Shout and tap   _____

        2. Check for pulse   _____

        3. Tilt the head to clear the airway   _____

        4. Look, listen, and feel for air   _____

        5. Give four quick breaths   _____

        6. Look, listen, and feel for air again _____

        7. Give 1 breath every 5 seconds   _____

                        _____
                        Signed (parent)

CONSUMER HEALTH

Objective. The student describes appeals that promote the sale of foods and medications used by children.

Level. Grades 4 to 6

Integration. Reading, language arts, creative expression, scientific observation

Vocabulary. Appeal, advertisement, claim, packaging

Content generalizations. Advertisements on television, radio, billboards, and in magazines use various techniques to appeal to children. Food products such as cereals, candy and gum, and medicines such as children's vitamins frequently have advertising aimed specifically at children. Even if the child does not purchase the item personally, he or she often has an influence on the parent's purchase of various items. Appeals to children's emotions and senses often will include enticements such as, "It is fun to use or eat; it is tasty or smells good; it is popular to do; it is attractive." Powerful words and claims also may be used by advertisers. Finally, the packaging of foods and medications used by children is important. Often games or toys are included with a product as an enticement.

Initiation. Coming Soon—A Great Taste Treat

A head of time, prepare a sign, advertisement, and package similar to the one in the *Advertisement Example*. Two days before the lesson post the sign, "Coming Soon—A Great Taste Treat," on the bulletin board. The day before beginning the lesson post the advertisement. Do not answer any questions about the signs. Tell students they will have to wait until we start the consumer health activities.

Write the word *advertising* on the board, and ask if anyone can tell what it means. Point to the signs on the bulletin board and the package, and explain that these are ways to advertise a product. Have students try to guess what it is. Then open the box, and display the product (a red apple). There may be some disappointment. Ask students what kind of product was expected. Use this opportunity to point out that often advertising gets us so excited about a product that we are disappointed when we try it because it is not what we expected.

ADVERTISEMENT EXAMPLE

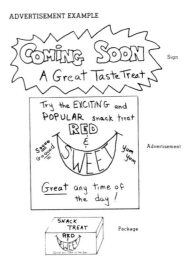

Consumer health

Materials

Teacher resource: *Advertisement Example* (p. 376)

Shoe box

Construction paper

Felt pens

Red apple

Then ask students, "What is the *purpose* of advertising?" (To get people to buy a product or service.) Tell them that it is very important to remember this purpose whenever they see or hear an advertisement and that advertisers never point out the bad or useless aspects of a product.

Activities

1. Commercials, commercials, commercials
   a. Ask students if they pay much attention to commercials on television. (They will probably say no.) Ask them what kinds of products are usually advertised on television shows for children. (Cereals, candy, beverages, fast-food restaurants, cookies, gum, vitamins, toys.)
   b. Divide the students into groups of five or six. Give each group a large piece of newsprint or butcher paper and a felt pen or crayon. Explain that they are going to see which team can recall the most *brand* names for foods and drugs that are advertised on *children's* television programs. Allow students 5 minutes to work on their lists. Then each group should post their list. Proclaim the "winner," and mention that we do remember products even though we *think* we are not paying attention to commercials.

   Materials
   Five or six sheets of butcher paper
   Felt pens or crayons

   c. Keep students in groups to continue some more activities with their lists. Have the groups retrieve the lists that were posted and consider the following for each product.
      (1) Is the product a food? If so mark an *F* after the product.
      (2) Is the product a drug? If so mark a *D* after the product.
      (3) Is the product high in sugar content? If so, circle the product.
      (4) Put a large *A* next to the products you think also might be advertised on adult shows.

d. After this has been done for each product, ask the groups to make some generalizations about the types of products that are advertised on children's programs. If students need further direction, ask if the products advertised on children's television programs are the following.
   (1) Mostly foods or mostly drugs
   (2) Low or high in sugar content
   (3) Seen more often on children's television shows or adult programs
e. If time allows, each group should report their findings (generalizations) to the class.

2. Advertising Appeals

   Explain to students that we will be focusing on products that are advertised to children, particularly foods and medications (such as vitamins).

   a. Write the word *appeal* on the board, and explain that advertisers use various methods to try to make a product *appeal* to us so that we will buy it. These methods are called advertising *appeals*.
      (1) *Fun:* Commercials often make using a product look like fun. The people or characters are shown having lots of fun, or the commercial is funny (such as a cartoon). The result is that the product looks like it is fun to use.
      (2) *Tasty:* Commercials often tell you how good the products taste. Remind students of their brainstorming activity in groups, and ask what kind of taste is advertised most often. (Sweet.)
      (3) *Popular:* Commercials often make the product look like it is popular to use. People in commercials are portrayed as popular and attractive with lots of friends. In other words, everybody who is anybody uses this product.

Consumer health

b. Tell students that they are going to practice identifying these appeals with real commercials. Play three or four previously recorded commercials for the class. (Videotape is preferable, but cassette recordings of television commercials work just as well.) After each commercial ask students which appeals they observed. To give all students a chance to think about their answers, have them record their ideas on paper before calling on a volunteer to share his or her answer.

NOTE: Because television advertising changes so frequently, it is not possible to provide examples of commercials using each appeal that still will be on television at the time of the lesson. The following are provided to give the teacher ideas.

(1) Trix cereal is a classic example of a commercial using appeals to *fun* and *taste*. The "silly" cartoon rabbit never gets the wonderfully tasting Trix cereal.

(2) Dr. Pepper and Coca Cola commercials have often used the *popular* appeal. Groups of attractive young adults convey the image that these beverages are used by the "in" crowd.

c. Refer back to the advertisement used in the initiation activity. Ask the students to identify the appeals used in this advertisement. (Taste and popularity.) Point out that another way to sell products is to use powerful words, or *power words*. Ask if anyone can identify a power word in the advertisement. Write the following power words on the board or on a sign hung on the bulletin board: wonderful, strong, great, super, new, exciting, and fun. Explain that these words often are used to attract attention to a product. Other power words also can be found in advertisements.

Materials

Television commercials (3 or 4 recorded on videotape or cassette recorder)

Materials

Teacher resource: *Advertisement Example* (p. 376)

3. What's the Appeal?
   a. As a homework assignment, hand out the worksheets, *What's the Appeal?* They are to watch television commercials about foods or medications and look at children's magazines to complete their assignment. The two worksheets should be used while viewing four television commercials and two printed advertisements. (A separate sheet will be needed for each commercial and advertisement.) The printed advertisements can be found in children's magazines, comics, or the comic section of the weekend newspaper.
   b. For each television commercial, the date, time of day observed, channel, and program are to be recorded. Explain that all scientific surveys involve gathering as much specific information as possible. The product that is being advertised must be listed, as well as a brief description of the advertisement. Then the advertising appeals observed should be listed including any power words.
   c. When the assignment is completed, put the students into their small groups to discuss their observations. What appeals were observed most often? What kind of products were observed most often? Were there many high-sugar foods? What power words were used most often? As time allows, the groups should report their findings to the class. Determine which appeal was observed most often by the entire class. Do the same for power words.

Evaluation. How Do They Sell That Product?
Have the groups act out one of the commercials observed, without mentioning the product name. The class should guess the type of product (and specific brand if possible). Tell each student to describe on paper the methods used to sell this product. Advertising appeals and power words should be identified in their descriptions.

Materials
Worksheet: *What's the Appeal? Television Commercials* (4 sheets per student) (p. 377); *Printed Advertisements* (2 sheets per student) (p. 378)

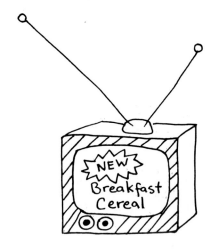

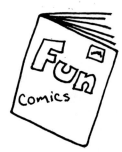

Consumer health

Teacher resource

ADVERTISEMENT EXAMPLE

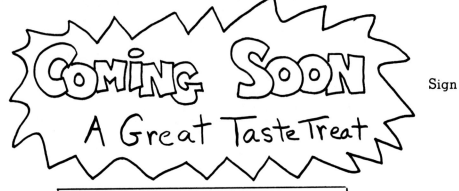

Sign

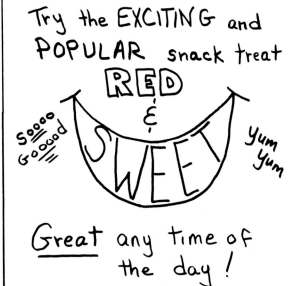

Advertisement

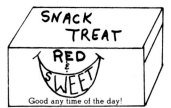

Package

Worksheet

WHAT'S THE APPEAL?
TELEVISION COMMERCIALS

Name _____

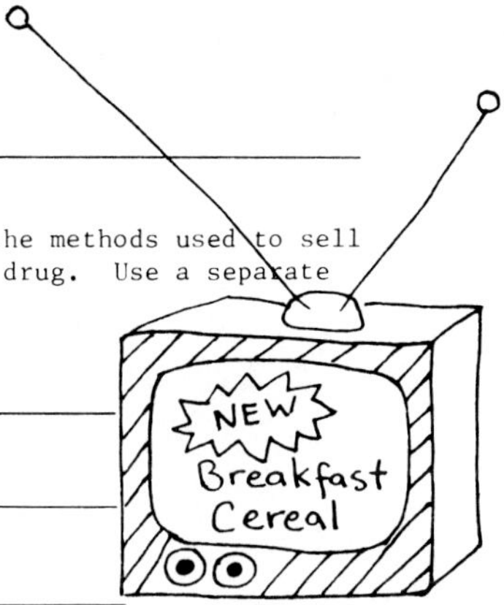

Directions: View four television commercials, and analyze the methods used to sell
a product to children that is either food or a drug. Use a separate
sheet for each commercial.

1.   Product name _____

2.   Television show where it was advertised _____

3.   Date and time viewed _____

4.   Channel _____

5.   Brief description of what happens in the commercial:

6.   Appeals used in the commercial _____

_____

7.   Power words used in the commercial _____

_____

8.   Is the product a FOOD or a MEDICATION?   (Circle one)

9.   Is the product high in sugar?   YES   NO   (Circle one)

Consumer health

Worksheet   Name _____

WHAT'S THE APPEAL?
PRINTED ADVERTISEMENTS

Directions: Find two printed advertisements in children's magazines, comics, or
              the comic section of the newspaper. Analyze the advertisements by
              answering the questions below. Complete a separate sheet for each
              advertisement.

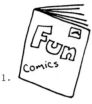

1.   Product name _____

2.   Newspaper or magazine where it was found _____

3.   Brief description of the advertisement (describe the picture or artwork):

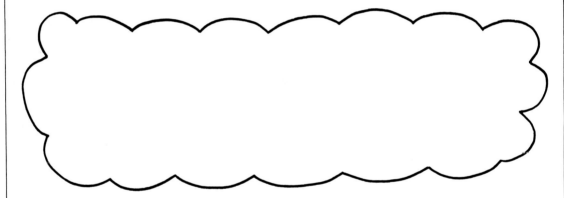

4.   Appeals used in the advertisement _____

     _____

5.   Power words used in the advertisement _____

     _____

6.   Was the advertisement about a   FOOD   or a   MEDICATION?   (Circle one)

7.   Was the product high in sugar?   YES   NO   (Circle one)

USE AND ABUSE OF DRUGS

Objective. The student explains reasons for laws regulating the use of drugs.

Level. Grades 4 to 6

Integration. Language arts, media, social studies

Vocabulary. Laws, legal, hazardous

Content generalizations. There are many laws that regulate the sale and use of drugs. These laws exist for the protection of the health and safety of all of society. Legal drugs are those that have passed rigorous testing to prove their safety and usefulness. These include drugs that are prescribed by a physician and those that are sold over-the-counter in drug stores without a prescription. Two other drugs that are not used to treat diseases or to promote health are alcohol and tobacco. These two drugs are recreational drugs that are legal for use by adults. However the sale and use of these drugs is controlled by state and local officials. In some places in the United States, the sale of alcohol is prohibited. And, many cities and local communities have passed laws to regulate cigarette smoking in public places.

Other drugs are thought to be unsafe and unhealthful and are not legal to use at all. Experts believe that illegal drugs such as marijuana, PCP, heroin, LSD, inhalants, cocaine and crack are dangerous and that safe and responsible use is not possible. The use of both legal and illegal drugs by young people is considered a serious problem in the United States.

Use and abuse
of drugs

Initiation. Drugs and the Law—Where Do You Stand?
Draw a line from one side of the board to the other. At one end of the line write the words, "More-Laws Larry" (or Lucy), and at the other end write "No-Laws Nelson" (or Nelli). Put a vertical line directly in the center of the long line.

Tell the students that the line represents all the attitudes about laws regulating drugs. The two mythical persons hold the *absolute* extreme attitudes on both ends. Explain to the students that you will be telling the class of these two persons' beliefs, and the students are to think of where their personal feelings are in relation to these two extremes.

Materials
Chalkboard with 15 or so small pieces of chalk in tray

Tell them, "More-Laws Larry thinks that all drugs should be available by prescription only. That includes aspirin, coffee, and cola drinks (because they contain caffeine). He thinks that alcohol and cigarettes should be totally against the law and that people caught with alcohol or cigarettes should be thrown in jail.

"No-Laws Nelson believes that there are already too many laws about drugs. People should be able to drink alcohol and smoke cigarettes whenever and wherever they please. There should be absolutely no age limits. In fact, he thinks kindergarten kids need to start drinking beer so they can learn how to hold their liquor. He thinks that all drugs should be legal and should be sold without a prescription, including marijuana, heroin, and crack."

Ask students to come to the board as a class and mark an *X* on the line where they think their beliefs lie regarding laws and drugs. Tell them that they cannot place their *X* on the center line. When the *X*'s have been marked, ask, "Where do most people's beliefs about laws lie?" (Most will be around the center, but there will be a range.) Ask if they have observed a difference in people's attitudes about laws regulating drugs.

Activities

1. And Now the News

   Involve the entire class in a project designed to find out about the laws related to drugs in your local area, the reasons for these laws, and the viewpoints of different people in the community about the laws.

   a. Tell the class that they will be putting on a full-scale television show (or radio show if videotape equipment is not available). It will be a program called *Drugs and the Law.* Several committees (teams) will be formed to accomplish the task. Suggested committee organization and responsibilities are as outlined as follows. Write the team name on the board as each is explained.

      (1) *Anchor host committee* (two cohosts) should provide leadership for the total production. They narrate the show and make certain all the teams are doing their jobs and will be on time for the taping.

      (2) *Production committee* (three to five members) is responsible for the actual taping. They must plan the staging and background props and make suggestions for costuming.

(3) *Reporter teams* (several committees of four to six students, based on the number of drugs and related laws studied) must research the stories, write the stories, take appropriate pictures to enhance the stories, and appoint reporter(s) to read the story on the air.

b. NOTE: The anchor hosts are very important. These might be elected by the students. Explain that responsible persons are essential in these positions. Given the criteria, students probably will elect capable persons to the positions.

c. After the anchor hosts are identified, allow students to sign up for positions on the other teams. The various reporter teams possible include the following.

   (1) Alcohol investigation team

   (2) Cigarette investigation team

   (3) Legal drugs investigation team (over-the-counter and prescription drugs)

   (4) Illegal drugs investigation team (such as heroin, crack, inhalants, PCP, LSD, and marijuana)

d. Put a sign up sheet for students to list a first and second choice. Divide the students equally among the groups.

e. When the committees and teams have been identified, have them meet in groups and elect a leader. The leaders will be in close contact with the anchor hosts regarding progress.

f. Give each reporter team a worksheet that correlates with their team. Allow them to study the ideas on the sheet and plan their strategy for the investigation.

g. The responsibilities for the reporter teams will generally be the following.

   (1) Identify the basic laws for that drug.

   (2) Find out why there are laws about that drug.

   (3) Find out how people in the community feel about the law and that drug.

   (4) Write an interesting script that tells all these findings.

   (5) Decide on a reporter(s) to be taped reading the script the team has written.

   (6) Practice and rehearse the script, and time it. Change the script if it is too long or too short for the minutes assigned by the production team.

Materials

Worksheets: *Investigating Alcohol/Investigating Cigarettes* (pp. 383–384); *Investigating Legal Drugs/Investigating Illegal Drugs* (pp. 385–386)

Use and abuse of drugs

h. Have the production committee meet with the anchor host committee to plan the strategy for the production. They will have to plan the general format of the show, decide how much time will be given to the various reports, and plan and write an introduction and ending for the show. It also would be a good idea to set up deadline schedules, rehearsals, and trial tapings.

i. Give the students class time every day to meet with their teams. Circulate and troubleshoot. Also make certain the anchor hosts are meeting regularly with the other committee and team leaders. All committees and teams will have to do script writing. The production committee will have to prepare sets and become familiar with any equipment they may be using. Two to three weeks is approximately the amount of time needed to prepare for the taping.

j. Have the students rehearse the production and tape it with a cassette tape. Allow the class to listen to the tape and critique it. Have the teams modify the show based on the suggestions and rehearse again if desired.

Materials
Casette tape recorder and tape

2. Lights, Camera, Action
Have students put on the production. After viewing the show, ask various students questions such as:
    a. Why are there laws about alcohol?
    b. Why are some drugs legal to buy and others not?
    c. Why are there age limits on certain drugs?
    d. Why are there laws relating to drinking and driving?

Materials
Videotape equipment, video monitor.

3. Parent Review
Invite parents to come to class and view the production. You may wish to have each team explain the part they played in the production process.

Evaluation. Why We Have Laws
Have students write an essay titled, "Why We Have Laws About Drugs in [name of city or state]."

Worksheet   Name _____
INVESTIGATING ALCOHOL

Reporter information:

You are investigating three basic questions about alcohol. Find several people in your community to interview. For each person interviewed, get their exact name, age, and type of job. Try to find different kinds of people to interview. The three areas you want to find out about are the following:

1. What are the basic laws regarding alcohol?
   a. What are the age laws regarding the purchase of alcohol?
   b. When can alcohol be sold (days of week and hours)?
   c. Where can it be sold? Where can it be consumed (where can people drink it)?
   d. What are the laws regarding driving under the influence of alcohol?
2. Why do we have these various laws about alcohol?
3. How do people feel about the laws?
   a. Are the age limits too high? Too low?
   b. Should alcohol be available for purchase more hours in the day than it is now? Fewer hours?
   c. Are the laws about drinking and driving too strong? Not strong enough?

Interview people in your community about these and other questions. Decide as a group who in the community should be interviewed. You may want to tape your interview on a cassette tape and take photographs. (Make certain you get permission to do this from the person being interviewed.) After the interviews work as a group to write a script for the program. Remember your three basic questions when writing the script. Decide on the readers for the script, practice, and rehearse. Keep in mind the time allowed for your part of the program. Check the time it takes your readers to read the script. Change the script if necessary to fit the time allotted.

Use and abuse
of drugs

Worksheet   Name_____

INVESTIGATING CIGARETTES

Reporter information:

You are investigating three basic questions about cigarettes. Find several people in your community to interview. These should be different kinds of people with different kinds of jobs and different ages. For each person interviewed get the exact name, age, and type of job. The three areas you want to find out about are the following:

1. What are the basic laws regarding cigarettes?
   a. What is the age limit for the sale of cigarettes?
   b. Where can they be sold?
   c. Are there laws about where you can and cannot smoke (that is, smoking and nonsmoking areas in public places)?
2. Why do we have laws about cigarettes?
3. How do people feel about the laws?
   a. Are the age limits too low? Too high?
   b. Should there be stronger laws about where they can be sold?
   c. Are the laws too strong about smoking and nonsmoking areas in public places? Not strong enough?

Interview people in your community about these and other questions. Decide as a group who in the community should be interviewed. You may want to tape your interview and take photographs. (Make certain you get permission to do this from the person being interviewed.) After the interview work as a group to write a script for the program. Remember your three basic questions when writing the script. Decide on readers for the script, practice, and rehearse. Keep in mind the time allowed for your part of the program. Check the time it takes your readers to read the script. Change the script to fit the time allotted, if necessary.

Worksheet   Name_____

INVESTIGATING LEGAL DRUGS

Reporter information:

You are investigating three basic questions about legal drugs. Find several people in your community who are familiar with these drugs. (Pharmacists, physicians, and nurses would be most helpful.) Get the exact name, age, and type of job for each person interviewed. The three areas you want to find out about are the following:

1. What are the basic laws regarding legal drugs?
   a. Who can buy over-the-counter drugs? Prescription drugs?
   b. Who can sell prescription drugs?
   c. Who can prescribe drugs?
2. Why do we have laws regarding over-the-counter drugs and prescription drugs?
   a. Why are certain drugs prescription drugs and others not?
   b. Why are some drugs that are legal in other countries not legal in the United States?
3. How do people feel about the laws regulating legal drugs?
   a. Are the laws too strong regarding prescription drugs? Should more drugs be available over the counter rather than by prescription?
   b. Should there be age limits on who can buy over-the-counter drugs?

Interview people in your community about these and other questions. Decide as a group who in the community should be interviewed. You may want to tape your interview on a cassette tape and take photographs. (Make certain you get permission to do this from the person being interviewed.) After the interviews work as a group to write a script for the program. Remember your three basic questions when writing the script. Decide on readers for the script, practice, and rehearse. Check the time it takes your readers to read the script. Change the script if necessary to fit the time allowed.

Use and abuse of drugs

Worksheet   Name_____

**INVESTIGATING ILLEGAL
DRUGS**

Reporter information:

You are investigating three basic questions about drugs that are illegal. Find several people in your community to interview. For each person interviewed, get their exact name, age, and type of job. These should be different kinds of people. You may want to start with someone on the police force in your community. The three areas that you want to find out about are the following:

1. What are the basic laws about illegal drugs?
    a. What drugs are illegal?
    b. Are there different laws regarding the sale and the possession of certain drugs?
2. Why do we have laws about these drugs? (Why are certain drugs legal to use and others not?)
3. How do people feel about the laws?
    a. Are the laws too harsh regarding illegal drugs? Too lenient?
    b. Should some of the drugs that are illegal be made legal? Should more drugs that are now legal be made illegal (for example, alcohol and cigarettes)?
    c. Should the penalties for using or possessing an illegal drug be stronger? Less harsh?

Interview people in your community about these and other questions. Decide as a group who in the community should be interviewed. You may want to tape your interview on a cassette tape and take photographs. (Make certain you get permission to do this from the person being interviewed.) After the interviews work as a group to write a script for the program. Remember your three basic questions when writing the script. Decide on readers for the script, practice, and rehearse. Check the time it takes your reader to read the script. Change the script if necessary to fit the time allotted.

ENVIRONMENTAL HEALTH

Objective. The student identifies causes of and ways to prevent environmental pollution.

Level. Grades 4 to 6

Intergration. Math, physical education, language arts, science, art

Content generalizations. People make an impact on their environment just by living in the world. Freeways, homes, factories, and office buildings noticeably modify the environment. An increase in the quality and comfort of life often is costly to the environment. Individuals can make choices in their daily lives that minimize personal contributions to environmental pollution.

There are several kinds of environmental pollution. Air pollution is caused largely by exhaust fumes from automobiles, airplanes, and factories. Walking or riding bicycles whenever possible is helpful in preventing air pollution. Water pollution often is caused by the use of water by industry and agriculture. Additionally, dumping trash and chemicals into lakes and streams will cause water pollution. Although industry causes much of the air and water pollution, individuals can help by doing their part to conserve water and not pollute water and air. Another kind of pollution is land pollution. This is caused by littering and the defacement of walls and other structures (graffiti). Individuals also can cause noise pollution. Being careful not to litter and to keep radios and stereos at a low level helps prevent these types of pollution.

Vocabulary. Environmental pollution, prevention, impact, cilia

Initiation. How much water do you use in a day? Display a gallon jug of water. Ask the students to think about all the water they use daily. Tell them that we need clean water to live. Ask them if they can name some of the reasons we need clean water. (Washing, drinking, bathing, cooking.) Explain that the class is going to have a contest to see who can come closest to guessing the number of gallons of water that the average person uses every day. Pass out slips of paper for the students to use to make their guesses. Have a student volunteer collect the papers

Materials

Gallon jug of water
Slips of paper
Envelope containing the correct answer (125 gallons)

Environmental
health

and arrange them in order from the highest number to the lowest number. Write the highest and lowest numbers guessed on the board. Then allow a student to open the envelope and read the correct answer (125 gallons). Compare the correct answer with the guesses made by class members. Declare the "winner."

Propose to the students that, if each one of us needs that much water every day, it must be important to make certain we keep our rivers, lakes, and oceans clean and pollution free. It also stands to reason that it is important not to waste water.

Activities

1. Environmental Journal

   Materials
   Construction paper
   Magazines
   Scissors
   Glue

   Have the students begin an "Environmental Journal." Explain that this will be a notebook in which to keep papers, notes, worksheets, ideas, and feelings about the environment and pollution. The notebooks should be collected and read periodically to check progress and participation. Students should look through magazines to find a picture they like that represents the word *environment* for them. The picture should be glued on the front of a folded piece of paper to make their "Environmental Journal."

   a. The first item that students should place in the journal is a sheet of lined paper to keep definitions of words. They can begin by defining the following words.

      (1) Environment   (4) Litter
      (2) Pollution   (5) Wastes
      (3) Impact   (6) Graffiti

   b. The dictionary can be consulted for help, but the definitions should be written in the student's own words.

   Materials
   Dictionaries

2. Environmental Health Survey

Tell the students they are going to take a personal survey to help them identify ways they contribute to environmental pollution. Explain that this survey is not for a grade. It is intended to provide information for personal use. The only way they will get an accurate idea about their personal impact on the environment is to be honest in answering the questions.

a. Hand out the worksheet, *Environmental Health Survey,* and allow the students to complete it. Provide help to students who need assistance in summation.

b. After all the students have completed their survey, tell them that a score of 50 is perfect; 45 to 49 is very good; 40 to 44 is good; 35 to 39 is fair; and below 35 is poor. Explain that these are all actions they can individually take to prevent or cause pollution.

c. Go over each statement on the survey orally with students. After each statement have the students write a letter to indicate the type of pollution they think it represents on the appropriate line. They should write an *A* for air pollution, *L* for land pollution, *W* for water pollution, *N* for noise pollution, and *C* for conservation. For each statement on the survey, ask students to speculate what the impact might be if everyone did that particular activity.

d. Have the students put their surveys into their journal. If time allows, they can write a poem on the prevention of pollution for their journal.

Materials

Worksheet: *Environmental Health Survey* (p. 392)

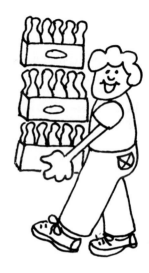

Environmental
health

3. Game: Stop That Pollutant
   a. Conduct a short discussion on air pollution. Ask students to list various causes of air pollution. (This discussion should be brief.) Tell them that the next activity will help them identify causes of air pollution and demonstrate the way the body reacts to air pollutants (dirty particles in the air).
   b. In preparation for this activity make three sets of signs from the patterns indicated in the margin. One set of signs will be needed for a third of the students in the class. Also make *dirty particle* labels. These are best done on pieces of masking tape. In the game a dirty particle label will be taped to a volleyball.
   c. Take the students outside to a playing field or to a gymnasium to play a game called "Stop That Pollutant." Divide the students into three teams. One group is the *dirty particle team*, another is the *cilia team*, and the third is the *lungs team*. Give the students signs for their team to wear around their neck.
   d. Briefly review the anatomy of the respiratory system. Explain that cilia are tiny hairlike projections in the bronchial tubes which sweep out dirty particles that are inhaled. But too much air pollution and cigarette smoking can damage the cilia.
   e. Arrange the teams as in the following illustration. The cilia team lines up in two lines between the dirty particles team (throwers) and the lungs team (catchers). The rules are as follows.

Materials

Teacher resource: *Game Directions: Stop That Pollutant* (p. 393)
Patterns: *Game Signs for Stop That Pollutant* (p. 394)
Masking tape
Construction paper
Crayons or felt pens
String
Game signs: "Lungs," "Cilia," and "Dirty Particles" (teacher made)
Volleyballs (3 to 5 balls)
Labels: "Dirty Particles" (30 labels, teacher made)

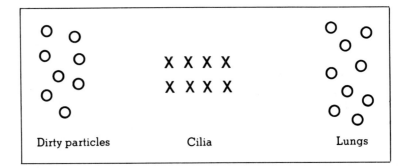

Dirty particles   Cilia   Lungs

(1) A member of the dirty particles team tapes a label on one volleyball and throws it.

(2) The dirty particle team members try to get the ball to the lungs team but must throw past the cilia team.

(3) Using one arm only, the cilia team members try to bat the ball back and keep it away from the lungs team.

(4) If the cilia team is successful, the dirty particles team must try again with that ball.

(5) If the ball gets past the cilia to the lungs, the member of the lungs team must take off and read the label on the ball. The label indicates the type of particle that has just gotten into the lungs (for example, car exhaust, cigarette smoke, factory waste, and fireplace smoke). After the type of pollutant is read, the lungs team should suggest a way that this type of pollution could be prevented.

(6) The object of the game is to see how many pollutants the dirty particles team can get into the lungs. The cilia and lungs teams are essentially on the same side. The cilia team tries to protect the lungs from the dirty particles, but once the ball gets past the cilia, a member of the lungs team *must* catch the ball.

(7) Have the teams trade roles.

Evaluation. Environmental mobile

Give the students four tagboard circles. On one side of each circle they should paste or draw a picture representing a cause for each type of pollution (air, land, noise, and water). On the other side of each circle they should write a sentence about how that type of pollution could be prevented.

Punch holes in the circles and suspend them from a hanger to make an environmental mobile. Others items that could be included on the mobile are poems about the environment and pictures of pleasant environments.

Materials

Tagboard circles (4 per student, approximately 5 inches in diameter)
Crayons or felt pens
String
Hole punch
Hangers (1 per student)

Environmental
health

Worksheet   Name _____

ENVIRONMENTAL HEALTH
SURVEY

Directions: Read each question. Think carefully about whether you do what is
              mentioned in the question. For each question, if you do that which
              is mentioned:

              Very often, circle 0
              Often, circle 1
              Sometimes, circle 3
              Never, circle 5

		Very often	Often	Sometimes	Never
1.	I let the water run while brushing my teeth.	0	1	3	5
2.	I spit chewing gum on the ground.	0	1	3	5
3.	I use only one side of a piece of writing paper.	0	1	3	5
4.	When walking, I drop food wrappers or paper on the side of the road.	0	1	3	5
5.	I write words on walls.	0	1	3	5
6.	I play my radio or stereo very loudly.	0	1	3	5
7.	I chew tobacco and spit it on the ground.	0	1	3	5
8.	When I am thirsty, I drink nonrecyclable canned or bottled soda pop.	0	1	3	5
9.	I ask Mom or Dad to take me in the car when I could ride my bicycle or walk instead.	0	1	3	5
10.	I throw in the trash usable toys or clothes when I no longer like them.	0	1	3	5

Now write the 10 numbers you circled and add them together.

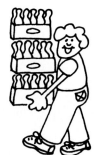

        1. ____
        2. ____
        3. ____
        4. ____
        5. ____
        6. ____
        7. ____
        8. ____
        9. ____
       10. _____

       [ ]   My score

Teacher resource

GAME DIRECTIONS: STOP THAT POLLUTANT

1. Make signs on tagboard for each team from sign patterns provided in this text. Each team will consist of a third of the students in the class. It may be useful to laminate the signs so they may be used over and over.

2. Make labels titled Dirty Particles. Use 1½- to 2-inch masking tape for the labels. Place a long section of tape onto a surface where the tape can be easily lifted off. Write the names of various air pollutants on the tape. Make about 30 labels using pollutant names over as necessary, such as the following:

    Car exhaust
    Truck exhaust
    Cigarette smoke
    Factory smoke
    Cigar smoke
    Fireplace smoke

3. Cut the labels from the long strip of tape, and mount them on a yardstick for easy access in the game.

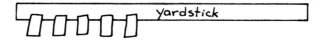

4. Organize the students outside or in a large gymnasium. Give each student a sign to wear indicating the team. Read the rules for the game as described in the activity section of this chapter. Trade off teams so that everyone has a chance to be on each team: lungs (catchers), cilia (one-handed defenders), and dirty particles (throwers).

Environmental
health

Patterns

GAME SIGNS FOR
STOP THAT POLLUTANT

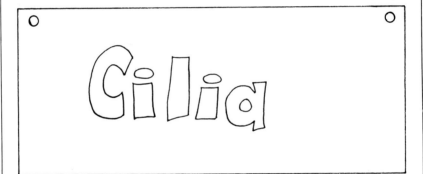

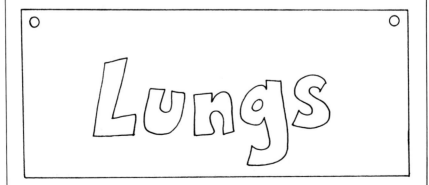

COMMUNITY HEALTH

Objective. The student identifies career opportunities in the health field.

Level. Grades 4 to 6 (most appropriate for grade 4)

Integration. Dictionary skills, language arts, listening skills

Content generalizations. There are many career opportunities in the health field available to students, including dentist, dental hygienist, pharmacist, nurse (hospital, surgical, and school), laboratory technician, medical researcher, health educator (community, school, and industry), and physician. As the field of medicine expands, individuals who pursue a career in medicine are becoming more highly specialized. The types of physicians that children are most likely to see include pediatricians, allergists, family practitioners, otologists, internists, surgeons, and psychiatrists.

Vocabulary. Nurse, dentist, pharmacist, researcher, technician, physician

Initiation. Health Careers That Interest Us

Conduct a brainstorming activity on the types of careers possible in the health field. Tell students to try to think of people who have helped them with their health. As ideas surface, write them on the board. If the students have difficulty, give clues such as the following:
1. What kind of people work at a dentist's office?
2. Who works in a hospital?
3. Is there someone here at school who helps you with your health?
4. What other kinds of doctors have you heard of?

When the brainstorming is finished, hand each student a strip of paper. Tell the students to print a health career on the paper that sounds interesting to them. They can copy the spelling off the board. They should print their name on the lower right corner of the paper. Mount the printed careers on a bulletin board entitled "Health Careers That Interest Us."

Materials

Strips of paper (approximately 12 inches long)

Bulletin board sign: "Health Careers That Interest Us"

Community health

Activities

1. Job Descriptions

    a. Have students use encyclopedias to look up the career they printed on the slip of paper. They should write a paragraph about that job and draw a picture of a person in that career. Students may need out-of-class time to complete this assignment. When it is finished, they are to mount their paragraph and picture on the bulletin board.

    b. Choose several career paragraphs to read aloud daily.

2. When Freddy Grows Up: A Play

    Tell the students that a play will be presented because "Freddy" is trying to decide what he wants to be when he grows up. Choose two students to read the parts. Change the gender as necessary.

    Option: Obtain two hand puppets and present the play as a puppet show. Or, have students present this play or puppet show to younger students in another class.

Materials

Encyclopedias
Paper
Crayons, felt pens, or colored pencils

Materials

Puppet stage (optional)
Two hand puppets that have the ability to grasp objects (optional)
Index cards with the following words printed (1 word on each card):
Doctor
Physician
Otologist
Dermatologist
Allergist
Pediatrician
Psychiatrist
Surgeon
Family practitioner
Internist
Telephone book

FREDDY WANTS A HEALTH CAREER

Freddy: I feel great! I am only 10 years old, and I know what I want to be when I grow up [whistles, cheers, etc.].

Frieda: [Enters stage] Freddy, you are shouting and cheering. What happened? Did you win the softball game?

Freddy: Oh! Hello Frieda. No, it is better than that. I know exactly what I am going to be when I grow up.

Frieda: Last week you said you wanted to be a video game expert. Will that be your profession?

Freddy: Nope. Video games are for entertainment only.

Frieda: A ball player, then; you are a great pitcher.

Freddy: I pitched that idea too. I know exactly what I am going to be when I grow up. *Exactly.* [To student audience] Can any of you guess what I am going to be?

Frieda: Now that everyone has guessed, tell us exactly what you want to be when you grow up.

Freddy: A doctor. D-O-C-T-O-R [waves card that say *doctor*].

Frieda: But exactly what kind of doctor?

Freddy: You know, a medical doctor, a physician [waves card that says *physician*]. A medical doctor is the same as a physician.

Frieda: Yes, that is true. But what *kind* of a *physician?*

Freddy: What do you mean?

Frieda: Well, my mom is a physician. She says that hardly any doctors take care of all the body parts—eyes, ears, feet—of all people, young and old. Doctors specialize in body parts or ages or diseases.

Freddy: Oh, doctors specialize in something. Then to know *exactly* what I am going to be I must know what *kind* of a doctor I am going to be.

Frieda: You have got the idea now. My mom is an ear doctor; she is an otologist [holds card that says *otologist*]. When people have trouble hearing, they see an otologist like my mom.

Freddy: An ear doctor is an otologist. Hmmm. No that is not for me. What other kinds of doctors are there?

Frieda: My brother goes to a dermatologist [holds up *dermatologist* card] because he sometimes has skin problems.

Freddy: That's a possibility. My sister goes to a dermatologist too.

Frieda: An allergist [holds *allergist* card] helps people who have allergies. People who break out in itchy bumps when they eat an orange or pet a cat see an allergy doctor—an allergist.

Freddy: Itchy bumps! That is not for me either. What else is there?

Frieda: The only other one I know of is a pediatrician [holds *pediatrician* card]. A pediatrician is a doctor who specializes in children. I am 10, and I go to a pediatrician.

Freddy: Let us look in the *Yellow Pages* of the telephone book to see what other kinds of physicians there are. There is one: psychiatrist [holds *psychiatrist* card]. A psychiatrist helps people with personal problems.

Frieda: Here is surgeon [holds *surgeon* card]. A surgeon operates to treat diseases or other problems.

Freddy: I found a family practitioner [holds *family practitioner* card]. They treat people of all ages.

Community health

Frieda: Internist [holds *internist* card]. An internist spe-
           cializes in organs inside people, like your heart
           and lungs, but usually does not operate.

Freddy: That is it! I know *exactly* what I will be. I will be an
           internist, and treat people's heart, lungs, and oth-
           er organs. Of course, I will tell them that if they
           keep healthy by playing baseball and sports and
           eating nutritious foods, they probably will not
           need an internist very often.

Frieda: [Asks students] Do you know the names of differ-
           ent types of physicians? See how many you can
Freddy   match to their job. Your teacher will give you a
and   worksheet. You can ask your teacher for help.
Frieda: Bye, good luck!

Ask the class, "If Freddy wants to have a health career when
he grows up, what other jobs could he do other than being a
physician?"

3. Different Kinds of Physicians

   After the play, hand out the worksheet, *Different Kinds of
   Physicians,* for students to complete. Review the worksheet, and have students correct mistakes.

Materials

Worksheet: *Different Kinds of Physicians* (p. 400)

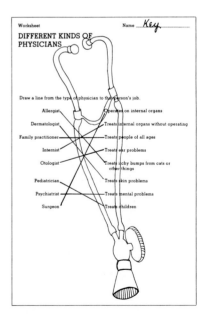

Evaluation. Who Does What?

Have the students complete the worksheet, *Who Does What?*, individually and without assistance. Tell them that this worksheet is very similar to the one they already did on different kinds of physicians. However, this time there are other careers in addition to physicians on the worksheet.

Materials

Worksheet: *Who Does What?* (p. 401)

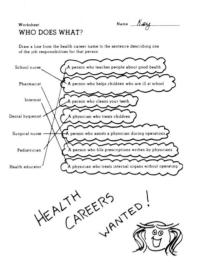

Worksheet   Name _____

DIFFERENT KINDS OF PHYSICIANS

Draw a line from the type of physician to that person's job.

Allergist   Operates on internal organs

Dermatologist   Treats internal organs without operating

Family practitioner   Treats people of all ages

Internist   Treats ear problems

Otologist   Treats itchy bumps from cats or other things

Pediatrician   Treats skin problems

Psychiatrist   Treats mental problems

Surgeon   Treats children

Worksheet   Name _____

WHO DOES WHAT?

Draw a line from the health career name to the sentence describing one
of the job responsibilities for that person.

School nurse   A person who teaches people about good health

Pharmacist   A person who helps children who are ill at school

Internist   A person who cleans your teeth

Dental hygienist   A physician who treats children

Surgical nurse   A person who assists a physician during operations

Pediatrician   A person who fills prescriptions written by physicians

Health educator   A physician who treats internal organs without operating

HEALTH CAREERS WANTED!

Community health

EXERCISES

1. Use a calendar with large spaces for the days, and plan the amount of time needed to teach one of the described teaching plans. The amount of time allotted to health each day will vary from teacher to teacher and school to school. Decide the number of minutes each day you will spend on health. Then write short descriptive phrases on the calendar, or on a piece of paper resembling a calendar, that will give you quick clues as to the activities students participate in each day, as in the box below.

SAMPLE DAILY LESSON PLAN **Forty minute class period**	**Monday** Introduction: Brainstorm types of careers. Post HEALTH CAREERS bulletin board. Assign paragraph on health career and have students begin work with encyclopedias or dictionaries. Integration: language arts, dictionary skills	**Tuesday** Students complete paragraph and drawing of health professional. Read 3-4 paragraphs and allow students to mount work on bulletin board. Integration: language arts, art
Wednesday Present puppet show "Freddie wants a Health Career." Students complete worksheet "Different Kinds of Doctors." Discuss and correct worksheets. Integration: listening skills	**Thursday** Culmination: Guest speaker; School Nurse Discuss job responsibilities and training	**Friday** Evaluation: Students complete worksheets, trade papers, discuss and correct.

2. Find out what teaching aids are available for grades 4 to 6 from local voluntary health agencies. Preview and write a review of at least one item.
3. Teach one of the learning opportunities (or a part of one) in a local school.
4. Develop a learning opportunity using an objective in Chapter 9 that was not used in Chapter 12. Use the plans in Chapter 12 as a model.

CHAPTER 14

Content Appropriate for Middle School Students

When you finish this chapter, you should be able to:

■ **Describe appropriate content in ten areas of health education for students in middle school.**

Middle school students in grades six, seven and eight are entering the formal operational stage and are able to understand the linkages between behavior and health outcomes; they can think of health and sickness as reciprocal components of the concept of "health." For adolescents in the seventh and eighth grades, peer groups are of extreme importance and have a profound effect upon the mental, emotional and social well-being of the individual. Because of these developmental characteristics, the middle school teacher has the opportunity to help shape students' attitudes and beliefs about self-reliance and the value of self-care at a time in their lives when self-responsibility is of extreme importance. This shaping process is most appropriate when health instruction is not "telling" about health and illness, but rather, providing the concepts and intellectual tools they need in order to build and sustain healthful lifestyles.

PERSONAL HEALTH

At the middle school level, students begin to assess personal health care habits and physical fitness activities. Students examine their eating habits, cleanliness habits, dental practices, and levels of physical activity in the context of both immediate and long-range outcomes. Additionally, the middle school years are an appropriate time to introduce the idea of setting and working toward personal health goals.

Acne

During puberty, the oil glands in the skin become more active and may manufacture more oil than is needed. When too much oil is produced, the ducts that transport the oil become clogged. This is called a "blackhead." The dark color is due to a chemical reaction that occurs when the oil is exposed to the air. If the excess oil remains in the oil gland and is not exposed to air, a "whitehead" is formed. In acne, the oil glands and ducts become swollen and infected, forming "pimples." The face, neck, shoulders, and back are common sites for acne because many oil glands exist there.

The best methods for minimizing acne are those that help to reduce the oiliness of the skin:

- Wash the affected areas with soap and water. Choose a soap that does not irritate the skin.
- Avoid any foods that seem to make acne worse. Authorities disagree on the role of diet in acne; however, there seem to be some foods that worsen acne in some persons (chocolate, nuts, fried foods, and rich desserts).
- Do not "pick" or squeeze blemishes. Squeezing can spread the infection to adjacent tissues and cause scarring.
- Get plenty of exercise, sleep, and eat a balanced diet (a variety of foods from the four food groups).
- Deal with daily stressors in a positive way.
- See a doctor for severe cases of acne.

Warts

Warts are caused by a virus that enters the skin and causes an increase in the number of skin cells. The hands and especially the fingers are common sites for the occurrence of warts during the teen years. Many warts will disappear without treatment; however, if they persist or cause discomfort, they may be removed by a doctor. Picking at warts to the point of bleeding can cause them to spread.

Malocclusion

Malocclusion is a condition in which the teeth are poorly aligned so that chewing ability and/or appearance is affected. Malocclusion results from hereditary factors or premature loss of deciduous or permanent teeth. Poorly aligned teeth can contribute to faulty nutrition, tooth decay and gum disease. Orthodontists are specially trained dentists who can correct occlusion problems by using wires, bands, tiny springs, and elastic devices. During orthodontic treatment, gentle pressure is exerted on the teeth to move them through the bone tissue until they are correctly aligned. This process takes from one to three years. While under orthodontic treatment, it is particularly important to practice good dental hygiene to keep the teeth and appliances free of food debris that can contribute to tooth decay and bad breath.

Sleep

Adequate sleep is necessary to keep mentally alert, to maintain a good disposition, to stay physically well, and to maintain proper growth. During adolescence, large amounts of the growth hormone are secreted by the pituitary gland during sleep. Sleep needs vary from one individual to the next; however, most people need from nine to ten hours of sleep during the teen years. A simple way to determine if you have had enough sleep is to see if you feel rested and energetic during the day.

Posture

Posture is a reflection of an individual's health status and is particularly important during adolescence because it is during this time that posture faults often develop. Poor posture is often seen in students who are self-conscious about height. However, some postural defects are physical in origin. "Scoliosis" (curvature of the spine) can cause defects in posture. Additionally, poor muscle tone resulting from a recent injury or illness may contribute to slouching or slumping. These types of posture defects can be

corrected under the advice of a physician through surgery, exercises, or a combination of surgery and exercise.

There is no one perfect standing, walking, or sitting posture for everyone because individuals differ in skeletal and muscular structure. Proper posture involves sitting, standing, and walking without appearing out of alignment by being slumped over, rigidly erect, or uncomfortable. Diet, fitness levels, and emotions affect posture so the best way to ensure good posture is to enhance health in general. Also, being conscious of one's posture and lifting heavy objects properly to avoid injury will aid in the development of good posture.

Fitness

Exercise is a necessary component for the maintenance and enhancement of personal health. Students should attempt to find physical activities that they enjoy and to establish exercise regimens that meet personal needs. The incorporation of fitness activities into adolescents' life styles increases the probability of making these positive health activities life-long habits. While individual definitions of fitness may vary, fitness has three basic components.

Flexibility is the range of motion that joints allow. As children develop, they become more flexible until adolescence, when gradual loss of joint mobility begins. Individual flexibility depends upon many factors; age, sex, posture, and fat/muscle distribution in the body. Flexibility can be increased through regular stretching exercises that are done properly. The safest way to stretch is "static" stretching which is a relaxed, gradual stretch that is held for a short time. When stretching, reach to the point of discomfort, then back off slightly, allowing the muscle to adjust for 20 to 30 seconds. Hold the stretch until the feeling of tension diminishes. Concentrate on the feeling of the stretch rather than the flexibility you want to attain. Some good exercises to increase flexibility include:

- Toe pull—Sit on the floor and bend your legs so that the soles of your feet touch. Pull on your toes while pressing your knees down with your elbows. Hold for 10 seconds and repeat at least five times.
- Knee-chest pull—Lie on your back, clasp one knee and pull it to your chest. Hold for 15 to 30 seconds then repeat with the other knee. Perform at least five repetitions with each knee.
- Wall stretch—Stand three feet from a wall with your feet slightly apart. Put your hands on the wall and lean forward slowly, keeping your heels on the ground. Hold the stretch for ten seconds then repeat five times.
- Seated toe touch—Sit on the floor with your legs extended to the front. Point your toes and slide your hands down your legs until you feel the stretch. Holding this position, slowly lean forward and try to touch your toes. Hold for ten seconds then repeat five times.
- Foot-buttocks roll—Lie on your stomach, reach back and grasp one foot. Bend your knee and pull your foot toward your buttocks. Hold the stretch for 15 to 30 seconds. Repeat with the other foot.

Cardiovascular stamina is the second component of fitness. It is maintained and increased through "aerobic" exercise that conditions the heart and lungs. Aerobic exercises are activities that utilize the large muscle groups of the body and that keep your pulse at the "target heart rate" for at least 20 minutes. Aerobic activities include:

walking
jogging
swimming
cycling
skipping rope
cross-country skiing
aerobic dance
skating

The best way to make sure that you are working hard enough but not overdoing is to use your heart rate as a guide. Calculate your target heart rate by using this formula:

$220 -$ your age $=$ maximum heart rate
maximum heart rate $\times 75\% =$
$$\text{target heart rate}$$

Find your pulse at the carotid artery by tilting your head slightly back and to one side. Slide your forefinger and middle finger into the groove to the side of your "Adam's apple" and feel for your pulse. Don't use your thumb because it has a pulse of its own. Learn to find your pulse quickly and easily.

About three minutes into your exercise, take your pulse for six seconds and multiply by ten. If your pulse rate is higher than your target heart rate, slow down. Speed up your exercise if your pulse rate is lower than your target heart rate zone. Monitor your pulse at several intervals during your workout to make sure that you are exercising at the proper intensity.

No matter which aerobic exercise you choose, your workout should follow the same steps:

- Warm up gradually to prepare your body for more vigorous exercise. Jogging in place is a good example. (5 minutes)
- Stretch to loosen your muscles and prevent injuries. (5 minutes)
- Exercise at your target heart rate. (20 minutes)
- Cool down by gradually decreasing your activity. (5 minutes)
- Stretch to prevent soreness. (5 minutes)

Muscular strength and endurance are the components of fitness that enable an individual to handle everyday tasks, like raking leaves. Exercising to increase muscular strength and endurance enables muscles to work efficiently and reliably and to give shape and tone to our bodies. Muscle tissue never stays the same. If it is used, it grows stronger. If it is unused, it breaks down. The only way to develop muscle tissue is to demand more work of it than it is used to performing.

Muscular exercises are classified as either "isometric" or "isotonic." Isometric exercises are those in which you pull or push against a stationary object. For example, pushing your ankles against the legs of a chair. Isotonic exercises involve moving a moderate load several times. Weightlifting and calisthenics are examples of isotonic exercises. Few repetitions of heavy weights are best for producing muscular strength. Low resistance and frequent repetitions are best for developing flexibility, coordination, and muscular endurance.

Weight Problems

Many adolescents feel that they either need to gain or lose weight. Before embarking on any program to alter body weight, it is important to have a physical examination by a physician to determine if a gain in body weight or a loss of body fat is warranted. Often the problem is an adolescent growth spurt that results in growing "out" before growing "up" or vice versa.

If the individual is truly underweight, the physician will try to determine physical causes that contribute to the condition. Glandular diseases, lack of proper diet, strong emotions, or failure to get enough sleep and rest can be contributing factors. If poor nutrition seems to be the cause, the doctor will suggest ways to increase the amount of nutrition taken into the body. Some helpful hints include:

- Eat breakfast daily.
- Eat healthful between-meal snacks.

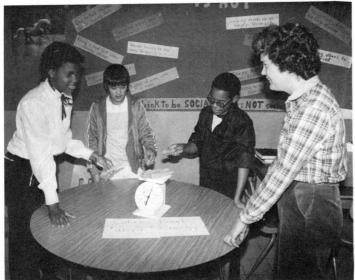

Don Merwin

- Drink milk instead of water.
- Get more sleep than you normally get.
- Eat second helpings.

A health examination is also important before a young person attempts to lose weight. Experts realize that body weight alone is not an accurate indicator of overweight. The amount of body fat is an important determinant of obesity. Altering diet at this age can be dangerous because, without a nutritious daily diet, the growing body may be deprived of essential nutrients needed for growth and development. Some helpful hints for decreasing body fat include:

- Eat three balanced meals each day.
- Do not take second helpings.
- Reduce the number of "empty" calorie foods in your diet.
- Increase exercise.

MENTAL HEALTH

The physical, mental, emotional, and social aspects of the individual are interrelated. What affects the individual physically most likely will affect him or her emotionally and socially as well. For example, a broken leg certainly has physical effects, but, in addition, during the physical mending process the individual cannot participate in normal social activities because it is more difficult to get around. Therefore emotional strain is expected. Although the health problem is physical, the ramifications to the whole person are mental, emotional, and social as well. This interrelationship can be seen in all health-related circumstances and choices.

Improving Mental Health

Mental health is built upon all experiences since birth. Future experiences will also contribute to mental health status. This means that it is possible to improve mental health through increased understanding of self and others. Some aids to improving mental health include:

- maintaining good relationships with family and friends.
- communicating with the people you care about.
- feeling good about yourself.
- becoming involved in activities that are interesting to you.
- appreciating individual differences.
- determining the personal values by which you want to live.

Personality

Personality is the combination of a person's physical, mental, and social traits which makes a person unique. Since everyone's personality is different, there is a wide range of personality traits. Personality is shown in how a person reacts to the people, things, and events in his or her environment. An individual's personality will change throughout life but most experts believe that the early years of a person's life are the most important. Heredity, personal experiences, self-concept, and the environment are factors that contribute to the formation of personality.

Setting Goals

It is important for adolescents to consider their hopes and dreams for the future and to stretch toward fulfilling their potential. In evaluating potential, it is important not to underestimate but to also be honest about abilities. Not all goals have to be on a grand scale. Focusing on a short-term goal, one that can be reached in a few weeks, allows more control in reaching the goal. And the more successful an individual is at setting and accomplishing small goals, the greater the experience and success in meeting long-range goals. For both short-term and long-term goals, it is important to chart out a step-by-step plan to accomplish the goal.

Stress

Stress is a normal part of life. It is both physical and mental tension. Stressful feelings occur when the unexpected happens, or when we face the unknown. Stress occurs during the more serious parts of life such as the death of a loved one or the divorce of parents, but it is not necessarily all bad. Sometimes stress can help us perform better in the face of a challenge. It is important that we learn what situations in our own lives produce stress and how we react in those situations. Coping with stressful situations successfully contributes to both mental and physical health.

When an individual is confronted with a stressful situation, the body reacts in several ways. The first response is one of alarm, sometimes called the "fight or flight" response. The body reacts physically with rapid breathing, increased pulse rate, tense muscles, and possibly a nervous feeling in the stomach. The body releases adrenaline in this stage to prepare for fight or flight. How one chooses to cope with the alarm response is significant. It can be constructive or destructive. One common destructive reaction to stress is the use of alcohol or other drugs to calm and mask the alarm response. Constructive ways to cope with stress include physical activity to work off the excess adrenaline, talking it out with a friend, taking one thing at a time, not trying to "win" every time, balancing work with play, taking a break, and practicing relaxation techniques. Learning how to systematically handle conflicts is also useful.

WAYS TO COPE

(1) *Physical activity:* Since the hormone adrenaline is released during stressful times and therefore muscles are tense, physical activity is useful in burning up the pent-up energy. Regular physical exercise programs have been shown to be useful in reducing stress levels. Ask the students what physical activities they think might be useful in reducing stress. (Aerobic exercises are of particular benefit.)

(2) *Talk things out:* Using a friend's ear just to get things off your chest can be very useful. It is not even necessary that the friend offer useful suggestions; just the chance to talk to someone about what is worrying you is helpful. (HINT: Suggest that the students find out about the technique called *active listening.*)

(3) *Take things one at a time:* When a problem seems overwhelming, break it into small pieces and consider one step at a time. For example, suppose that you have a very messy room. The closet is a mess, your drawers are messed up, and you have dirty clothes all over the floor. Tackle the problem in parts. How could you take care of your messy room in parts?

(4) *Do not try to win every time:* Life has ups and downs. We cannot always have things our way. Accepting the fact that sometimes things do not work out the way you want them to is one way of coping with stress. Even the best football or basketball teams lose games.

Continued.

WAYS TO COPE—cont'd

(5) *Balance play with work:* You will create a stressful situation if you ignore responsibilities and go off and play. However, it is just as stressful to work all day in school and go home and do homework all evening. A balance is needed.

(6) *Take a break for yourself:* It is a good idea to plan a certain amount of time each day for yourself—15 to 20 minutes to do something you like to do, such as read a magazine, listen to music, watch a favorite television show, or do some special relaxation exercises. It might even be day-dreaming for a few minutes, but it should be planned time for yourself.

Coping Mechanisms

Everyone wants to feel at ease, so, from time to time, everyone uses "coping mechanisms" to protect herself or himself from uncomfortable thoughts or feelings. Some of the ways we defend ourselves are by:

- repression—keeping threatening memories, feelings, or wishes from becoming conscious. For example, "forgetting" to feed the dog after once being bitten.
- denial—refusing to accept a painful fact. For example, refusing to believe that someone you love is dying of cancer.
- rationalization—substituting "good" reasons for the real motivations of behavior. For example, saying you can't come to a friend's house because you have to study when the real reason you don't go to her house is because you are angry at something she said.
- projection—attributing your own unacceptable feelings to someone else. For example, saying that your girlfriend or boyfriend broke up with you because she or he wanted to date someone else when you were really the one who wanted to date other people.

- displacement—redirecting feelings from their true object to a substitute. For example, snapping at your best friend when you are really angry with your teacher.

Suicide Prevention

The American Psychiatric Association estimates that there has been more than a threefold increase in the rate of suicide among adolescents in the past 25 years. Usually, a person considering suicide gives clues that can serve as warning signals. Among young persons, common signals of suicide are:

- increased moodiness
- seeming depressed or uncommunicative
- feelings of worthlessness
- withdrawal from normal activities
- writing and/or talking about death
- specific suicide threats
- breaking off friendships
- failure or poor school performance
- increased drug and alcohol use
- failed love relationship
- giving away prized possessions

If someone exhibits signs of suicide, talk to them and show them that you care. Suggest possible solutions to their problems and make future plans. Have your friend promise that he or she won't do anything to harm himself or herself without calling you first. If your friend calls, get to them immediately. Suggest that you and your friend talk to a professional who can help. A teacher, school nurse, or school counselor can provide the help your friend needs.

FAMILY LIFE

Adolescence is a time of great change in all dimensions related to health. Physically, it is a time when students gain sexual maturity. Rapid periods of growth are accompanied by new sexual feelings. All of this change requires mental and emotional adjustments to the person the adolescent is becoming. It is common for adolescents to experience depression, confusion, and sometimes loneliness and isolation. The high rate of teenage suicide can be related to this difficult emotional time. Socially, teenagers commonly have conflicts with parents relating to their desire for independence from parental constraints. As the acceptance by peers becomes all important, conflicts between familial values and peer pressures commonly arise.

Friendships

Friendship is a universal and satisfying experience for persons in all age groups and cultures. In American society, friends may include classmates, neighbors, or persons you grow up with. Even though it is normal to occasionally become angry with the people we consider friends, everyone has the need to maintain long-term friendships. In order to make and keep friends, a person must exhibit the qualities that friendships build and nurture—respect, tolerance, and loyalty.

Peer Pressure

Peer pressure is perhaps the single most important influence in the life of the adolescent and can have a significant effect on health choices, either positive or negative. Common peer-influenced health choices include use or nonuse of drugs, eating healthful or unhealthful snacks, being active or sedentary, and taking or not taking risks. Students at this level can learn to recognize peer pressure and take steps to consciously resist pressure when they wish to do so.

Dating

The purpose of dating is to allow persons to interact and become better acquainted with each other. Dating also provides an opportunity to learn how to make conversation and to share feelings and opinions. An individual's definition of an ideal date may change from one month to the next as the person experiences dates with persons exhibiting a variety of traits.

Dating also provides an opportunity to explore sexual identity. This is why it is not unusual for adolescents to choose a date by appearance alone. Sexual attraction brings couples together where they may discover commonalities or may break up after the initial attraction cools. It is often difficult to sort out emotional feelings from sexual desires but eventually each person must make decisions about sexual behavior in relationships. The first step in making a responsible decision is respecting your own sexual values and those of your partner.

Reproduction

Reproduction is an important and natural part of life. It begins with two cells: the sperm cell from the male and the egg cell (ovum) from the female. These two cells come together inside the female after millions of sperm cells are deposited inside her body (vagina) during sexual intercourse. Conception occurs if an egg cell is present. Since the female ovulates about once every 28 days, the egg cell is not always present, so conception does not always result from sexual intercourse. If an egg cell is present, however, it is highly likely that conception will occur. The fertilized egg is called a zygote and later a blastocyst as it travels to the uterus and implants on the wall. It is called an embryo from about the first to the twelfth week. The embryo grows and is nourished by the mother. It begins to change from a ball of cells to a form looking somewhat like a tiny human. After the twelfth week (third month) it is called a fetus (although some call it a fetus at all stages of development). The fetus continues to grow until it is fully developed. Then birth occurs, and a new baby (infant) is brought into the world. Pregnancy lasts approximately 9 months. When the baby is ready to be born, the mother feels contractions, sometimes called labor pains. She then knows that the baby is ready to be delivered. In a normal birth the baby comes out through the vagina head first, face up. Sometimes babies are born feet first. This is called a breech birth. In complicated births it is sometimes necessary to do an incision on the abdomen of the mother and deliver the baby surgically. This is called a caesarean section.

The birth of a baby is usually a happy time for parents and other family members. Now it is common for the father to be present during the birth of his child, and in some hospitals brothers and sisters may be there as well. The birth of a baby signifies a big change in the lives of the mother, father, and entire family.

Contraception

Various contraceptive methods are available to prevent unwanted pregnancies: birth control pills; contraceptive sponges; diaphragms; condoms; spermicides; and natural family planning methods. The best way to prevent a pregnancy is abstinence. In many situations the need for middle school students to be aware of contraceptive methods is great. However, it is important to follow district guidelines and policies when teaching about reproduction and contraception.

Prenatal Health

Most adolescents expect to be parents at some time during their lives. Because the outcome of a pregnancy is influenced by the health status of the parents before conception, it is important that adolescents become aware of the effect their health habits have upon future childbearing. Additionally, knowledge of prenatal care is an important aspect of health instruction for the intermediate student.

- nutrition—Eating a well-balanced diet is critical for the development of the unborn baby and the health of the mother. No vitamin supplement can replace the nutrients that a varied diet can provide. It is recommended that the mother gain from 24 to 27 pounds during the course of the pregnancy.
- exercise—Exercise is recommended for the pregnant woman throughout the pregnancy. As a general rule, women should engage in the same activities they enjoyed before becoming pregnant (swimming, jogging, and playing tennis are examples). As the uterus enlarges, some women may find vigorous activities to be uncomfortable and may substitute brisk walking.
- rest—It is important for the pregnant woman to get adequate rest. If frequent urination during the night or other discomforts keep the woman from getting enough sleep, she may need to nap or schedule rest periods during the day.
- smoking—Women who smoke during pregnancy increase their risk of having a miscarriage or delivering a baby who is premature. The more cigarettes that are smoked, the greater the risks.

- alcohol—When consumed by a pregnant woman, alcohol passes through the placenta and into the baby's bloodstream. Children who are born to mothers who have drunk heavily during pregnancy are at risk for "fetal alcohol syndrome." These babies suffer low birthweight, mental retardation, cardiovascular disorders, and specific facial characteristics. There is no safe level of alcohol consumption for pregnant women; therefore, health professionals recommend that women who are pregnant, or are trying to become pregnant, avoid alcohol.
- drugs—Any drug that is taken into the body of a pregnant woman can affect the baby in some way. In order to avoid the risks of birth defects and complications surrounding delivery, drugs should be avoided unless prescribed by a physician who is aware of the pregnancy.
- age—The "best" time to have a healthy baby is between the ages of 25 and 29. Teenage mothers and their babies are at increased risk of physical and psychological problems. Pregnant teens are more likely to have premature babies and to have difficult labors. Newborn babies of teenage mothers are less likely to survive.
- environmental risks—High levels of radiation and pollutants have been associated with birth defects. As research continues in this area, women are advised to be cautious about environmental conditions that constitute hazards to unborn children.

NUTRITION

The amount of energy that foods provide is measured in terms of calories. Different foods have different caloric values, depending on the energy potential of that food. All foods have cal-ories. Some foods, such as cakes, candies, frostings, and gravy, are high in calories and low in nutrients. Others, such as meats and nuts, are high in calories and also high in nutrients.

The body needs a certain amount of calories a day to function. Every activity of life from jogging to breathing requires energy. This energy is measured in calories. *Basal metabolism* refers to the minimum amount of energy required to maintain vital body functions and muscle tone at rest. Exact energy requirements vary from individual to individual because of differences in their basal metabolism and daily activities. Most teenagers require between 2400 and 2800 calories per day to maintain their weight. If an individual is balancing the calories eaten daily with the calories used daily, body weight will stay the same. If more calories are eaten than are used daily, weight will increase. The body stores the excess energy in the form of fat. If fewer calories are eaten than are used, the body uses the energy stored in the fat cells, and weight decreases.

Comparing personal food choices with recommended servings in each of the four food groups is one way to analyze eating habits. Often teenagers find that they eat too few servings in one or two of the groups. Or they may be eating foods with a lower nutritional quality within a food group. For example, ice cream is classified in the milk group, but it is of lower quality nutritionally than milk. Teenagers may also find that they are eating several extra foods that are not in a food group at all and are taking in "empty" calories. Extra foods may be problematic for persons desiring a weight loss. Often individuals who want to lose weight engage in fad diets that can be dangerous to the health.

Fad Diets

Despite their popularity and sales appeal, fad diets simply don't work. Not only do they fail,

THE FOUR FOOD GROUPS—SERVINGS PER DAY FOR TEENS

Food	Amount per serving	Servings per day for teenagers
Milk Group		
Milk	8 ounces (1 cup)	
Yogurt, plain	1 cup	
Hard cheese	1¼ ounces	
Cheese spread	2 ounces	4
Ice cream	1½ cups	
Cottage cheese	2 cups	
Protein and Meat Group		
Meat, lean	2 to 3 ounces cooked	
Poultry	2 to 3 ounces	
Fish	2 to 3 ounces	
Hard Cheese	2 to 3 ounces	
Eggs	2 to 3	2
Cottage cheese	½ cup	
Dry beans and peas	1 to 1½ cups cooked	
Nuts and seeds	½ to ¾ cup	
Peanut butter	4 tablespoons	
Vegetable and Fruit Group		
Vegetables, cut up	½ cup	
Fruits, cut up	½ cup	
Grapefruit	½ medium	
Melon	½ medium	
Orange	1	4
Potato	1 medium	
Salad	1 bowl	
Lettuce	1 wedge	
Bread and Cereal Group		
Bread	1 slice	
Cooked cereal	½ to ¾ cup	
Pasta	½ to ¾ cup	4
Rice	½ to ¾ cup	
Dry cereal	1 ounce	

Based on amounts established by the U.S. Department of Agriculture.

they can also cause health problems.

- low-protein diets—These diets lack essential minerals and force the body to break down its own muscle tissue for protein. A person using this diet will lose muscle tissue as well as fat. In cases of extreme dieting, dieters develop diarrhea, shock, or heart irregularities.
- low-carbohydrate/high protein diets—These diets limit fruits and vegetables and therefore, many vitamins and minerals. The excess protein that is promoted in these diets force the kidneys and liver to work harder.
- fasting—Fasting can be hazardous to health by contributing to feelings of depression, loss of muscle tissue, and heart rhythm abnormalities. When an individual fasts, the body's metabolism slows down to conserve energy. So during a fast, you lose weight slowly, if at all.

Eating Disorders

When dieting is taken to extremes or psychological problems accompany the desire to be thin, eating disorders may develop. Increasing numbers of people, especially young females, are exhibiting eating disorders. The most common are anorexia nervosa and bulimia.

- anorexia nervosa—This is a psychological condition in which the victims, usually middle- to upper-class women in their teens and twenties, view themselves as overweight no matter how thin they become. They may stop eating completely and throw up any food that is forced on them. In addition to dieting, the anorectic may exercise strenuously and use large amounts of laxatives. The victims become emaciated and malnourished. Heart problems can occur and result in an untimely death.

SYMPTOMS OF EATING DISORDERS*

Suspect an eating disorder when there is one or more of the following symptoms:

abnormal weight loss
refusal to eat, except for tiny portions
binge eating
vomiting
abuse of laxatives, diuretics, emetics, or diet pills
denial of hunger
excessive exercise
distorted body image (seeing self as fat though actually thin)
preoccupation with food
absent or irregular menstruation in women
depression

School counselors, the community hospital, or health services may give information, referrals to medical professionals and self-help groups. For more information write to NAAS (The National Anorexic Aid Society) 5496 Karl Road, Columbus, OH. HOTLINE NUMBER 614-436-1112.

*From the National Anorexic Aid Society, Inc. Newsletter, vol. XI, Issue 4.

- bulimia—Like anorexia, bulimia primarily affects adolescent and young adult women. Bulimics rapidly consume large amounts of high calorie foods and then vomit to control their weight. Bulimics may also use laxatives.

DISEASE PREVENTION AND CONTROL

Around the turn of the century the leading causes of death in the United States were largely infectious diseases such as pneumonia, influenza, and tuberculosis. Medical science has progressed greatly. We have learned the importance of cleanliness and isolation from infectious microbes in preventing and controlling many diseases. The average life expectancy has increased dramatically since 1900. Now more people die from noninfectious diseases such as cardiovascular diseases, cancer, and stroke. The chances of getting one of these diseases (and others, such as cirrhosis of the liver) are related to the health habits established early in life and to heredity. Most of these diseases attack people later in life. Even though the part that heredity plays has not been entirely determined yet, personal life style choices involving good nutrition, exercise, avoidance of smoking, and good stress management can help prevent cardiovascular diseases. Cirrhosis of the liver is related to alcohol abuse, skin cancer to overexposure to the sun, and lung cancer to cigarette smoking. Hypertension, which is chronic high blood pressure, sometimes is controlled by lowering salt intake, not smoking, good nutrition (including eating less fatty foods), and regular aerobic exercise.

Studies on the relationship of life style choices to the prevention of disease are continuing, and the information changes as new facts are learned. Most experts believe that the following factors contribute to longevity: (1) regular exercise (sustained aerobic exercise for at least 20 minutes, at least 3 times a week), (2) good nutritional habits (low in fats, sugar, and salt; high in fresh vegetables and fruits), (3) not smoking, (4) regular use of seat belts, (5) successful management of stress, (6) abstinence or moderation in alcohol use, and (7) maintenance of a normal weight (less than 20% overweight or underweight).

Chronic Diseases

Certain illnesses may last a long time or recur often. These illnesses are called chronic diseases. Most chronic diseases develop as a result of health-related behaviors and are not caused by pathogens. These diseases often cannot be cured, only controlled; therefore, prevention of these diseases is particularly important.

Allergies are the most widespread chronic condition among young people. When a person has a reaction to a substance that most other people do not react to, she or he is said to be ''allergic.'' The most common sites for allergic reactions are the skin, eyes, digestive tract, and air passages, although a reaction may take place in almost any part of the body.

Epilepsy is a disorder that is characterized by ''seizures'' (sudden attacks, loss of consciousness, or loss of muscle control). Seizures are caused by excessive discharges of energy in the brain. Seizures may be caused by infection, brain injury, growths in the brain, or unknown causes.

Emphysema is common in adults that have smoked cigarettes or have been exposed to other lung irritants. In emphysema, the air sacs of the lungs lose their elasticity; therefore, the body must work much harder to get the oxygen it needs. Persons with emphysema cough, wheeze, become dizzy, and experience shortness of breath.

Ulcers are breaks in the inner lining of the stomach or small intestine that are thought to be caused by nervous tension. When a person is under pressure, the stomach may form too much acid that can eat away parts of the linings of the organs of the digestive tract. Persons with ulcers experience pain deep in the stomach and/or back.

Cardiovascular disease is another chronic

SEVEN WARNING SIGNS OF CANCER

The seven warning signs of cancer can alert an individual to possible cancerous growths.
- Change in bowel or bladder habits.
- A sore that does not heal.
- Unusual bleeding or discharge.
- Thickening or lump in the breast or elsewhere.
- Indigestion or difficulty swallowing.
- Obvious change in a wart or mole.
- Nagging cough or hoarseness.

---

disorder that primarily affects adults although the behaviors that influence the development of these conditions begin early in life. Cardiovascular diseases are disorders of the heart and blood vessels and include: high blood pressure; atherosclerosis; angina pectoris; heart attack; stroke; and congestive heart failure.

Cancer is a disease of the cell in which the mechanism that regulates cell growth goes out of control. Even though cancer is the most feared chronic disease, it is also the most curable. The key to cancer cure is early detection and treatment.

Sexually Transmitted Diseases

The incidence of sexually transmitted diseases has increased in the United States to epidemic proportions. These are diseases which are spread mainly through intimate sexual contact. The most common are chlamydia, gonorrhea, herpes (both herpes simplex 1 and 2 can be transmitted sexually), and syphilis. In many cases the symptoms of certain sexually transmitted diseases are not noticed. Females usually do not notice the symptoms of gonorrhea,

syphilis, or chlamydia. Males usually have painful urination and a discharge with gonorrhea and chlamydia and have noticeable although painless sores with syphilis. Herpes is a very painful disease for both men and women. Herpes is characterized by painful sores in the genital area that flare up, subside, and then flare up again. The recurrent outbreaks often are related to stress in the life of the victim. The herpes sores are infectious and will transmit the virus to sexual partners. There is currently no cure for herpes. It is possible, however, to effectively treat gonorrhea, syphilis, and chlamydia with drugs. Early medical treatment is essential to avoid permanent damage from these diseases.

AIDS (Acquired Immune Deficiency Syndrome) is the most deadly and mysterious sexually transmitted disease. AIDS victims suffer from impaired immune systems that leave the individual at risk for infections and cancer. In addition, AIDS victims may experience damage to the nervous system. All persons who carry the AIDS virus are infectious even though they do not all develop full-blown AIDS. The HIV virus, which causes AIDS, can be transmitted in any of three ways; through sexual contact with an infected partner, through using contaminated needles (IV drugs), and from an infected mother to her baby.

The best way to deal with STDs is to prevent them. There are many ways to lessen the chances of contracting such a disease. *The most effective is to abstain from sexual activity*. With some diseases the only way a female ever knows that she has been infected is if she is informed by her male partner.

NOTE: When teaching about sexually transmitted diseases, the teacher must be certain to follow district guidelines and recommendations.

AIDS EDUCATION CONTENT AS RECOMMENDED BY THE CENTERS FOR DISEASE CONTROL*

Late Elementary/Middle School

Education about AIDS for students in late elementary/middle school grades should be designed with consideration for the following information.

Viruses are living organisms too small to be seen by the unaided eye.

Viruses can be transmitted from an infected person to an uninfected person through various means.

Some viruses cause disease among people.

Persons who are infected with some viruses that cause disease may not have any signs or symptoms of disease.

*AIDS (an abbreviation for **a**cquired **i**mmuno**d**eficiency **s**yndrome) is caused by a virus that weakens the ability of infected individuals to fight off disease.*

People who have AIDS often develop a rare type of severe pneumonia, a cancer called Kaposi's sarcoma, and certain other diseases that healthy people normally do not get.

About 1 to 1.5 million of the total population of approximately 240 million Americans currently are infected with the AIDS virus and consequently are capable of infecting others.

People who are infected with the AIDS virus live in every state in the United States and in most other countries of the world. Infected people live in cities as well as in suburbs, small towns, and rural areas. Although most infected people are adults, teenagers can also become infected. Females as well as males are infected. People of every race are infected, including whites, blacks, Hispanics, Native Americans, and Asian/Pacific Islanders.

The AIDS virus can be transmitted by sexual contact with an infected person; by using needles and other injection equipment that an infected person has used; and from an infected mother to her infant before or during birth.

A small number of doctors, nurses, and other medical personnel have been infected when they were directly exposed to infected blood.

It sometimes takes several years after becoming infected with the AIDS virus before symptoms of the disease appear. Thus, people who are infected with the virus can infect other people—even though the people who transmit the infection do not feel or look sick.

Most infected people who develop symptoms of AIDS only live about 2 years after their symptoms are diagnosed.

The AIDS virus cannot be caught by touching someone who is infected, by being in the same room with an infected person, or by donating blood.

*Guidelines for effective school health education to prevent the spread of AIDS, MMWR Supplement, January 29, 1988, Centers for Disease Control, Atlanta.

ACCIDENT PREVENTION AND SAFETY

Many home accidents can be prevented if hazards are reduced and emergency plans have been made. Hazards exist in all rooms of the home. Typical hazards in the home include the following:

1. Improper storage of poisonous or flammable chemicals, knives, and medicine
2. Overloaded electrical outlets
3. Open cupborad doors and drawers
4. Improper storage of electrical appliances and tools
5. Loose throw rugs (without a rubberized backing)
6. Poor lighting
7. Clutter (particularly on steps)
8. Handles on pots and pans on the stove that protrude

Correcting such hazards can be a part of a home safety program. Being prepared for emergencies also can add to the safety of the home. This involves having appropriate emergency numbers posted near the telephone, including the telephone number of the police, fire department, poison control center, and ambulance. All members of the family should know where the numbers are located and how to call. Every home should have a basic first-aid kit, including small bandages, sterile pads (2 × 2 inches), antiseptic, tape, large bandages (roller gauze, 2 inches in width), tongue depressors, alcohol, and possibly a triangular bandage. Other items that are important to have available in case of an emergency include a flashlight with extra batteries, candles and matches, battery-operated radio, and bottled water. A fire escape plan should be developed. Every family member should know the best route out of the house in case of fire. It is a good idea to have smoke alarms. Reducing hazards and planning for possible emergencies make the home a safer place to live.

First-aid

Artificial respiration—The only way to save the life of someone who has stopped breathing is to get air into and out of her or his lungs. The best way to do this is by mouth-to-mouth breathing.

1. Clear the victim's mouth of any foreign matter.
2. Tilt the head back by lifting the lower jaw.
3. Look, listen, and feel for breathing.
4. Inflate the victim's lungs by sealing your mouth over her or his and breathing forcefully. Pinch her or his nostrils shut to prevent air leakage.
5. Remove your mouth to let the victim exhale passively.
6. Check for a pulse at the carotid artery.
7. Continue ventilations at the rate of about 12 breaths/minute.

Choking—When a foreign object lodges in the air passage, choking results. If the victim is unable to cough or speak, administer six to ten abdominal thrusts by placing the thumb side of your fist slightly above the victims navel. Stand behind the victim and cover your fist with your other hand (you will be encircling the victim with your arms). Pull sharply back and up to force the object out of the victim's air passage.

Severe bleeding—If someone is bleeding profusely from a wound:

1. Apply direct pressure with a sterile or clean cloth.
2. Elevate the wound.
3. Apply pressure on the pressure point (the brachial or femoral).
4. Use a tourniquet (only as a last resort).

Shock—Persons who have been injured or become ill must be treated for shock as a preventive measure. Treatment for shock includes:

1. Positioning the victim to improve circulation (usually with the legs and feet elevated).
2. Insuring an open airway.
3. Maintaining body heat (by lightly covering the victim).

Poisoning—In case of poisoning by mouth for a conscious victim:

1. Dilute the poison with water or milk.
2. Induce vomiting (unless the poison is a strong acid base, or petroleum product).
3. Get medical help.

Fainting—Fainting is the result of inadequate oxygen supply to the brain. If you feel faint, sit down with your head between your knees. This position increases blood flow to the brain. First-aid for someone who has fainted consists of keeping him or her in a flat position. Get medical help if the person does not regain consciousness almost immediately.

Seizure—Persons who are victims of seizures may harm themselves if they hit their head as they lose consciousness or bump into obstacles during the seizure. First-aid for a seizure includes:

1. Clear all obstacles away from the area.
2. Do NOT restrain the victim.
3. Do NOT put anything into the victim's mouth.
4. Stay with the victim after the seizure is over or until he or she regains composure.
5. Reassure the victim.
6. Get medical help if the seizure lasts longer than 10 minutes or is followed immediately by another.

Accident Prevention

One of the major reasons for accidents, particularly among young people, relates to risk-taking behaviors. Showing off for friends on bicycles, skateboards, roller skates, and even in cars can result in accidents. This type of behavior commonly is induced by peer pressure or the desire for attention. It is unlikely that adolescents will ever cease involvement in risk-taking behavior, but they can be made to understand the hazardous nature of certain actions.

CONSUMER HEALTH

Informed consumers know how to choose food, clothing, cosmetics, and other products that are marketed. Evaluating the quality of the products and evaluating advertisements allow the consumer to get the greatest value and satisfaction from the money spent.

Advertising

There are many methods used to promote the sale of products and services that affect health. Advertising on television, on radio, and in magazines often is directed at adolescents. Often attractive people are portrayed enjoying life with a specified product, the idea being that use of the product will somehow make life as wonderful as shown in the advertisement. Cigarette and smokeless tobacco advertisements often show young, active people having fun. Many times cigarettes or smokeless tobacco are not even in use by those portrayed. It is important for students to learn to look critically at advertisements, keeping in mind that the purpose is to sell a product or service. For obvious reasons the negative aspects of the product or service will not be advertised. However, laws require cautionary statements to accompany some advertisements. Usually advertising appeals are more emotional than rational. For example, statements such as, ''Nine out of ten doctors recommend...,'' should be examined to see if there is enough information given in the advertisement to indicate that an actual study was conducted, who conducted it, how many doctors were involved and whether they were physicians.

Fads

Fads are often the motivation for the use of products that are health-related, particularly for middle school students. If "everyone" else is using or doing something, adolescents tend to follow suit. This is true of their choice in clothes, activities, food, and acne remedies. Choosing acne remedies, other over-the-counter medications, soaps, and shampoos, based on scientific information is a much more reliable method.

Medical Fraud

When information about health is needed, it is important to be able to find an adviser who is capable of providing accurate information. The first source of help for the selection of health advisers is usually ones parents. Because of previous experience with health professionals, parents often can provide a referral to an appropriate adviser. School nurses also are qualified to provide certain health information and to refer students to appropriate health advisers when necessary. An appropriate health adviser is one who has the credentials for providing the health services needed. This usually means a degree from a college and a license to provide their services. The credentials of particular physicians, dentists or other health professionals usually can be verified by contacting the local medical society, dental society, or state licensing board. It is a good idea to locate a general practitioner or a family physician who can answer most health questions and treat most health problems. They also will refer patients with complicated health problems to a qualified specialist.

To avoid medical fraud, sometimes called *health quackery,* do not take advice from some-

one who (1) offers medical advice or treatment that is not available anywhere else, (2) discourages a second opinion from other medical personnel, (3) sells remedies door to door, through public lectures, or through advertisements in magazines, television, or newspapers, (4) uses testimonials, coupons, or guarantees, and (5) makes the service or product seem too good to be true. Common sense is often the best way to detect fraud. Ask yourself, "Is it really possible to lose 25 pounds in 2 weeks? Can creams and tonics really cause hair to grow on a bald head?"

Generally, select a health adviser who is trained to provide the information required and who is able and willing to refer you to another practitioner who may be more qualified to provide particular health services.

Government Agencies

Various governmental and volunteer agencies and organizations monitor laws that are designed to protect the consumer. Government enforcement agencies include the Food and Drug Administration (FDA), which requires that all medical drugs, food additives, cosmetics, and other devices pass tough tests to be certain they are safe and effective for public use and sale. The Federal Trade Commission (FTC) monitors advertising misrepresentation, price fixing, and other unfair business practices. The U.S. Postal Service is responsible for protecting the public from mail fraud, including the sale and transportation of worthless or dangerous health remedies through the mail. The U.S. Department of Agriculture (USDA) ensures that food is safely processed. The Consumer Product Safety Commission (CPSC) enforces uniform safety standards for products where injuries or illness could occur. An example of the importance of the CPSC is the enforcement of standards for children's sleepwear requiring products to be flame retardant before they can be sold in the United States.

DRUG USE AND ABUSE

Why people use and abuse drugs, the physiological effects of types of drugs, and local resources for drug abuse treatment are significant topics for middle school students. Many factors influence drug use or abuse, including family, culture, and religion. The beliefs and actions of friends and family have a profound effect on personal use or abuse of drugs. Peers are particularly influential in the lives of adolescents, and adolescents often abuse drugs to be accepted by peers.

Peer pressure is considered the single most important factor contributing to adolescent use and abuse of drugs. Adolescents are very concerned about being accepted by group members. It is normal for adolescents to form groups of friends who dress similarly, are involved in the same activities, and explore new activities together. If these groups are involved in using drugs, there usually is a great deal of peer pressure for everyone to participate. Often this pressure is so great that adolescents will participate despite the wishes and values of their parents or themselves. Additionally, knowing the health risks related to the abuse of drugs does not necessarily act as a deterrent when peer pressure is involved.

It is helpful for adolescents to know what peer pressure is and that it is a normal part of growing up. In fact peer pressure is a part of adult life as well, although it is not as significant in influencing important adult decisions as for adolescents. Adolescents need help in understanding that it is all right to be different and that, if they are not interested in certain activities in which their friends are involved, perhaps they should find new friends.

Teenage problem drinking and alcoholism are becoming more prevalent in the United States and therefore demand particular attention among adolescents. The concept of responsible drinking can be introduced in middle school. If the decision is made to use alcohol, it should be used in a responsible way. That includes avoiding driving or riding a bicycle while under the influence, avoiding riding with a driver who has been drinking, being aware of alcohol habits, and not overdoing it. Drinking can be paced to allow the body time to metabolize the alcohol. It is always a good idea to eat food when consuming alcohol. Some people choose not to drink alcohol at all; their choice should be respected and they should not be pushed into drinking.

Types of Psychoactive Drugs

Stimulants act on the central nervous system to increase pulse rate, blood pressure, strength of heart contractions, and muscle tension. Caffeine, amphetamines, cocaine, and nicotine are examples of stimulant drugs.

Depressants are drugs that slow down the central nervous system. Alcohol is the most commonly used depressant drug. Others are tranquilizers and barbiturates. Effects of these drugs include lowering of inhibitions, sedation, and sleep; in higher doses, effects include coma and death.

Psychedelics and hallucinogens change the perceptions in some way. Peyote, psilocybin, LSD, PCP, and mescaline are examples of drugs that are categorized in this group.

Narcotics provide pain-relief and induce sleep. Examples of narcotics include opium, morphine, codeine, heroin, meperidine, and methadone.

Cannabis is a plant that is processed and sold as marijuana and hashish. The active ingredient in all cannabis products is THC (tetrahydrocannabinol). At low dosage levels, THC produces effects similar to the depressant drugs. At higher levels, hallucinogenic effects are experienced including sensory distortion and vivid hallucinations.

Effects of Drug Use

Because they are usually in good health it is often difficult for young people to see the health hazards related to the use of tobacco, alcohol and other "social" drugs. Also they see peers using these drugs with no ill effects. Most of the physical diseases related to drugs take years to develop. In the case of tobacco and cardiovascular disease, the disease most often linked to cigarette smoking, it may take 20 to 30 years before any symptoms or problems appear. Cirrhosis of the liver, commonly linked to alcohol abuse, also takes years to develop. With chewing tobacco, more problems related to the gums (including cancer) are being found. It is helpful for young people to see some immediate effects. The effect of nicotine can be observed by testing pulse rate, blood pressure and fine motor skills. A tobacco user will find it difficult to hold the hand as steady after using tobacco as before. Individuals who use smokeless tobacco can see changes in the soft tissues of the mouth in the area where the tobacco is "held." Staining of the teeth, recession of the gum tissue, and sensitivity to hot and cold are also signs of tobacco's effects.

Drug Abuse

An important consideration in the use of any drug is the question of dependency. Some adolescents find themselves depending upon drugs to cope with feelings of fear, anxiety, and emotional pain. Since adolescence is a time of great emotional insecurity, dependency may develop for those persons who use drugs to escape pres-

sures and problems in life. When drugs are used as coping mechanisms, the adolescent does not develop the skills and emotional tools needed to become an emotionally stable adult.

Treating Drug Abuse

Treatment of drug abuse is difficult and requires that the drug user admit that he or she has a problem and needs help. It is important to realize that drug abuse affects not only the person who uses the drug(s) but also the family and friends of that person. The basic approaches to drug abuse treatment are:

1. Detoxification—The supervised withdrawal from drug dependence.
2. Therapeutic communities—Controlled environments where drug abusers live and participate in counseling as they learn to develop drug-free lifestyles.
3. Outpatient drug-free programs—Groups that emphasize various forms of counseling and support systems. Alcoholics Anonymous (AA) is an example of such an organization that is made up of alcoholics and recovered alcoholics. Other organizations have been formed to help persons with other drug-related problems (Narcotics Anonymous) and to help the families and friends of persons with drug dependencies (Alanon and Alateen). Other groups, like the American Cancer Society and the American Lung Association, offer programs for the cessation of tobacco use.

ENVIRONMENTAL HEALTH

The environment is a crucial factor in individual health. Everything in the environment, from the air we breathe to the number of persons inhabiting the earth, plays a role in our well-being. There are many community groups and agencies interested in the protection and preservation of the environment. Laws have been enacted and enforced that protect the environment and therefore the individual's health. However, communities and agencies cannot provide a clean and safe environment alone. The individual must do his or her part in working toward this objective. Middle school students can become active in groups that recycle trash or clean up litter along local highways. These activities can demonstrate to students the importance of community members working together for the betterment of all.

Government

Nationally, the Environmental Protection Agency (EPA) was formed by the federal government to set standards, monitor and enforce regulations regarding the protection of the environment. The EPA has been partially responsible for the improvements in the nation's air and water in recent years. Another group formed by the U.S. government is the Council on Environmental Quality. The council makes recommendations about ways in which environmental problems should be handled. States and local governments also take measures to protect the environment by enacting laws that limit the amount of pollution from different sources.

Industries

Industries can help to fight environmental problems by adhering to the laws seeking to regulate the amount of pollutants given off as industrial by-products. They can experiment with ways to burn cleaner fuels and can engage in and promote recycling of solid waste materials. Industries can also research methods to make wiser use of existing natural resources.

Other Groups

In addition to the government and industry, other groups are trying to fight problems that affect the quality of the environment. Such groups include national citizens' organizations that have provided education, lobbying, or actual clean-up work. The Sierra Club, National Wildlife Federation, Izaak Walton League, and the Audubon Society are examples of groups that have raised money for research and management of pollution problems.

Individuals

In reality, it is up to individuals to take steps to ensure the quality of the environment. Such practices include:

- Using soaps, paper products, and other materials that are biodegradable.
- Using water sparingly.
- Using electricity (lights and appliances) only when necessary.
- Cutting down on disposable items.
- Recycling materials (paper and aluminum cans).
- Walking or bicycling for short trips.
- Keeping cars, trucks, and motorcycles in good operating condition.
- Promoting and supporting legislation that protects the environment.

COMMUNITY HEALTH

Many health problems must be handled by the community as a whole. These include the environmental problems addressed previously and the prevention of the spread of communicable diseases. For any community health activity to be successful, the participation and cooperation of individuals within the community are essential. Communication among health professionals, school officials, and elected officials will hasten the identification of health problems and help in the determination of their solutions. However, not only professionals must become involved; citizens must also take responsibility for personal action and recognize that certain health problems cannot be solved without their assistance. This assistance can be in many forms, including volunteer work, financial donations, and the political support of candidates concerned about the health problems of the community.

Communicable Disease Control

In many states children must have certain vaccinations before entering school. Local communities often provide free or inexpensive clinics for the inoculation of children against communicable diseases common in the area. The national incidence of sexually transmitted diseases is considered epidemic. Local communities have a responsibility to provide health services for those with sexually transmitted diseases. This usually involves detection services, treatment, and an educational program. Health departments often work with schools to develop an educational program that is aimed at the prevention of communicable diseases. Certainly the best way to deal with any communicable disease is to prevent it, and education is often the key.

Career Opportunities

Careers in the health field are varied. One major group of health workers are caregivers who provide direct health services and products to those with health problems or emotional concerns. Some examples of direct-care health workers are dentists, physicians, nurses, dental hygienists, pharmacists, optometrists, physical therapists, and mental health counselors. Another category of health careers includes workers in the administration of health institutions or other facilities. These people administer the employees' services and policies of hospitals, voluntary health agencies, mental health facilities, nursing homes, and health departments.

Education is the primary function of health educators. Some work in the community and conduct educational programs through hospitals, health departments, clinics, voluntary health agencies, and even businesses and industries. School health educators are credentialed teachers of health in schools and universities.

Research in the health field is very important and is constantly being conducted in the areas of disease prevention and the discovery and testing of new drugs and medical devices. Individuals interested in laboratory sciences can find a career in the health field as well. Medical laboratory technicians and assistants perform tests to determine the absence, presence, or extent of a disease. There are general laboratory technicians and ones who specialize in fields such as chemistry, hematology, and microbiology.

Those interested in the science and preparation of food might be interested in becoming a dietician or nutritionist. Others interested in journalism or art can become medical writers or illustrators. Careers in sales also can be found in the health field, usually involving the sale or marketing of new products or drugs to medical practitioners so they in turn will recommend these products to patients. Since the careers available in the health field are so varied, it is likely that individuals can find one to suit their interest and ability.

Health Agencies and Organizations

Most communities have many organizations both public and private that are interested in the health of community members. The various types of organizations include voluntary health agencies (such as the American Cancer Society, American Lung Association, American Heart Association, and American Red Cross), official governmental organizations (such as the public health department and public hospitals), private industry (such as privately owned hospitals, local drug stores, private physicians, and other health professionals in private practice), professional organizations (such as local chapters of the American Medical Association [AMA], AMA Auxiliary, American Dental Association, and American Public Health Association), and service clubs (such as the Kiwanis, Rotary Club, and Lions Club). In most cases these organizations require individual voluntary participation to effectively carry out health activities in the community. Voluntary help and contributions are essential if these organizations are to accomplish their goals.

REFERENCES

American National Red Cross: Standard first aid and personal safety, Garden City, NY, 1979, Doubleday & Company, Inc.

Bailey C: Fit or fat? Boston, 1977, Houghton Mifflin.

Brody J: Jane Brody's the new york times guide to personal health, New York, 1982, New York Times Books.

Centers for Disease Control: Guidelines for effective school health education to prevent the spread of AIDS, Atlanta, 1988, US Dept of Health and Human Services.

Chiras D: Environmental science: a framework for decision-making, Menlo Park, Cal, 1985, Addison-Wesley.

Hales D and Williams B: An invitation to health, Menlo Park Cal, 1986, The Benjamin/Cummings Publishing Company, Inc.

Johnson P et al: Sport, exercise, and you, New York, 1975, Holt, Rinehart and Winston.

Julien R: A primer of drug action, San Francisco, 1981, WH Freeman and Company.

Mirkin G: Getting thin, Boston, 1983, Little, Brown.

Newman P and Halvorson P: Anorexia nervosa and bulimia, New York, 1983, Van Nostrand Reinhold.

Pregnancy basics, Bethesda, MD, National Institute of Child Health and Human Development.

Smith L: Diet plan for teenagers, New York, 1987, McGraw-Hill.

United States Department of Education: What works: schools without drugs, Washington DC, 1986

Waldinger R: Psychiatry for medical students, Washington, DC, 1984, American Psychiatric Press.

CHAPTER 15

Middle School Teaching Activity Ideas

When you finish this chapter, you should be able to:

- **Develop learning opportunities in health education for the middle school level which appropriately provide for practice with the behavior and content specified in an objective.**

Middle school students range from 11 to 14 years of age. Teaching students at this level can be particularly difficult, sometimes called "challenging," or particularly rewarding, but in most cases it is the latter. Students in middle school change rapidly both physically and socially. They seem to go through puberty practically before the teacher's eyes. It is this rapid physical change which makes this level "difficult."

Since students are so preoccupied with the changes in their body and in their social situation, health education is often a subject of high interest. They are eager to learn about ways that their actions will affect the development of their body and their health in later life. A good health education class can be an exciting and meaningful experience for these students. To be effective, the teacher must always keep in mind the physical and social influences that affect students. Peer pressure is probably the single most important factor in these young people's lives. Being accepted and not being different are crucial. A good teacher will not make a student look bad in front of friends. Discipline is most effective on a one-to-one basis away from peers. Being firm yet warm and understanding is effective. It is important for students to know that there are standards and rules but that the teacher is approachable. It is equally important for the teacher to remember that his or her role is that of teacher, not parent or best friend. Middle school students can be loyal, fun, and hardworking when there is a sincere and patient teacher.

Health education at this level is found in many different forms. It may be integrated into other subjects such as home economics, social studies, or science. It may be taught on rainy days in physical education class, or it may be a separate class. A separate class is the most desirable, but health can be effectively integrated into other subjects by a skilled teacher. However, it is doubtful that teaching health on a rainy day to large physical education classes in the gymnasium will be worthwhile. This situation is usually disliked by the students and teacher.

A principal who is personally interested in a good health program in the school is the key to success. He or she is ultimately responsible for what is taught in the classroom. It is important to keep the principal informed and involved, particularly since some topics in health can be sensitive and controversial. In addition, the principal should keep the teacher informed as to the district policy regarding these topics. It is essential that the teacher follow the guidelines outlined by the principal and the school district. The quickest way to lose favor with an administrator is to have a parent call about topics covered in a health class of which the principal has no knowledge. The teacher should always strive for an open honest relationship with the principal. The more trust and respect the principal has for the teacher, the greater the support for the health program.

This chapter has 10 different teaching plans for middle school students developed from objectives in the scope and sequence plan in Chapter 9. Students at this level are more sophisticated and can do more work on their own. They are involved in many research activities and cooperative learning activities designed to make them think at the higher levels of cognition described by Bloom, et al., 1956.* Analysis and evaluation are required, and stu-

---

*Bloom, B. S.: Taxonomy of objectives, Handbook I: Cognitive domain, New York, 1956, McKay Co. Inc.

dents must come to conclusions on their own. Often there will not be a ''right'' answer because students are dealing with content that is more abstract and subjective than in the lower levels.

The teaching plans include an objective, content generalization, initiation, several activities including a culmination, and evaluation activity. These activities are not the only way to accomplish the stated objective, but only an example of one way. The teacher will need several days to teach each set of activities, but the actual time will vary depending on the length of the classroom periods and the pace of the individual teacher and students. A good health education class can be exciting and interesting. These teaching plans serve as examples of ways to make health the class students can hardly wait to attend.

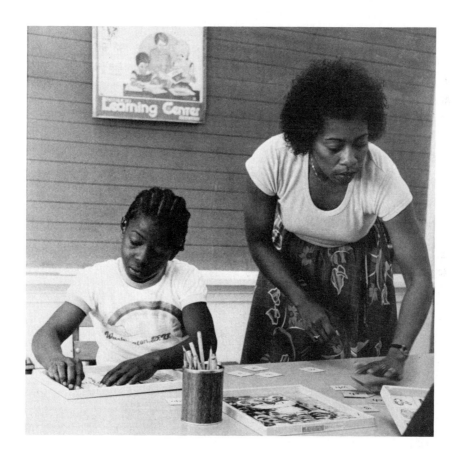

PERSONAL HEALTH AND FITNESS

Objective. The student proposes individual health care and
fitness programs to meet individual needs and interests.

Level. Grades 6 to 8

Content generalizations. Often people take better care of
their automobiles than they do of their body. Personal
health care habits contribute to social attractiveness, as
well as physical and mental health. Proper care of teeth,
eyes, ears, and skin will enhance attractiveness and contribute to physical and mental well-being. Adequate
amounts of sleep and exercise are needed as well for mental and physical fitness. An important aspect in the success of a program of personal health care and fitness is that
it must be valued by the individual. Exercises that the
individual enjoys and health practices that he or she views
as important are more likely to be incorporated into a life
style.

Vocabulary. Life style, fitness, aerobic

Initiation. My Ideal
  Ask the class to identify an adult who most students in the
  class consider "ideal." Ask, "Who in sports, on television,
  or in the movies is particularly attractive? Who is the 'picture of health?' " Write the names of persons who students
  identify on the board. Tell the students to look in magazines and cut out pictures of these people or of any person
  they think looks attractive and healthy.

Materials
Magazines (brought in by students)
Scissors

Activities
1. Picture of Health
   a. Tell the students to use the picture they recently cut
      out to observe healthy characteristics. Explain that
      people are attractive for many reasons, and different
      people think different traits make a person attractive.
      Most people think that being and looking healthy
      makes a person look attractive. Tell students to look at
      the pictures and try to determine why these particular
      people look attractive and healthy.
   b. Write the words *heredity* and *life style* on the board.
      Explain that certain factors influencing our health are
      inherited from our parents, and others are the result of
      the way we live.

c. Hand out the worksheet, *Picture of Health*. For each question on the worksheet, have students check the box that they think most contributed to the attractiveness and health of the person in their picture. Explain that they may not know exactly in each case, but they should guess. It is possible that both heredity and life style will apply to many questions.

d. After students have attempted to judge which characteristics were caused mostly by heredity or life style, review each question. Have students make corrections on their worksheets, as necessary. Emphasize that these worksheets are for awareness and reference; they were not expected to know the correct answers to all questions. The answers are as follows.

(1) Color of eyes is hereditary.

(2) Sheen of hair is both, but largely life style. Clean hair shines.

(3) Color of skin is largely hereditary, but tans are a factor of life style.

(4) Complexion is both. However, life style habits of cleanliness and proper nutrition usually can help even the most difficult complexion problems.

(5) Clean teeth are due to life style. Brushing and flossing teeth regularly not only help teeth look clean but also remove plaque that causes tooth decay.

(6) Build of body is both. You inherit a basic body type, but exercise and eating habits will determine the muscle development and shape of the body.

(7) Cavity-free teeth are both. You inherit a tendency toward cavities or not, but eating habits, brushing, flossing, and regular visits to the dentist also are important.

(8) Clean body is life style. Washing removes dirt, oil and germs that cause odor and disease. Being clean is both attractive and healthful.

Materials

Worksheets: *Picture of Health* (p. 435)

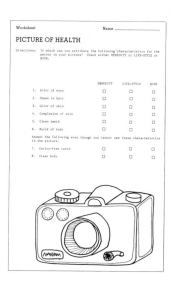

e. Have students look at all the items that have *life style* or *both* checked. Explain that all these characteristics are ones we *can* control in our lives. We can choose a life style that contributes to health and appearance. Ask if there is one important health habit that was not mentioned. (Sleep.) Ask them if they think getting enough sleep also can contribute to attractiveness and why or why not.

2. What A Workout!

Explain to students that a good exercise program is planned and tailor made for the individual. To achieve cardiorespiratory gains (increased heart and lung capacity), it is necessary for your heart to beat hard continuously for at least 20 minutes. Tell them they are going to check their pulse rate before, immediately after, and 3 minutes after exercise.

a. Tell students to put two fingers (not the thumb) on the side of their neck and feel for a pulse. When they have all found their pulse, check the pulse rates. Tell students to count the beats of their pulse to themselves while the teacher times exactly 30 seconds on a stopwatch or watch with a second hand. Say "stop" when the 30 seconds have passed. Ask the students to multiply the number of beats counted by 2 to determine their resting pulse rate.

Materials
Stopwatch or watch with a second hand

b. Pass out the worksheet, *What a Workout!* Have students record their resting pulse rate on the worksheet. Then ask them to run in place for 1 minute. Have them check their pulse rate the same way by counting the beats for 30 seconds and multiplying by 2. Have them record that number on the worksheet as well. Then have them rest for 3 minutes and take the pulse rate again. Tell the students that the faster your pulse rate returns to normal after exercising, the better. The heart should work hard during exercise but should return to normal quickly. Pass out the worksheet, *Step Test,* and suggest they try it with their parents at home. This test is an adaptation of the Harvard step test.

c. Find out from students what the highest and lowest pulse rates were for the three measurements. Record the highest and lowest rates on the board. Point out that this range shows the individual differences that exist in one class. It reinforces the point that all programs should be tailored to individual needs.

Materials

Worksheets: *What a Workout!* (p. 436);
Step Test (p. 437)

Worksheet   Name _____

WHAT A WORKOUT!

PULSE RATE: Resting _____ After exercise _____

3 Minutes after exercise _____

PULSE RATE

1. My resting pulse rate was _____ beats per minute.

2. My pulse rate immediately after exercise was _____ beats per minute.

3. My pulse rate 3 minutes after exercise was _____ beats per minute.

4. Did your pulse rate drop 10 to 15 beats per minute after 3 minutes? _____

THE PARTS OF A WORKOUT

1. _____ exercises such as _____

for _____ minutes

2. _____ exercises such as _____

for _____ minutes

3. _____ exercises such as _____

for _____ minutes

4. _____ exercises such as _____

for _____ minutes

WORKING OUT FOR 2 WEEKS

On the back of this worksheet draw a calendar for 2 weeks, and fill in your progress as in the example below. (Record the aerobic exercise only, but do warm up and cool down.)

Monday	Tuesday	Wednesday	Thursday	Friday	Saturday	Sunday
After-school jog, 20 minutes						

STEP TEST   Modified from the Harvard step test.

Test your heart's capacity to adapt to and recover from strenuous exercise.

1. Use a platform 14 to 17 inches high. Step up and down 30 times per minute for 4 minutes.

2. Start by placing the left foot on the platform at the command up. Then step up with the other foot, so both feet are on the platform. Then step down, using the same rhythm. Use a marching count: up, 2, 3, 4. The signal up comes every 2 seconds.

3. Exercise for 4 minutes. Then sit down and remain quiet.

4. One minute later the pulse rate is taken for 30 seconds.

5. Two minutes after exercising the pulse rate is taken for 30 seconds.

6. Three minutes after exercising the pulse rate is taken for 30 seconds.

7. Add the total of all three 30-second counts.

RECOVERY INDEX

Total count	Index	Your response
199 or more	60 or less	Poor
171 to 198	61 to 70	Fair
150 to 170	71 to 80	Good
133 to 149	81 to 90	Very good
132 or less	91 or more	Excellent

This test taxes the cardiorespiratory resources of the individual and is approved by the American Medical Association.

d. Review the kinds of exercises that students indicated they enjoy. Record them on the board. Ask if there are any on the board that get the heart working hard. (Jogging, dancing, basketball, swimming, skating, bicycle riding, jumping rope.) Explain that these are called *aerobic* exercises and should be done at least three times a week. Have the students fill in the worksheet *What a Workout!*, as you explain that during a workout one should do the following.

  (1) Warm-up exercises (stretching) such as touching toes and stretching arms to the sky for 5 to 10 minutes

  (2) Some endurance and strength exercises such as pushups, sit-ups, and possibly weight lifting for 5 to 10 minutes

  (3) Some aerobic exercises such as swimming, running, dancing, jumping rope, bicycle riding, and quick walking for 15 to 20 minutes

  (4) Some cool-down exercises like the warm-up exercises for 5 to 10 minutes

Materials

Worksheet: *What a Workout!* (p. 436)

Evaluation. Checking Myself

Hand out the worksheet, *Checking Myself.* Explain that this is very personal. They have learned a great deal on health care habits and exercise. This worksheet is a way to see how well they personally do with various health habits. These papers should be checked only to see if the assignment was completed, not for correct responses. Encourage students to be honest in this activity. Tell them that this is a 2-week project. Give them about 2 minutes each day in class to work on these worksheets. Allow students to choose one person in the class as a partner. It should be someone with whom they feel comfortable. Allow the pairs to talk to each other about their findings. Tell the students that they only need to share information they feel comfortable sharing. Have the students talk with their partner regarding health care habits that may need improving and develop a written plan about how to do so. Students should review their success in the exercise program with their partners.

Materials

Worksheet: *Checking Myself* (p. 438)

CHECKING MYSELF

Directions: This worksheet is a personal record to help you see how well you do with various health care habits. Simply put a check mark in the box for the days that you did those activities. It is not necessary to do all activities every day to have good personal health habits. Some are daily habits; others are not. This will help you see how often you perform each habit. Then you can determine whether it is often enough.

	Date									
1. Brushed teeth										
2. Flossed teeth										
3. Slept 8 to 9 hours										
4. Washed hair										
5. Washed clothes										
6. Changed sheets										
7. Changed towels										
8. Scrubbed fingernails										
9. Clipped toenails										
10. Washed face										
11. Showered or bathed										

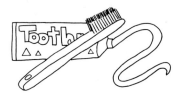

Worksheet   Name _____

PICTURE OF HEALTH

Directions: To which can you attribute the following characteristics for the
person in your picture? Check either HEREDITY or LIFE-STYLE or
BOTH.

		HEREDITY	LIFE-STYLE	BOTH
1.	Color of eyes	☐	☐	☐
2.	Sheen in hair	☐	☐	☐
3.	Color of skin	☐	☐	☐
4.	Complexion of skin	☐	☐	☐
5.	Clean teeth	☐	☐	☐
6.	Build of body	☐	☐	☐

Answer the following even though you cannot see these characteristics
in the picture.

7.	Cavity-free teeth	☐	☐	☐
8.	Clean body	☐	☐	☐

Worksheet   Name _____

WHAT A WORKOUT!

PULSE RATE: Resting _____ After exercise _____

3 Minutes after exercise _____

PULSE RATE

1. My resting pulse rate was _____ beats per minute.

2. My pulse rate immediately after exercise was _____ beats per minute.

3. My pulse rate 3 minutes after exercise was _____ beats per minute.

4. Did your pulse rate drop 10 to 15 beats per minute after 3 minutes? _____

THE PARTS OF A WORKOUT

1. _____ exercises such as _____ _ _ _____

   _____

   for _____ minutes

2. _____ exercises such as _____

   _____

   for _____ minutes

3. _____ exercises such as _____

   _____

   for _____ minutes

4. _____ exercises such as _____

   _____

   for _____ minutes

WORKING OUT FOR 2 WEEKS

On the back of this worksheet draw a calendar for 2 weeks, and fill in your progress as in the example below. (Record the aerobic exercise only, but do warm up and cool down.)

Monday	Tuesday	Wednesday	Thursday	Friday	Saturday	Sunday
After-school jog, 20 minutes						

Worksheet   Name _____

STEP TEST   Modified from the Harvard step test.

Test your heart's capacity to adapt to and recover from strenuous exercise.

1. Use a platform 14 to 17 inches high. Step up and down 30 times per minute for 4 minutes.

2. Start by placing the left foot on the platform at the command up. Then step up with the other foot, so both feet are on the platform. Then step down, using the same rhythm. Use a marching count: up, 2, 3, 4. The signal up comes every 2 seconds.

3. Exercise for 4 minutes. Then sit down and remain quiet.

4. One minute later the pulse rate is taken for 30 seconds.

5. Two minutes after exercising the pulse rate is taken for 30 seconds.

6. Three minutes after exercising the pulse rate is taken for 30 seconds.

7. Add the total of all three 30-second counts.

RECOVERY INDEX

Total count	Index	Your response
199 or more	60 or less	Poor
171 to 198	61 to 70	Fair
150 to 170	71 to 80	Good
133 to 149	81 to 90	Very good
132 or less	91 or more	Excellent

This test taxes the cardiorespiratory resources of the individual and is approved by the American Medical Association.

Worksheet   Name _____

CHECKING MYSELF

Directions: This worksheet is a personal record to help you see how well you do
             with various health care habits. Simply put a check mark in the box
             for the days that you did those activities. It is not necessary to
             do all activities every day to have good personal health habits.
             Some are daily habits; others are not. This will help you see how
             often you perform each habit. Then you can determine whether it is
             often enough.

Date										
1. Brushed teeth										
2. Flossed teeth										
3. Slept 8 to 9 hours										
4. Washed hair										
5. Washed clothes										
6. Changed sheets										
7. Changed towels										
8. Scrubbed fingernails										
9. Clipped toenails										
10. Washed face										
11. Showered or bathed										

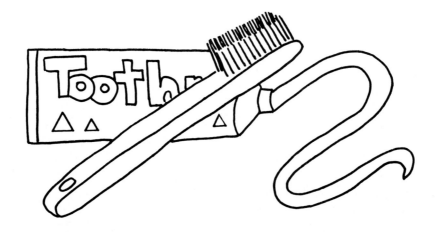

MENTAL AND EMOTIONAL HEALTH

Objective. The student identifies constructive ways to manage stress.

Level. Grades 6 to 8

Mental and
emotional health

Content generalizations. Stress is a normal part of life. It is an outcome of both physical and mental tension. Stress occurs during the more serious parts of life such as death of a loved one or the divorce of parents, but it is not necessarily all bad. Sometimes stress can help us perform better in the face of a challenge. It is important that we learn what situations in our own lives produce stress and how we react in those situations. Successfully coping with stressful situations contributes to both mental and physical health.

Vocabulary. Stress, coping, adrenaline, conflict

Initiation. Stress—What Does It Feel Like?

Write the word *stress* on the board. Tell the students that we will be spending some time talking about stress. Ask them to look up the word in a dictionary and write a definition of it in their own words. Inform them that this is to be a quiet activity.

Materials
Dictionaries

While the students are concentrating on their work, set up one of the following situations to produce "stress" in their lives at that moment. Two options are suggested:

1. Walk to the back of the classroom. Make certain that no one is looking, then make a sudden loud noise by slamming a door or dropping tin cans or books on the floor. Practice ahead of time with several items to see what makes a good loud noise.

2. Announce to the class that a very important test will be given the next day. It will be several pages long and involve at least two essay questions that will have to be a full written page in length.

   Tell the students of your hoax. Then ask what physical feelings they experienced. Write them on the board. Such reactions will include fear, pumping heart, butterflies in stomach, and anger at teacher. Tell the students that they have just experienced a stressful situation and that the reactions they are describing are normal responses to stress.

Activities

1. Cope With Stress

   Using a transparency and worksheet, explain various ways to deal with stress. Hand out the worksheet, *Stress—Don't Let It Get You Down*. Tell the students to write the various ways to deal with stress on their worksheets as they are explained in class. Use the transparency, *Cope With Stress*, as an aid in the brief lecture.

   • *Physical activity*
   • *Talk things out*
   • *Take things one at a time*
   • *Do not try to win every time*
   • *Balance play with work*
   • *Take a break for yourself*

   After explaining each of these coping strategies, ask students if they can think of any others. Tell them to go home and ask parents and other adults how they cope with stressful situations. They should record ideas on their worksheets as they are discovered.

Materials

Worksheet: *Stress—Don't Let It Get You Down* (p. 443)
Transparency: *Cope with Stress* (p. 444)

COPE WITH STRESS

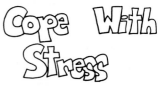

1. Get some physical activity.

2. Talk things out.

3. Take things one at a time.

4. Don't try to win every time.

5. Balance play with work.

6. Take a break for yourself.

2. Stress—Don't Let It Get You Down

Allow students to work in pairs to complete this activity. Explain that you will be telling them about two stressful situations. Each pair of students should discuss ways to deal with stress in that particular situation and either draw or write a suggested course of action. It may be helpful to the students to write the situations on a transparency and project them on the screen while they are working.

SITUATION A

Andrea had a large report due in her social studies class. She was so nervous about the report that she did not play after school or watch television. She forced herself to work instead, but she just sat in her room staring at her books. She had butterflies in her stomach and was having a hard time sleeping. What could she do?

SITUATION B

Stevie's friend Dave was having a party. Everyone important would be there, but Stevie did not get an invitation. When he thought about it, his heart started pounding. He knew that he should never have loaned his favorite record to Dave. What can he do?

When the students are finished, ask each pair what suggestions they have for Andrea and Stevie.

Materials

Worksheet: *Stress—Don't Let It Get You Down* (partially completed by students) (p. 443)
Blank transparency
Transparency pen
Overhead projector

Mental and emotional health

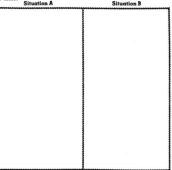

Worksheet   Name _____

**STRESS—DON'T LET IT
GET YOU DOWN**

Part I

Fill in ways to deal with stress below as they are discussed in class:

1. _____   6. _____
2. _____   7. _____
3. _____   8. _____
4. _____   9. _____
5. _____   10. _____

Part II

Draw or write a way to deal with the stressful situations explained in class.

Situation A	Situation B

3. Stress Test

Hand out the worksheet, *Stress Test,* and allow the students to chart their personal reaction to various potentially stressful situations. Emphasize that stress is a normal part of life. (There is no correct answer for this test. It is designed to help them see how stressful their life is and to see what situations cause the most stress.) Then ask the students to brainstorm other potentially stressful situations. Choose a few to discuss in class.

Materials

Worksheet: *Stress Test* (p. 445)

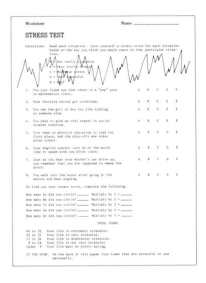

Evaluation. Dealing With Stress

Hand out plain paper to the students. Have them divide the paper into four equal sections. Use the eight situations in the *Stress Test,* or make up eight new ones for this evaluation. Ask students to identify a way to deal with each stressful situation. They can either draw or write about a coping strategy for each situation. Tell them that they may choose to use a strategy more than once. It is important, however, that they identify a coping strategy they would personally use.

An option is to have the students use two pieces of paper, putting four drawings on each piece. Then they can cut out the drawings and staple them together in a booklet. They should put a title page on the booklet, such as ''Dealing With Stress,'' and take it home to their parents.

Materials

Plain paper

Felt pens, crayons or colored pencils

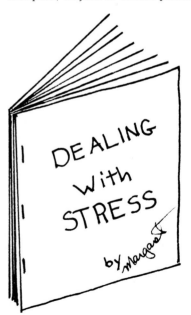

Worksheet   Name _____

STRESS—DON'T LET IT
GET YOU DOWN

Part I

Fill in ways to deal with stress below as they are discussed in class:

1. _____   6. _____

2. _____   7. _____

3. _____   8. _____

4. _____   9. _____

5. _____   10. _____

Part II

Draw or write a way to deal with the stressful situations explained
in class.

Situation A	**Situation B**

Transparency master

COPE WITH STRESS

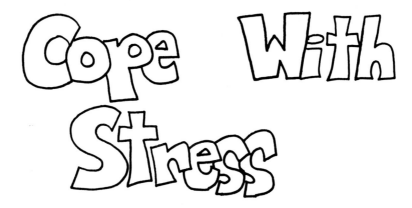

1. Get some physical activity.

2. Talk things out.

3. Take things one at a time.

4. Don't try to win every time.

5. Balance play with work.

6. Take a break for yourself.

Worksheet   Name _____

STRESS TEST

Directions: Read each situation. Give yourself a stress score for each situation
              based on the way you think you would react to that particular situa-
              tion.

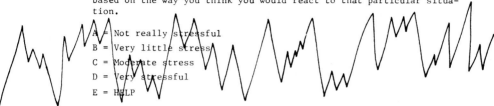

              A = Not really stressful
              B = Very little stress
              C = Moderate stress
              D = Very stressful
              E = HELP

1. You just found out that there is a "pop" quiz   A   B   C   D   E
    in mathematics class.

2. Your favorite record got scratched.   A   B   C   D   E

3. You see the girl or boy you like talking   A   B   C   D   E
    to someone else.

4. You have to give an oral report in social   A   B   C   D   E
    studies tomorrow.

5. Your team in physical education is tied for   A   B   C   D   E
    first place, and the play-offs are today
    after school.

6. Your English teacher says he or she would   A   B   C   D   E
    like to speak with you after class.

7. Just as you hear your mother's car drive up,   A   B   C   D   E
    you remember that you are supposed to sweep the
    porch.

8. You walk into the house after going to the   A   B   C   D   E
    movies and hear arguing.

To find out your stress score, complete the following:

How many As did you circle?_____ Multiply by 1 = _____
How many Bs did you circle?_____ Multiply by 2 = _____
How many Cs did you circle?_____ Multiply by 3 = _____
How many Ds did you circle?_____ Multiply by 4 = _____
How many Es did you circle?_____ Multiply by 5 = _____

                          TOTAL SCORE

40 to 33   Your life is extremely stressful.
25 to 32   Your life is very stressful.
17 to 24   Your life is moderately stressful.
 9 to 16   Your life is not very stressful.
Under 9   Your life must be pretty boring.

IF YOU WISH: On the back of this paper list items that are stressful to you
              personally.

FAMILY LIFE

Objective. The student describes the reproductive processes.

Level. Grades 6 to 8

Content generalizations. Reproduction is a complicated process involving the production of egg cells in women and sperm cells in men. The fertilization of the ovum by a sperm cell is called "conception." The fertilized egg implants in the uterus and grows as a fetus in the body of a pregnant woman. In approximately nine months childbirth occurs, and a baby is born.

NOTE: When teaching about reproduction, it is important to be fully aware of the recommendations and guidelines for your school or district. The activities presented here are conservative and simply designed. Traditional teaching methods involving lectures, discussions, books, and audiovisual materials are the most effective and appropriate approach. However, it cannot be emphasized enough that any books, films, filmstrips, charts, or transparencies used in teaching about reproduction should be submitted to review by parents.

Vocabulary. Reproduction, ovum (ova), sperm, fertilization, conception, embryo, fetus

Initiation. Parent letter

Explain to the students that the class will be studying about human reproduction and birth. Tell them that you would like them to invite their parents to a meeting where they can meet the teacher and talk about the program. Explain that it is often hard for parents and children to talk about this subject. Possibly, if reproduction is discussed with the parents at school, it will be easier for parents and children to talk about it at home.

Materials

Teacher resource: *Sample Parent Letter* (p. 451)

SAMPLE PARENT LETTER

Dear Parent:

In a few weeks we will begin our family life unit in health class. This unit was carefully designed to fit the needs of the students in our school district. A curriculum committee consisting of teachers, parents, administrators, and community members was involved in the development of the program.

We would like to invite you to a meeting at the school on the evening of _____ at _____ P.M. At this time you will have the opportunity to view the films and filmstrips used in the program and review all other materials. It will also give you a chance to meet and talk with your child's teacher.

We encourage every student to participate in the family life program. Nevertheless, it is voluntary. If you do not wish your child to be involved in the classroom activities, complete the bottom portion of this letter, and send it back to school. We will remove your son or daughter from health class during the unit and involve him or her in an independent study activity dealing with some other aspect of health.

Sincerely,

_____
(Principal)

_____
(Teacher)

To the Principal of _____ School:

I do not wish my son or daughter _____ to
                                    (Name)
participate in the family life unit in health class. Please remove him or her from class during those activities and assign an independent study assignment on some other aspect of health. Thank you.

Signed _____
        (Parent)

Date _____

Hand out a letter from the teacher for students to take home to their parents. Use the *Sample Parent Letter* for a reference. It is suggested that parents be asked to respond to the letter in one of two ways. (The way that parents should respond already may be a specified guideline for your state or district.)

1. Ask the parents to sign and return the letter if they *do* give their permission for their child to be in class during the discussions on reproduction. In other words, only allow a student to stay in the class if you have written permission from the parents.

2. Ask the parents to sign and return the letter if they *do not* give their permission for their child to be in class during discussions of reproduction.

Suggest to the students that they ask their parents a few questions about their own birth, such as the following:

• Was my birth normal, breech, or caesarean?
• Was my father present at the birth?
• How long was mother in labor?

NOTE: Teachers should be sensitive to the differences in families and the presence of adopted children in class. Therefore the questions to ask parents should be voluntary.

Activities

1. The question box

   Explain that a *question box* will be a part of the activities for the next several days. Display a question box you have prepared. (A decorated shoe box with a slot at the top or any other decorated box of similar size will work well.) Explain that the box will be used every day to collect questions they may have. These questions will be answered the following day in class. All students will get an index card (or a slip of paper) each day. If the students have a question, they are to write it on the card and put it in the box. If they do not have a question, they are to put a blank card into the box. This method ensures that the questions are anonymous.

Materials

Question box (decorated shoe box, teacher-made)
Index cards or slips of paper

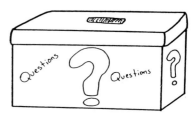

Family life

Each day read the questions and prepare answers for the next day in class. Some questions may not be suitable for answering in a full group situation. In those cases tell the class, ''There were a few questions that we did not have time to address in class. If you are concerned that your question was not answered, please see me after class or after school, and I will attempt to provide an answer.'' This process helps the teacher sort out the questions that are ''planted'' to embarrass him or her (which does happen). Also, you may get questions like, ''Hi!'' ''How are you?'' and ''This class is boring!'' Deal with these in a light and friendly manner.

After a few days of using the question box students may become comfortable asking questions aloud in class. You need to decide then whether to field these questions openly in class or ask students to continue to put their questions in the question box. This will depend entirely on the skill, experience, and confidence of the teacher.

2. Film or Filmstrip or Video

Show a film or filmstrip on reproduction. The school or district may have titles that are recommended. Tell students to note questions after the film for the question box.

If the students have not yet been exposed to activities regarding growth and puberty, it may be wise to address these topics now.

Materials

Film/filmstrip/video: district approved titles

Film/filmstrip projector or video monitor

3. Male and Female Reproductive Systems

   Review the anatomy of the male and female reproductive systems, using the transparencies indicated in the margin. Hand out worksheets, and have the students record the anatomical locations on their worksheets as each system is reviewed.

Materials

Worksheets and transparencies: *The Female Reproductive System* (p. 452); *The Male Reproductive System* (p. 453)

Overhead projector

Transparency pen

Family life

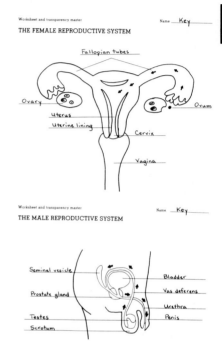

Worksheet and transparency master   Name Key

THE FEMALE REPRODUCTIVE SYSTEM

Fallopian tubes, Ovary, Ovum, Uterus, Uterine lining, Cervix, Vagina

Worksheet and transparency master   Name Key

THE MALE REPRODUCTIVE SYSTEM

Seminal vesicle, Prostate gland, Testes, Scrotum, Bladder, Vas deferens, Urethra, Penis

4. Mini-lecture on Pregnancy and Birth

   Address the following points in a lecture on pregnancy and birth. Use whatever visual aids possible to dramatize these points.

   NOTE: Students are often interested in the topics of pregnancy and birth. They certainly will ask questions about abnormal births. Try to avoid long discussions on abnormalities, and emphasize that most births are normal.

   • *Fertilization,* or conception, occurs when a male sperm cell enters a female ovum. This happens after a man and woman have had *sexual intercourse:* an erect male penis is placed into the woman's vagina. Sperm is ejaculated out of the man's body into the woman's body.

   One of the first signs that a woman may be pregnant is the skipping of a menstrual period.

- The fertilized egg is first called a *zygote,* then, as it multiplies, a *blastocyst,* and then an *embryo.* It grows very rapidly. The embryo implants onto the wall of the uterus and continues to grow. The growing organism is called an embryo for the first 3 months of pregnancy.
- The life-support system that connects the baby and mother is called the *placenta.* It is a large organ housing many blood vessels that is attached to the wall of the uterus. Through the placenta, nutrients and oxygen are provided to the embryo, and waste products are taken away. Drugs, including nicotine, alcohol, and caffeine, also can pass through the placenta to the developing embryo.
- About the fourth month the developing baby is approximately 3 inches long. It now is called a *fetus.*
- Movement of the fetus can be felt around the fifth month. The heartbeat usually can be heard by a physician earlier than the fifth month. By the end of the sixth month the fetus is about 12 to 14 inches long.
- During the last 3 months of pregnancy the fetus grows rapidly. A *premature* baby (one born too soon, whose weight is less than normal) may survive if born during the last 3 months of pregnancy.
- *Birth* is the process when the baby moves out of the mother's uterus through the birth canal (vagina) into the world.
- There are three basic stages of birth. In the first stage contractions begin, and the cervix opens wide enough to allow the baby's head to pass. In the second stage the baby is pushed completely out of the uterus, and in the third stage the placenta is expelled from the uterus. This is called the *afterbirth.*
- There can be complications during birth. Sometimes caesarean births are necessary, where surgery is used to remove the baby from the uterus. There also are breech births, which means the baby is not born head first.

Evaluation. "Where Did I Come From?"
Ask the students to write a report answering the question, "Where did I come from?" Tell students to pretend they have to explain reproduction to a young child. It must be done simply but factually. Suggest that they visit their local library and read a few books about this subject written for young children. In evaluating the reports, look for descriptions of fertilization of an egg cell, implantation in the wall of the uterus, growth of an embryo and fetus, and birth.

Teacher resource

SAMPLE PARENT LETTER

Dear Parent:

In a few weeks we will begin our family life unit in health class. This unit was carefully designed to fit the needs of the students in our school district. A curriculum committee consisting of teachers, parents, administrators, and community members was involved in the development of the program.

We would like to invite you to a meeting at the school on the evening of _____ at _____ P.M. At this time you will have the opportunity to view the films and filmstrips used in the program and review all other materials. It will also give you a chance to meet and talk with your child's teacher.

We encourage every student to participate in the family life program. Nevertheless, it is voluntary. If you do not wish your child to be involved in the classroom activities, complete the bottom portion of this letter, and send it back to school. We will remove your son or daughter from health class during the unit and involve him or her in an independent study activity dealing with some other aspect of health.

Sincerely,

_____

(Principal)

_____

(Teacher)

To the Principal of _____ School:

I do not wish my son or daughter _____ to
(Name)
participate in the family life unit in health class. Please remove him or her from class during those activities and assign an independent study assignment on some other aspect of health. Thank you.

Signed _____
(Parent)

Date _____

Name_____

THE FEMALE REPRODUCTIVE SYSTEM

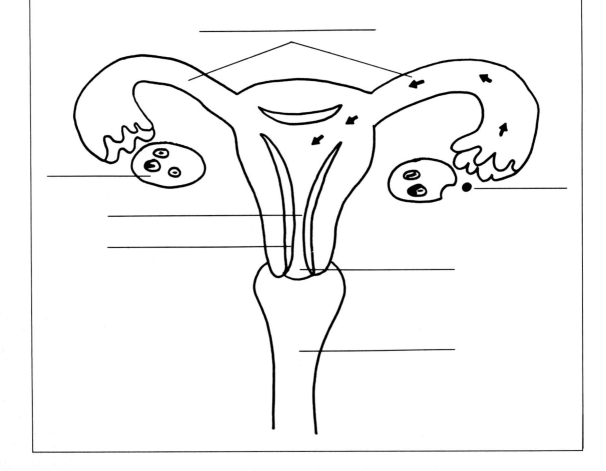

Worksheet and transparency master

Name _____

THE MALE REPRODUCTIVE SYSTEM

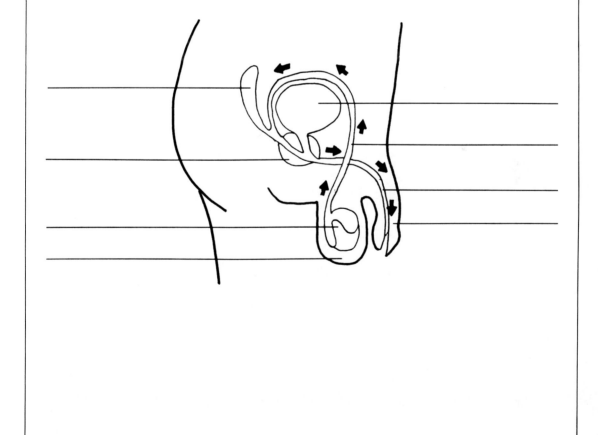

NUTRITION

Objective. The student explains the relationship between calorie intake and level of activity to body weight.

Level. Grades 7 and 8

Content generalizations. The amount of energy that foods provide is measured in terms of calories. Different foods have different caloric values, depending on the energy potential of that food. All foods have calories. The body needs a certain amount of calories a day to function. Every activity of life from jogging to breathing requires energy. This energy is measured in calories. *Basal metabolism* refers to the minimum amount of energy required to maintain vital body functions and muscle tone at rest. If an individual is balancing the calories eaten daily with the calories used daily, body weight will stay the same. If more calories are eaten than are used daily, weight will increase.

Vocabulary. Calorie, balance, basal metabolism

Initiation. What is a calorie?

Hold up a large fresh carrot for the class to view. Ask, "What are some ways to measure this carrot?" Students should be able to come up with various ways to measure the carrot, including weighing it and measuring its length, circumference, and diameter.

As each way to measure the carrot is suggested, ask a volunteer to actually measure the carrot and record the measurement on the board.

Suggest that there is one more measurement we have not yet done. We have not measured the food energy potential of the carrot. In other words, we have not determined the number of calories in the carrot.

Using the transparency, *What Is a Calorie?* explain that calories are a measure of energy. All foods have calories. The number of calories depends on how much energy it takes the body to burn up the food.

Tell the student that the average carrot has 35 calories and have a student record the calorie measurement for the carrot on the board.

Materials

Carrot (1 large, fresh)
Transparency: *What Is a Calorie?* (p. 457)
Measuring tape
Food scale (optional)

WHAT IS A CALORIE?

Calories are units of measure

8 inches: Measures the length of this carrot

35 calories: Measures the amount of heat energy this food can provide

Activities

1. The Calories Are Right—A Game

   To help students become more familiar with calories in foods, have them work in small groups to make various flash cards. On the front of the card they should place a picture of a food. (Pictures can be cut from magazines or drawn.) On the back of the card they should write the number of calories provided by that food. Students must look up the calories in a book. It is optimum to have one calorie equivalent book per group, but one book can be shared by all the groups. Using the flash cards, play "The Calories Are Right" game. This game is similar to the television game, *The Price is Right;* however, instead of guessing the correct price of items, students "bid" on the correct calories of different foods. Ask for four or five volunteers to be contestants. Show a picture of a food to the class and the contestants. Ask for bids on the number of calories from the contestants only. Contestants should write their bids on the board. Then the teacher can ask the rest of the class which bid they think is the closest answer without going over the correct calorie amount. Reveal the correct answer, and declare a winner for that round. The winner of the round stays for the next round, and new contestants are chosen. Continue playing the game until everyone has had an opportunity to be a contestant. The contestant who has won the most rounds is the class winner.

2. A Balancing Act

   Write the word *balance* on the board, and explain that the next activity is based on the concept of balance in calorie intake and expenditure. Tell the students, "Each person has individual calorie requirements, depending on his or her energy demands. During periods of growth, more calories usually are needed. Students your age often are active and require more calories. Your estimated calorie requirements are between 2400 and 2800 calories per day. These numbers can be higher or lower depending on the individual and how active he or she is."

   Hand out the worksheet, *A Balancing Act.* Use a transparency made from the worksheet. Read number 1 on the worksheet, and tell the students to complete the answer to item a. Ask for a volunteer to share his or her answer. Explain that our calorie needs are related directly to the amount of energy we use. When we eat more calories than we use, the body stores the excess as fat. When we eat fewer calories than we use, the body uses the stored

Materials

Magazines

Scissors

Glue

Index cards (several per student)

Books: Several calorie equivalent books (purchased in drug stores or super-markets)

Materials

Worksheet and transparency: *A Balancing Act* (p. 458)

Transparency pen

A BALANCING ACT

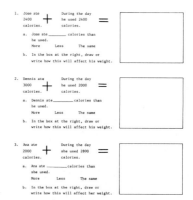

fat for energy. Ask the students to answer item 1.b. on their worksheet, and then discuss it. Ask, ''What will happen to Jose's weight?'' (It will stay the same.) Have the students finish the worksheet individually, then discuss numbers 2 and 3. Ask, ''What will happen to Dennis' weight?'' (It will increase.) ''What about Sara's weight?'' (It will decrease.)

Explain to the students that this is a gradual process, that over time a person who eats more calories than he or she uses will gain weight, and a person who eats less calories than those used will lose weight.

3. Burn Up Those Calories

Have the students consult the library or health texts to find out which activities burn more or less calories. They should list the activities they like, then find out the number of calories burned per hour for each activity. Tell them to include watching television as an activity if it is something they do often in their leisure time.

Then have students complete the worksheet, *Burn Up Those Calories*. Students are to find or draw a picture of their favorite snack, then find out the calorie equivalent for that snack and record it. They should figure out how long it will take to burn off that snack by participating in one of the activities they listed previously.

Materials

Library resource books
Worksheet: *Burn Up Those Calories* (p. 459)

BURN UP THOSE CALORIES

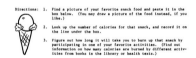

Directions:　1.　Find a picture of your favorite snack food and paste it in the box below. (You may draw a picture of the food instead, if you like.)
　　　　　　　2.　Look up the number of calories for that snack, and record it on the line under the box.
　　　　　　　3.　Figure out how long it will take you to burn up that snack by participating in one of your favorite activities. (Find out information on how many calories are burned by different activities from books in the library or health texts.)

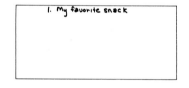

1. My favorite snack

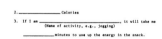

2. _____ Calories

3. If I am _____, it will take me
　　　　　　(Name of activity, e.g., jogging)

_____ minutes to use up the energy in the snack.

Evaluation. Dear Barry . . .

Read the following story to the students, and have them respond in writing.

Barry is a good student. He spends most of his time after school doing homework. When he is done with his homework, he likes to watch television. He has noticed lately that he has gained some weight. It is not very much, but he is a little worried. He wonders why this is happening. Explain to Barry why this is happening, and offer a suggestion as to how he can avoid a further weight gain.

In the responses to the story, students should explain to Barry that he is probably eating more calories than he is using. They could suggest that Barry get involved in something more active than watching television after school.

Transparency master

WHAT IS A CALORIE?

Calories
are units of
measure

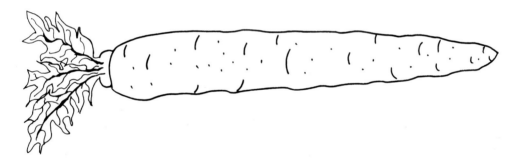

8 inches: Measures the length
                   of this carrot

35 calories: Measures the amount
                of heat energy this
                food can provide

Worksheet   Name _____

A BALANCING ACT

1. Jose ate   ✚   During the day   ═   [ ]
    2400   he used 2400
    calories.   calories.

    a. Jose ate _____ calories than
        he used.
        More   Less   The same

    b. In the box at the right, draw or
        write how this will affect his weight.

2. Dennis ate   ✚   During the day   ═   [ ]
    3000   he used 2000
    calories.   calories.

    a. Dennis ate _____ calories than
        he used.
        More   Less   The same

    b. In the box at the right, draw or
        write how this will affect his weight.

3. Ana ate   ✚   During the day   ═   [ ]
    2000   she used 2800
    calories.   calories.

    a. Ana ate _____ calories than
        she used.
        More   Less   The same

    b. In the box at the right, draw or
        write how this will affect her weight.

Worksheet   Name _____

BURN UP THOSE CALORIES

Directions: 1. Find a picture of your favorite snack food and paste it in the box below. (You may draw a picture of the food instead, if you like.)

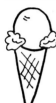

2. Look up the number of calories for that snack, and record it on the line under the box.

3. Figure out how long it will take you to burn up that snack by participating in one of your favorite activities. (Find out information on how many calories are burned by different activities from books in the library or health texts.)

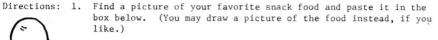

1. My favorite snack

2. _____ Calories

3. If I am _____, it will take me
              (Name of activity, e.g., jogging)

   _____minutes to use up the energy in the snack.

DISEASE PREVENTION AND CONTROL

Objective. The student analyzes the relationship of personal life style choices to disease prevention.

Level. Grades 6 to 8

Content generalizations. People who get regular exercise, eat nutritious diets, avoid tobacco use, manage stress, and maintain an ideal weight increase their resistance to disease. It is also important to avoid contact with communicable diseases. All of these behaviors are life style choices that each person must make individually. Some choices will contribute to health and help prevent disease, whereas others will increase the risks of developing a disease.

Vocabulary. Cardiovascular disease, hypertension, cancer, cirrhosis, life style

Initiation. Life Style Quiz

Write the words *life style choices* on the board, and ask the students what they mean. (The choices that we make regarding habits that affect our health.) Explain to students that habits established now can help prevent disease and prolong life. Hand out the worksheet, *Life Style Quiz.* Explain that this quiz is personal and will not be collected or graded. It is a way to look at current life style choices to get an idea of the risk we have of contracting a disease as an adult.

Materials
Worksheet: *Life Style Quiz* (pp. 462-463)

Activities

1. Case Studies

   Tell the students that they will be researching various diseases which are particularly affected by life style choices. They are to do this research in groups and report their findings to the rest of the class. Each group will be given a case study about a person with a certain disease. The groups should do the following.
   - Find out about the disease that affects the person in their case study.
   - Identify the health habit choices of the person in their case study that may have contributed to the disease.
   - Find out what, if any, treatment or changes in health habits can help this condition.

• List the various life style choices that teenagers can make which could help to prevent this disease.

Hand out the worksheet, *Case Studies,* and allow class and library time to work on the reports. Tell the groups that they may want to prepare visual aids such as transparencies or posters for their reports. As each group presents a report, tell the rest of the class to record the health life style choices discussed. When all the reports are finished, review the lists of choices accumulated, and summarize them on the board. They should include the following.

(1) Do not smoke.
(2) Get good nutrition (limit fatty foods, salt and sugar; eat more fresh fruits and vegetables).
(3) Get regular exercise.
(4) Control weight.
(5) Avoid overexposure to the sun.
(6) Abstain or limit use of alcohol.
(7) Learn how to manage stress.

2. Talking With Parents

Have the students rewrite the *Life Style Quiz* so that it is appropriate for adults. Suggest that they give it to their parents. (Giving the quiz to parents should be optional.)

Materials
Worksheet: *Case Studies* (one case study per group) (pp. 464-466)

Evaluation. How's Your Life Style?

Ask the students to analyze the life style choices of two hypothetical teenagers in the worksheet, *How's Your Life Style?* Hand out a worksheet to each student, and explain the directions. They are to read about the life styles of each person and then determine if the choices are *excellent, average,* or *poor* for preventing disease later in life. Students also must explain why they think the life style is excellent, average, or poor based on what they have learned about habits that promote or harm health.

Materials
Worksheet: *How's Your Life Style?* (p. 467)

Disease prevention and control

Worksheet

LIFE-STYLE QUIZ

Directions: In each of the areas below, circle the number that best describes your
             habits. Then total the number for each area, and find out what your
             scores mean on the next page.

CIGARETTE SMOKING

If you never smoke, enter a score of 10 and go on.

		Always	Sometimes	Almost never
1.	I avoid smoking cigarettes.	10	1	0

SMOKING SCORE _____

ALCOHOL AND DRUGS

		Always	Sometimes	Almost never
1.	I avoid drinking alcoholic beverages.	4	1	0
2.	I avoid using drugs (especially illegal drugs) as a way to handle problems.	2	1	0
3.	I do not drink alcohol or take other medicines.	2	1	0
4.	I read the label and follow the directions on all medicines.	2	1	0

ALCOHOL AND DRUG SCORE _____

EATING HABITS

		Always	Sometimes	Almost never
1.	I eat a variety of foods from each of the four food groups.	4	1	0
2.	I limit the amount of fatty foods I eat, such as butter, fat on meat, eggs, and shortening.	2	1	0
3.	I limit the amount of salt that I eat by not putting it on food at the table, not cooking with it, and not eating salty snacks.	2	1	0
4.	I avoid eating too much sugar (especially candy and soft drinks).	2	1	0

EATING HABITS SCORE _____

EXERCISE AND FITNESS

		Always	Sometimes	Almost never
1.	I maintain a desired weight and am not overweight or underweight.	3	1	0
2.	I do hard exercise for 15 to 30 minutes at least three times a week (like running, swimming, or hard bicycle riding).	3	1	0
3.	I do strength exercises for muscle tone for 15 to 30 minutes at least three times a week (like calisthenics, weight lifting, or yoga).	2	1	0
4.	I use part of my leisure time for participating in sports activities.	2	1	0

EXERCISE AND FITNESS SCORE _____

Modified from Healthstyle: a self test, U.S. Public Health Service.

Worksheet

LIFE-STYLE QUIZ (CONT.)

STRESS CONTROL

		Always	Sometimes	Almost never
1.	I enjoy school or have a hobby I enjoy.	2	1	0
2.	It is easy for me to relax and express my feelings.	2	1	0
3.	I know what kind of situations make me feel stress.	2	1	0
4.	I have close friends or relatives to talk to about my problems.	2	1	0
5.	I belong to a club or have a group of friends that I enjoy.	2	1	0

STRESS CONTROL SCORE _____

SAFETY

		Always	Sometimes	Almost never
1.	I wear a seat belt when riding in a car.	3	1	0
2.	I avoid riding in cars with drivers who are under the influence of drugs or alcohol.	3	1	0
3.	I obey traffic rules when riding a bicycle or walking.	2	1	0
4.	I am careful when using potentially dangerous products or substances such as household cleansers, poisons, and electrical devices.	2	1	0

SAFETY SCORE _____

What your scores mean to YOU

Scores of 9 and 10
     Excellent. Your answers show that you are aware of the importance of this area
to your health. More important, you are putting your knowledge to work for you by
practicing good health habits. As long as you continue to do so, this area should
not pose a serious health risk. It's likely that you are setting an example for your
family and friends to follow. Since you got a very high test score on this part of
the test, you may want to consider other areas where your scores indicate room for
improvement.

Scores of 6 to 8
     Your health practices in this area are good, but there is room for improvement.
Look again at the items you answered with a "Sometimes" or "Almost Never." What
changes can you make to improve your score? Even a small change can often help you
achieve better health.

Scores of 3 to 5
     Your health risks are showing! Would you like more information about the risks
you are facing and about why it is important for you to change these behaviors? Perhaps you need help in deciding how to successfully make the changes you desire. In
either case, help is available.

Scores of 0 to 2
     Obviously, you were concerned enough about your health to take the test, but
your answers show that you may be taking serious and unnecessary risks with your
health. Perhaps you are not aware of the risks and what to do about them. You can
easily get the information and help you need to improve, if you wish. The next step
is up to you.

Disease preven-
tion and control

Worksheet

CASE STUDIES

Lewis has just found out that he has hypertension.* He is 40 years old with a wife and two sons. He has a good job working in a bank. His boss does get on his nerves sometimes, and Lewis comes home in a bad mood. Lewis loves to eat steak and big batches of french fries with lots of salt. His wife fixes this meal often because it helps Lewis get out of his bad mood. Even though Lewis likes all kinds of sports, he spends more time watching them on television than actually participating. Therefore he has put on a few extra pounds in the last few years. He is really not certain what hypertension is and what he can do about it. Help Lewis out.

1. Find out what hypertension is. What does this disease do to the body?
2. What habits does Lewis have that may make the disease worse?
3. What can be done about the disease (treatments and changes in habits)?
4. What life-style choices can teenagers make that could help prevent this disease?

* Contact the American Heart Association for information on hypertension.

Jayne has skin cancer.* She is a very active woman of 38 years. She seems to be outdoors most of the time, both at work and at home. She loves to snow ski, garden, jog, and play tennis. Everyone is jealous of her wonderful year-round tan. She eats well, avoiding fatty and salty foods. She is also at her ideal weight. Jayne is a bit confused about why she has cancer. She lives such a healthy life. She would not think of smoking a cigarette, so why does she have cancer?

1. Find out what skin cancer is. What does it do to the body?
2. What life-style choices in Jayne's life could be the reason for her cancer?
3. What can be done about the disease (treatments and changes in habits)?
4. What life-style choices can teenagers make to help prevent this disease?

* Contact the American Cancer Society for information on skin cancer.

Worksheet

CASE STUDIES (CONT.)

Harry has just suffered from a mild heart attack.* The physician said he
needs to change some habits to prevent another attack. After all, he is only 42
years old with a daughter in junior high school. He has a good job as a stock broker.
There is often a lot of pressure in the job, which is why he likes to come home and
collapse in the chair with a drink, a cigarette, and some pretzels. Harry admits
that he smokes too much, but it helps calm him down from his demanding job. He says
he does not have time to exercise because of his job, his daughter, and his wife.
The only free time he has is on Sundays, and then he likes to watch sports on television with the guys and eat chips, hamburgers, and beer.

1. What is a heart attack? What happens to the body?

2. What habits does Harry have that may have caused the heart attack?

3. What can be done about someone who has a heart attack (treatments and
    changes in habits)?

4. What choices in their life-styles can teenagers make to prevent heart
    attacks?

* Contact the American Heart Association for information on heart attacks.

Shelia has emphysema.* She is 50 years old and has smoked cigarettes
since she was 16. When she started smoking, it was very popular with her friends.
She always thought she could quit whenever she really wanted to. Now her physician
says she has to stop smoking cigarettes. Shelia is not certain she has the will-
power to do it now. Cutting back to one pack a day has not seemed to help her
gasping for air. It is still very difficult to breathe. She wonders, "Why bother
to stop smoking all together?"

1. What is emphysema? What does it do to the body?

2. What habits does Shelia have that may be related to the disease?

3. What can be done about the disease (treatments and changes in habits)?

4. What choices can teenagers make in their life-style that can help prevent
    this disease?

* Contact the American Lung Association for information on emphysema.

**Disease preven-
tion and control**

Worksheet
CASE STUDIES (CONT.)

Dennis has just been to the physician and found out that he has lung cancer.* He is 64 years old and is almost ready to retire. He has always been healthy—you have to be to work in construction. The only time he can even remember being sick was a few years ago when he had the flu. That is why he was never worried that he smokes two packs of cigarettes a day. His father smoked until he died of a heart attack at age 69. Dennis has always watched his weight and his diet. He does not eat salty foods and prefers fish and chicken to steak. He thinks the physician must be mistaken and that he is too healthy to have cancer.

  1. What is lung cancer? What does it do to the body?

  2. What habits does Dennis have that may have caused the disease?

  3. What can be done about the disease (treatments and changes in habits)?

  4. What life-style choices can teenagers make to avoid getting lung cancer?

* Contact your local American Cancer Society for information on lung cancer.

Douglas has cirrhosis of the liver. He has always been a sociable guy. Everyone likes him. He usually stops by the local bar after work and has a few drinks with friends before going home. When he gets home, he has a few beers and watches television. Because he is single, he usually does not cook dinner for himself. He eats whatever he can find in the house. That often means hot dogs, potato chips, and beer. Sometimes he only has the beer. Douglas has never had a problem with his weight, even though he does not exercise. Why does he have cirrhosis of the liver?

  1. What is cirrhosis of the liver? What does it do to the body?

  2. What habits does Douglas have that may have caused the disease?

  3. What can be done about the disease (treatments or changes in behavior)?

  4. What life-style choices can teenagers make to prevent this disease?

Worksheet   Name _____

HOW'S YOUR LIFE-STYLE?

Directions: Read the following life-style choices for Mary and Steve. Decide if
the choices are excellent, average, or poor for preventing diseases
later in life. Explain why.

Mary is 16 years old. She is a good athlete and plays on several school teams. She also jogs and rides her bicycle regularly with her father. Sometimes she plays tennis with her mother. She enjoys being active. Mary and her friends like to go to the movies and roller skating. Once in a while some of her friends smoke cigarettes and drink. Mary tried it one time, but did not like it, so she drinks cola instead of beer.

Mary watches what she eats. When she eats at home, she gets lots of fresh fruits and vegetables, and her family has learned to enjoy foods without adding salt. When she goes out to eat with her friends, she does eat fatty foods like french fries, hamburgers, and milkshakes.

How do you think Mary's life-style rates for preventing diseases later in life?
(Circle one)

EXCELLENT   AVERAGE   POOR

Explain why:

Steve is 15 years old. He loves fried foods with lots of salt. He has the menus of all the fast-food restaurants in town memorized! All his friends hang out at the hamburger stand near school. Often they smoke cigarettes and drink colas all afternoon. Steve usually meets his friends there except during baseball season. Then he plays on the school team. Baseball is really the only sport Steve is interested in. He is a good catcher.

Steve likes to go to the movies too. Sometimes he and his friends sneak beer into the theater. One time they got caught, and the theater manager called their parents. Steve's mom was really mad, so he does not do it much anymore.

How do you think Steve's life-style rates for preventing diseases later in life?
(Circle one)

EXCELLENT   AVERAGE   POOR

Explain why:

Disease prevention and control

ACCIDENT PREVENTION AND SAFETY

Objective. The student proposes a home safety program.

Level. Grades 6 to 8

Content generalizations. Many home accidents can be prevented if hazards are reduced and emergency plans have been made. Hazards exist in all rooms of the home. Correcting such hazards can be a part of a home safety program. Reducing hazards and planning for possible emergencies make the home a safer place to live.

Vocabulary. Accident, hazard, emergency

Initiation. A Hazard Looking for an Accident

Using a great deal of dramatic flair, enter the classroom with a sign "A Hazard Looking for an Accident." Wear a large sloppy coat whose pockets are bulging with items that could be hazardous in the home, such as a plastic bag from the dry cleaners, frayed electrical cord, small throw rug without a rubberized backing, bottle of cleaning fluid, or any other item that could be stuffed in the coat or put somewhere on your body. Dramatically pull out one item at a time, and tell a story about an accident that happened with the item. Make up the stories, and make them funny with nothing serious happening to the victims described. At the end of the "show" explain that the reason we can laugh at these stories about accidents is because no one was really hurt in the accidents described. This, of course, is not always the case.

Write the words *accident* and *hazard* on the board. Have the students look up these words and find out the difference between them (possibly for homework).

Materials

Coat with lots of pockets

Items to represent hazards:
   Plastic dry-cleaning bag
   Frayed electrical cord
   Pot with handle
   Throw rug without rubberized backing

Sign: "A Hazard Looking for an Accident" (teacher-made)

Activities

1. Home Safety Checklist
   Hand out the worksheet, *Home Safety Checklist*. Explain that they are to use to check their home for hazards. Read through the *Home Safety Checklist* with the students. For each item on the checklist, ask them why the situation described could be hazardous. Have them take home the worksheet and analyze their own home.

Materials

Worksheet: *Home Safety Checklist* (p. 472)

HOME SAFETY CHECKLIST

Directions: Use the following list to check and correct hazards in your home. Do nothing on items that you have checked yes. Try to correct those where you have checked no.

STORAGE OF POISONOUS SUBSTANCES	YES	NO	CORRECTED
Medicines are out of reach of children.			
Labels are left on medicines and poisonous chemicals.			
Poisonous substances are always stored in original containers. (Do not put gasoline in a cola bottle for storage.)			
Household cleaners and chemicals are not stored on the same shelf as or a shelf above food.			
Kerosene, gasoline, and other flammable fluids are stored away from heat sources.			

PROPER USE AND STORAGE OF ELECTRICAL APPLIANCES			
All electrical cords are in good condition and not frayed.			
Electrical outlets are not overloaded.			
Extension cords are not under carpets, through doors, or over nails.			
Electrical appliances are used away from water.			
When not in use, electrical appliances and tools are stored neatly out of the reach of children.			

Accident prevention and safety

2. "Hazards" Pictures
   Ask the students to take a picture of a hazard that they found in their own home. If a camera is not available, ask them to draw the hazard. Students then should correct the hazard and take or draw another picture of the situation. These pictures can be posted on a bulletin board, "Don't Let a Hazard Become an Accident." It may be necessary to rotate student pictures if several classes are involved in this activity.

3. In Case of Fire
   Ask the students, "What is the purpose of fire drills at school?" (To practice the proper way to proceed if a fire occurs at school.) Ask them to describe the proper way to exit your classroom should a fire occur. Explain that it is important to be prepared for a possible fire at home as well.

Materials

Camera and film for use by students in their own home (if available) or drawing paper and felt pens
Bulletin board: "Don't Let a Hazard Become an Accident"

Hand out the worksheet, *In Case of Fire*. Tell the students that this is a floor plan of a house. Using the transparency on the overhead projector, mark the normal exit route from the bedrooms to the outside. Ask the students, "What should be done if a fire in the hallway blocks an exit from the bedrooms?" (The door to the hallway should be closed, and a secondary exit should be taken. The family should have a prearranged meeting spot outside the home.) Ask students to locate a secondary exit route from each bedroom on their worksheet. Then discuss the routes, and draw them on the transparency.

Materials

Worksheet and transparency: *In Case of Fire* (p. 473)
Overhead projector
Transparency pens (2 colors)

IN CASE OF FIRE

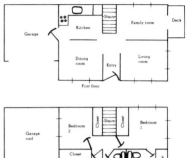

Directions: With the help of the teacher you will be locating the primary and secondary exit routes from the bedrooms of this house in case of fire.

Evaluation. Be Prepared—Firstaid at Home

Ask the students to check at home for a first-aid kit and for a list of emergency numbers posted near the telephone. Hand out the worksheet, *Be Prepared*. Explain that their assignment is to find out the emergency telephone numbers appropriate for their area and record them on the worksheet. Suggest that students look in the front pages of the telephone book for help in locating emergency numbers. The bottom part of the worksheet deals with the assembly of a first-aid kit and the gathering of a few items that could be necessary in an emergency. Suggest that students work together with parents to gather items for the first-aid kit and for possible emergencies. Set up a display of all the items indicated on the worksheet. Allow the students several weeks to complete this project. Tell them to get help from family members. It may be useful to discuss the problems students may be having in putting together first-aid kits for their homes. The discussions could be as a total class or in small groups. Encourage the students to help each other work out problems.

Materials

Worksheet: *Be Prepared* (p. 474)

Telephone book

Items for first-aid kit: bandages (several sizes and roller gauze), sterile pads (2 × 2 inches), antiseptic, adhesive tape, alcohol, tongue depressor, triangular bandages

Other items for emergency situations: flashlight with extra batteries, candles and matches, battery-operated radio, bottled water

Worksheet   Name _____

BE PREPARED

Directions: Find the following emergency telephone numbers for your community. Then cut out along the dotted line and mount it on a 5 × 8 index card or a piece of tagboard cut to the correct size. Place your *be prepared* sign near the telephone in your home. If you have more than one telephone, make other signs.

EMERGENCY TELEPHONE NUMBERS

Police _____

Fire _____

Ambulance _____

Poison control center _____

Work with your parents to assemble a first-aid kit for your home. Include the following items. Check them off as you assemble the kit.

___ Bandages, several sizes   ___ Tongue depressor
___ Sterile pad, 2 X 2 inches   ___ Triangular bandage
___ Roller gauze   ___ Optional items: flashlight,
___ Antiseptic   batteries, candles, matches,
___ Adhesive tape   bottled water, battery-
___ Alcohol   operated radio

Accident prevention and safety

Worksheet   Name _____

HOME SAFETY CHECKLIST

Directions: Use the following list to check and correct hazards in your home.

Do nothing on items that you have checked yes. Try to correct those where you have checked no.

STORAGE OF POISONOUS SUBSTANCES	YES	NO	CORRECTED
Medicines are out of reach of children.			
Labels are left on medicines and poisonous chemicals.			
Poisonous substances are always stored in original containers. (Do not put gasoline in a cola bottle for storage.)			
Household cleaners and chemicals are not stored on the same shelf as or a shelf above food.			
Kerosene, gasoline, and other flammable fluids are stored away from heat sources.			
PROPER USE AND STORAGE OF ELECTRICAL APPLIANCES			
All electrical cords are in good condition and not frayed.			
Electrical outlets are not overloaded.			
Extension cords are not under carpets, through doors, or over nails.			
Electrical appliances are used away from water.			
When not in use, electrical appliances and tools are stored neatly out of the reach of children.			
SAFETY AROUND THE HOUSE	YES	NO	CORRECTED
Hallways and stairs are well lit.			
Throw rugs have rubberized backing.			
Floors and steps are not cluttered.			
Water or grease on floors is quickly wiped up.			
Cupboard doors, closet doors, and drawers are kept closed.			
Stairways have handrails.			
Smoke detectors are in the home.			
SAFETY AROUND THE KITCHEN			
Pots and pans are used with handles not protruding from stove.			
Curtains are not near the stove.			
The kitchen has a fire extinguisher.			
Knives are stored separately from other utensils and away from children.			
Matches are out of the reach of children.			

Worksheet   Name _____

IN CASE OF FIRE

Directions: With the help of the teacher you will be locating the primary
and secondary exit routes from the bedrooms of this house in case
of fire.

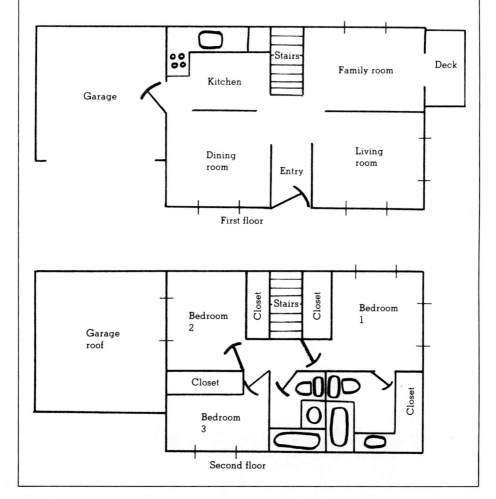

Accident prevention
and safety

Worksheet   Name _____

BE PREPARED

Directions: Find the following emergency telephone numbers for your community.
Then cut out along the dotted line and mount it on a 5 × 8 index card or
a piece of tagboard cut to the correct size. Place your *be prepared*
sign near the telephone in your home. If you have more than one telephone,
make other signs.

EMERGENCY TELEPHONE NUMBERS

Police _____

Fire _____

Ambulance _____

Poison control center _____

Work with your parents to assemble a first-aid kit for your home. Include the
following items. Check them off as you assemble the kit.

___ Bandages, several sizes	___ Tongue depressor
___ Sterile pad, 2 X 2 inches	___ Triangular bandage
___ Roller gauze	___ Optional items: flashlight,
___ Antiseptic	batteries, candles, matches,
___ Adhesive tape	bottled water, battery-
___ Alcohol	operated radio

CONSUMER HEALTH

Objective. The student identifies criteria for the selection of an appropriate health adviser.

Level. Grades 6 to 8

Content generalizations. The first source of help for the selection of health advisers is usually parents. Generally, select a health adviser who is trained to provide the information required and who is able and willing to refer you to another practitioner who may be more qualified to provide particular health services.

Vocabulary. Advice, quackery, fraud, testimonials

Initiation. Advice
Write the word *advice* on the board. Ask the students to define the word. (A recommendation about what to do about a problem.)

Ask the students if they ever ask for advice from other people. Ask, "Why do people need advice? Do we ever get bad advice? What might be some examples of bad advice?"

Activities

1. What's Wrong Here?
   Hand out the worksheet, *What's Wrong Here?* Review the directions with students. Explain that they are to read a story about someone who was seeking advice on a problem. Students are to write a short explanation of what each person did wrong in seeking advice. When they have finished the worksheets individually, ask them to share their responses with one or two others in the class. Then discuss the situations as a whole class. Ask the following questions.
   (1) What is wrong with Peter asking his dentist to fix his car? (Peter has no idea if the dentist knows anything about cars. The dentist is not qualified to fix cars, only teeth.)
   (2) What is wrong with Vicki asking her neighbor to fix her faucet? (Her neighbor is not qualified to fix plumbing. If he tries and something goes wrong, it may end up being a bigger problem.)
   (3) What is wrong with Ken asking Bruce what to do about his cold and sore throat? (Bruce is not qualified to answer medical questions.)

Materials
Worksheet: *What's Wrong Here?*
(p. 477)

Worksheet   Name _____
WHAT'S WRONG HERE?

Directions: Below are several stories about people who needed advice. Read the
story, then write an explanation about what the person did wrong in
seeking advice on the problem.

1. Peter had car problems. Every time he started the car, black smoke would come
   out of the exhaust, and the car would make clunking noises. He had a problem,
   so he called his dentist. After all, his dentist was the smartest person he
   knew; certainly he could fix the car if Peter offered to pay him.

2. Vicki had a sink that dripped water from the faucet even when it was turned
   off. Her water bills were higher than normal, and the constant dripping noise
   was driving her crazy. So she called her neighbor Sam. He was an accountant,
   but he had a few tools.

3. Ken was sneezing and coughing. He felt terrible. So he asked his best friend
   Bruce what he should do about his cold and sore throat. Bruce's mother was a
   nurse, so certainly he would know what to do.

After discussing each situation ask the students, "What is the most important factor to think about in seeking advice?" (Is the person qualified?) Remind the students that people may be qualified to give advice in some areas but not in others. For example, Peter's dentist certainly could give advice on care of the teeth but not on cars.

2. Criteria for Qualified Advisors

Ask the students if they have any idea how to choose someone to advise them on health matters. Ask "How do you know if a person is qualified?" After they have offered suggestions, explain that most people qualified to give health advice have been to school and have special training. Often the state requires that health professionals take a special test to get a license to practice in that state.

Write the following criteria on the board, and have the students copy it.

(1) Qualified health advisers have:

• Special training (for example, 8 to 15 years of schooling for medical doctors)

• A license from the state

(2) Qualified health advisers do not:

• Offer a secret cure that only they can provide

• Say that you do not need another adviser's opinion

• Sell products from door to door, in magazines, or on television

• Use testimonials, coupons, or guarantees

3. Reading the Fine Print

Have the students cut out advertisements from magazines about cures for problems such as baldness and obesity. Students should look for advertisements that seem too good to be true. Explain the importance of reading the fine print. Post them all on a bulletin board. From time to time during the activities on consumer health, ask for volunteers to share an advertisement they found particularly questionable.

Evaluation. Good Advice—Bad Advice

Give each student a copy of the worksheet, *Good Advice—Bad Advice*. Tell them to circle *yes* if they think the advice will be from a qualified health adviser or *no* if they think the person may not be qualified.

After everyone has had a chance to circle their answers, go over each item orally in class. Ask for volunteers to share their responses and explain the reason for the choice.

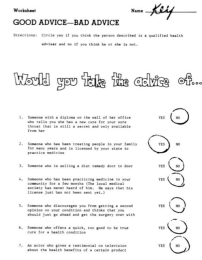

Worksheet   Name ___Key___

GOOD ADVICE—BAD ADVICE

Directions: Circle yes if you think the person described is a qualified health
             adviser and no if you think he or she is not.

Would you take the advice of...

1. Someone with a diploma on the wall of her office
   who tells you she has a new cure for your sore
   throat that is still a secret and only available
   from her   YES   (NO)

2. Someone who has been treating people in your family
   for many years and is licensed by your state to
   practice medicine   (YES)   NO

3. Someone who is selling a diet remedy door to door   YES   (NO)

4. Someone who has been practicing medicine in your
   community for a few months (The local medical
   society has never heard of him. He says that his
   license just has not been sent yet.)   YES   (NO)

5. Someone who discourages you from getting a second
   opinion on your condition and thinks that you
   should just go ahead and get the surgery over with   YES   (NO)

6. Someone who offers a quick, too good to be true
   cure for a health condition   YES   (NO)

7. An actor who gives a testimonial on television
   about the health benefits of a certain product   YES   (NO)

Materials

Worksheet: *Good Advice—Bad Advice*
   (p. 478)

Worksheet   Name _____

WHAT'S WRONG HERE?

Directions: Below are several stories about people who needed advice. Read the

story, then write an explanation about what the person did wrong in

seeking advice on the problem.

1. Peter had car problems. Every time he started the car, black smoke would come
    out of the exhaust, and the car would make clunking noises. He had a problem,
    so he called his dentist. After all, his dentist was the smartest person he
    knew; certainly he could fix the car if Peter offered to pay him.

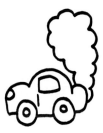

2. Vicki had a sink that dripped water from the faucet even when it was turned
    off. Her water bills were higher than normal, and the constant dripping noise
    was driving her crazy. So she called her neighbor Sam. He was an accountant,
    but he had a few tools.

3. Ken was sneezing and coughing. He felt terrible. So he asked his best friend
    Bruce what he should do about his cold and sore throat. Bruce's mother was a
    nurse, so certainly he would know what to do.

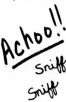

Worksheet   Name _____

GOOD ADVICE—BAD ADVICE

Directions: Circle yes if you think the person described is a qualified health

adviser and no if you think he or she is not.

Would you take the advice of...

1. Someone with a diploma on the wall of her office   YES   NO
    who tells you she has a new cure for your sore
    throat that is still a secret and only available
    from her

2. Someone who has been treating people in your family   YES   NO
    for many years and is licensed by your state to
    practice medicine

3. Someone who is selling a diet remedy door to door   YES   NO

4. Someone who has been practicing medicine in your   YES   NO
    community for a few months (The local medical
    society has never heard of him. He says that his
    license just has not been sent yet.)

5. Someone who discourages you from getting a second   YES   NO
    opinion on your condition and thinks that you
    should just go ahead and get the surgery over with

6. Someone who offers a quick, too good to be true   YES   NO
    cure for a health condition

7. An actor who gives a testimonial on television   YES   NO
    about the health benefits of a certain product

USE AND ABUSE OF DRUGS

Objective. The student evaluates the significance of peer pressure on the decision to abuse drugs.

Level. Grades 6 to 8

Content generalizations. Peer pressure is considered the single most important factor contributing to adolescent use and abuse of drugs. Adolescents are very concerned about being accepted by group members. It is normal for adolescents to form groups of friends who dress similarly, are involved in the same activities, and explore new activities together. If these groups are involved in using drugs, there usually is a great deal of peer pressure for everyone to participate. Often this pressure is so great that adolescents will participate despite the wishes and values of their parents or themselves. Additionally, knowing the health risks related to the abuse of drugs does not necessarily act as a deterrent when peer pressure is involved.

It is helpful for adolescents to know what peer pressure is and that it is a normal part of growing up. In fact peer pressure is a part of adult life as well, although it is not as significant in influencing important adult decisions as for adolescents. Adolescents need help in understanding that it is all right to be different and that, if they are not interested in certain activities in which their friends are involved, perhaps they should find new friends.

Vocabulary. Peer pressure

Initiation. It's "In"

Find something to wear to class that will look strange to the students. It should be some mode of dress that is different from your normal attire. It should not be too bizarre, but it should be noticeable.

When the students remark on your new attire, and they will, tell them that this is the new "in" thing for teachers. Convince them that soon they will be seeing this type of attire on every teacher in the school. End your "act" by saying, "If any of the other teachers want to hang around with me, they're going to wear clothes like this." Then move immediately into activity 1.

Materials
Unusual clothing that will cause students to remark on your appearance, such as:
Hat
New tie
Shoes

Use and abuse
of drugs

Activities

1. Me and My Friends

   Tell the students to just think "yes" or "no" answers to the following questions but not to answer aloud: "Are there certain kinds of clothes you and your friends wear? Are there certain activities that you and your friends like to do? Are there activities you have done that you probably would not have done unless your friends were there doing it too? Have you ever done something you wouldn't normally do, but one of your friends dared you to do it?" Ask them to raise their hands if they could answer yes to any of the questions. Tell the class as a whole, "Congratulations, you are all normal teenagers [or preteens]."

   Hand out the worksheet, *Me and My Friends,* and ask the students to complete it as directed. The questions are similar to those previously asked in class, and students are to provide examples of activities influenced by their friends.

   NOTE: Up to this point the discussions regarding peer pressure should have been general. The relationship of drug usage to peer pressure will be brought in gradually as it surfaces in discussions and on worksheets. The last item on the worksheet asks a simple yes or no question, "Do any of your friends smoke or drink?"

   After the students have finished the worksheets, have them divide into groups to discuss their worksheets and to consider the question, "Are friends important in affecting the way you act and dress?" A representative from each group should share the group's ideas with the entire class at the end of the activity.

Materials

Worksheet: *Me and My Friends* (p. 483)

Worksheet   Name _____

ME AND MY FRIENDS

Directions: Read the questions below, and list what you do with or because of your friends.

1. What kind of clothes are "in" with your group of friends?

2. What do you like to do with your friends?

3. Do you have different friends at home than at school? If so, do you do different activities with these friends? List the activities you do.

4. Are there things you probably would not have done unless your friends were doing them also? List them.

5. Do any of your friends smoke cigarettes? (Circle one)   YES   NO

   Do any of your friends drink alcoholic beverages? (Circle one)   YES   NO

2. Survey Sheet—Peer Pressure
   Tell the students that they are to participate in a survey. Each student will use the worksheet, *Survey Sheet,* to ask an adult smoker some questions about when he or she started smoking. Explain to the students that the purpose of this survey is to find out if peer pressure was involved in that person's decision to start smoking. Review the questions on the *Survey Sheet,* and allow the students several days to complete the survey.

3. Tally Sheet—Peer Pressure Survey
   Using butcher paper, make and post a large *Tally Sheet* for use in analyzing the data collected from the student surveys. As each student returns a completed survey, allow him or her to record the findings on the large class *Tally Sheet.* (One *Tally Sheet* could be used to collect data from several classes.)

4. Practice Saying ''No''
   Allow each student to practice ''saying no'' to peer pressure. Go around to each student in the class, and offer a cigarette to each. Tell them they must resist your pressure to smoke. Suggest that they give answers such as, ''No thanks, I don't want lung cancer,'' ''Are you kidding, those things are coffin nails,'' ''No thanks, athletes don't smoke,'' or, ''My mom would kill me, and I'm too young to die!'' A more humorous response could be, ''No thanks, I like clean breath and white teeth,'' or, ''Are you kidding? I love to play tennis without breathing problems so I can get a natural high.''

   You may wish to repeat this activity several times during different class periods. It is important, however, that every student in the class has a chance to respond. Ham it up as the pressurer.

   NOTE: In this activity it is important that the teacher apply the pressure. Students should receive practice in *resisting* pressure, not *applying* pressure.

Materials

Worksheet: *Survey Sheet* (p. 484)

Worksheet   Name _____
SURVEY SHEET

Directions: Use the questions on this worksheet to interview an adult about
           cigarette smoking. Ask a smoker when and why he or she started
           smoking cigarettes. The responses on your survey will be com-
           bined with the responses that other class members collect.

1. Name of adult smoker _____

2. Age of smoker (Circle one)
   19 to 25 years, 26 to 35 years, 36 to 50 years, over 50 years

3. Questions
   a. How old were you when you first started smoking cigarettes? (Circle one)
      Under 10 years, 11 to 13 years, 14 to 16 years, 17 to 21 years, over 21 years

   b. Why did you start smoking?

   c. Did any of your friends smoke or start smoking at the same time you started?

   d. When you started smoking, did either of your parents smoke cigarettes?
      If the answer is yes, indicate if it was the mother, father, or both.

   e. Did you know the health hazards of cigarette smoking before you started?

   f. Have you ever tried to quit smoking?

   g. Do you have any advice for young people who have not yet made the decision of whether to smoke or not?

Materials

Teacher resource: *Tally Sheet* (p. 485)
Butcher paper
Felt pens

Use and abuse of drugs

Teacher resource
TALLY SHEET

Directions: Use a large sheet like the one shown here to tally the responses to
           the smoking survey. Several classes' responses could be recorded on
           one tally sheet posted in the classroom.

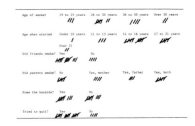

Evaluation. In My Opinion—Essay

Have the students write an essay describing their opinions on the question, "How important is peer pressure in the decision to smoke cigarettes or use drugs?" You may wish to provide students the option of taping their opinions on a cassette tape. In either case students should explain the reasons for their opinions.

Worksheet   Name _____

ME AND MY FRIENDS

Directions: Read the questions below, and list what you do with or because of
            your friends.

----

1. What kind of clothes are "in" with your group of friends?

2. What do you like to do with your friends?

3. Do you have different friends at home than at school? If so, do you do different
    activities with these friends? List the activities you do.

4. Are there things you probably would not have done unless your friends were doing
    them also? List them.

5. Do any of your friends smoke cigarettes? (Circle one)   YES   NO

    Do any of your friends drink alcoholic beverages? (Circle one)   YES   NO

Use and abuse
of drugs

Worksheet   Name _____

SURVEY SHEET

Directions: Use the questions on this worksheet to interview an adult about
             cigarette smoking. Ask a smoker when and why he or she started
             smoking cigarettes. The responses on your survey will be com-
             bined with the responses that other class members collect.

1. Name of adult smoker _____

2. Age of smoker (Circle one)

        19 to 25 years, 26 to 35 years, 36 to 50 years, over 50 years

3. Questions

    a. How old were you when you first started smoking cigarettes? (Circle one)

        Under 10 years, 11 to 13 years, 14 to 16 years, 17 to 21 years, over 21 years

    b. Why did you start smoking?

    c. Did any of your friends smoke or start smoking at the same time you
        started?

    d. When you started smoking, did either of your parents smoke cigarettes?

        If the answer is yes, indicate if it was the mother, father, or both.

    e. Did you know the health hazards of cigarette smoking before you started?

    f. Have you ever tried to quit smoking?

    g. Do you have any advice for young people who have not yet made the decision
        of whether to smoke or not?

Teacher resource

TALLY SHEET

Directions: Use a large sheet like the one shown here to tally the responses to
the smoking survey. Several classes' responses could be recorded on
one tally sheet posted in the classroom.

Age of smoker	19 to 25 years	26 to 35 years	36 to 50 years	Over 50 years
	///	ЖИ //	////	//

Age when started	Under 10 years	11 to 13 years	14 to 16 years	17 to 21 years
	/	///	ЖИ ЖИ	ЖИ
	Over 21			
	//			

Did friends smoke?	Yes	No		
	ЖИ ЖИ ///	////		

Did parents smoke?	No	Yes, mother	Yes, father	Yes, both
	ЖИ	////	///	ЖИ

Knew the hazards?	Yes	No		
	ЖИ ///	ЖИ ///		

Tried to quit?	Yes	No		
	ЖИ ЖИ ЖИ	////		

Use and abuse
of drugs

ENVIRONMENTAL HEALTH

Objective. The student evaluates the efforts of community groups and agencies in improving and protecting the environment.

Level. Grades 6 to 8

Content generalizations. The individual is ultimately responsible for the health of the environment. For example, an individual can take personal responsibility for not polluting the air. However, if no one else in the community takes action to avoid pollution, the air still will be polluted. With environmental health concerns, in particular, it is necessary for people to work together to protect the environment. Several types of groups exist: official governmental agencies such as the public health department and the state environmental protection agency; voluntary agencies such as the American Lung Association; and special interest groups such as the Sierra Club, National Audubon Society, National Wildlife Federation, and American Camping Association. The individual can help protect the environment by participating in groups such as these and by following recommendations and laws designed to help the environment.

Vocabulary. Official agency, voluntary agency, community, environment

Initiation. Clean, Safe Water

Display a large pitcher of water and paper cups. Ask if anyone wants a drink of water. Tell students that it is tap water and safe to drink. If there is a faucet in your classroom, fill the water pitcher in front of students to prove it is tap water.

After a few students have tasted the water, ask a few questions:
1. How does it taste?
2. Is it clean?
3. How do you know?
4. Can we trust the tap water to be safe in this city, state, or country?
5. Would you trust the tap water to be safe in other countries?

Materials
Water pitcher filled with tap water
Paper cups

Explain to students that we often take for granted the clean water that comes out of the tap. In many places in the world, and sometimes even in the United States, the water that comes out of the tap is not safe to drink. The reason that we usually can trust our water is because we have groups of people in our community that work together to make certain our water is clean. (Typical groups in communities that do this are the public health department, water and power department, department of sanitation, and local ecology groups.)

Activities

1. Mini-Lecture—Pollution
   Write the words *land, air,* and *water* on the board. Ask the students to brainstorm actions that individuals can take to protect these valuable resources. This can be done in groups or as a full class. The students' list might include avoid littering, recycle glassware and aluminum, do not waste water, avoid polluting streams and lakes, walk or ride bicycles rather than use automobiles, and make certain all automobiles have proper equipment to filter exhaust fumes.

   Explain to the students that it is important for individuals to do their part in protecting the environment; however, often certain problems must be solved by groups of people. It is also important that individuals support the work of community groups to protect the environment.

2. Protecting the Environment
   Divide students into groups to do research on various groups that work to protect the environment. Hand out the worksheet, *Protecting the Environment,* and review the directions with students.

   a. Instruct each group to visit the library to identify an environmental issue (environmental concern in the community) they would like to study.
   b. Once an issue has been identified, students should locate various groups that may be involved. The groups may be official (governmental), voluntary, or special interest.
   c. The students should contact each group with a letter asking *specific* questions.
   d. When the students get the correspondence back, they should prepare an oral report that describes the issue they have chosen and the work done by various groups in the community; they should evaluate how well the groups are doing in protecting the environment.

Materials

Worksheet: *Protecting the Environment* (p. 489)

Environmental health

Encourage the students to use charts and other visual aids for their group presentation. Tell students that they may have to wait several weeks for a reply from the various agencies. If they do not hear from the agencies contacted, have them prepare a presentation without the letters.

NOTE: Review the issues chosen by groups and the lists of agencies that each plans to contact. It may be necessary to change the issues addressed to avoid sending too many letters to one agency.

3. Field Trip

Take a field trip to a local agency concerned with protecting the environment, such as one of the following.

(1) Water treatment plant
(2) Sanitation site
(3) Public health department
(4) State environmental protection agency

Contact the agency first, and ask for a guide who can explain the operation and the way that they work to protect the environment. Ask that the guide have suggestions for individuals that could make the agency's work easier. After the field trip ask the students to describe what that particular agency does to protect the environment. Also ask if they think the agency is doing a good job.

Evaluation. Certificate of Appreciation

List on the board all the agencies nominated by the class for a certificate of appreciation. Tell the students they must decide which agencies from the list should receive a certificate of appreciation from the class. For each agency a sentence or two describing why the award is deserved should be written by the group nominating it.

Have a committee of students tally the votes and determine which agencies will be awarded the certificate. Announce the winners to the class, and ask student volunteers to help in filling in and mailing the certificates.

Materials.

Teacher resource: *Certificate of Appreciation* (p. 490)

Teacher resource
CERTIFICATE OF APPRECIATION

Directions: After the class has determined which agencies are doing a good job protecting the environment, have a committee mail out certificates to these agencies. An example is provided below.

CERTIFICATE OF APPRECIATION

The _____ class at _____ School

is awarding this special certificate of appreciation to

_____
(Name of agency)

for outstanding efforts in protection of the environment in our community.

_____ Signed _____
(Date)   (Teacher)

Certificate of Appreciation Committee

_____   _____
_____   _____
_____   _____

Worksheet   Name_____

PROTECTING THE ENVIRONMENT

Directions: In your groups you will be researching an environmental concern. You
              will be studying groups that are working to help the environment and
              try to figure out if they are doing a good job of protecting the en-
              vironment. As a group, follow the steps outlined below. Your group
              will be responsible for an oral presentation after you have done your
              research.

1. As a group, identify an environmental issue you would like to study. You may
    have to visit the library and talk to the librarian for help in this task.

    The environmental issue we will study is _____

2. Find out what groups are interested in the same environmental issue. Ask the
    librarian for help. Find out if the groups are governmental, voluntary, or
    special interest. You may have to look these words up in a dictionary first.

    The groups concerned with this issue are:

    _____   _____

    _____   _____

3. As a group, write a neat letter to each group identified in 2. Ask some spe-
    cific questions such as: (1) what does your group do about (issue)? (2) what
    are some of the problems that your agency has dealing with (issue)? (3) are
    there things that your agency would like to do about (issue) but for some
    reason cannot do at this time? (4) what can individuals in the community do
    about (issue)?

    All members in the group should sign the letter. Make certain that all words
    are spelled correctly and that you have indicated a return address. It might
    be a good idea to enclose a self-addressed stamped envelope.

4. When you have heard from all the agencies that you contacted, prepare an oral
    report that analyzes the effectiveness of the groups in protecting the environ-
    ment. In other words, "Are they doing a good job or not?"

    In your presentation you should have some visual aids prepared to add interest.

Environmental
health

Teacher resource

CERTIFICATE OF APPRECIATION

Directions: After the class has determined which agencies are doing a good job
              protecting the environment, have a committee mail out certificates
              to these agencies. An example is provided below.

CERTIFICATE OF APPRECIATION

The_____ class at _____ School

is awarding this special certificate of appreciation to

_____
(Name of agency)

for outstanding efforts in protection of the environment in our community.

_____Signed_____
(Date)   (Teacher)

Certificate of Appreciation Committee

_____   _____

_____   _____

_____   _____

COMMUNITY HEALTH

Objective. The student concludes that individual participation is essential if community health activities are to be successful.

Level. Grades 6 to 8

Content generalizations. Most communities have many organizations both public and private that are interested in the health of community members. The various types of organizations include voluntary health agencies (such as the American Cancer Society, American Lung Association, American Heart Association, and American Red Cross), official governmental organizations (such as the public health department and public hospitals), private industry (such as privately owned hospitals, local drug stores, private physicians, and other health professionals in private practice), professional organizations (such as local chapters of the American Medical Association [AMA], AMA Auxiliary, American Dental Association, and American Public Health Association), and service clubs (such as the Kiwanis, Rotary Club, and Lions Club). In most cases these organizations require individual voluntary participation to effectively carry out health activities in the community. Voluntary help and contributions are essential if these organizations are to accomplish their goals.

Vocabulary. Volunteer, professions, organizations

Initiation. Are You a Health Volunteer?
Write the word *volunteer* on the board, and ask the students if they have ever volunteered to do something for an organization or for school. As students suggest activities, write or have a student write them on the board. Volunteer work they may have done includes collecting money for the American Red Cross or another organization; participating in a Walk-A-Thon or Bike-A-Thon for a voluntary agency, a club, or a cause; or participating in a recycling program with a club or the school.

Explain to students that in each case their voluntary help was probably very important. Often it takes many people working together to accomplish something. Voluntary participation is particularly important in community health activities. Many community health organizations would not be able to function without individual volunteers.

Community health

Activities

1. Health Fair

   Ask the students to help organize a health fair for the school. Explain that several health organizations will be invited to come to school and tell what they do for the health of the community and how they use volunteers. Booths or tables will be set up, and students can visit the different organization representatives to find out about their work.

2. Community Health Volunteers

   Give each student a copy of the worksheet, *Community Health Volunteers*. Go over the worksheet with students to explain its use during the health fair. Students are to ask representatives from each organization a few questions about volunteer work. (It is a good idea to tell the representatives that students will be asking certain questions.) It may be helpful to rotate students around to the booths in small groups so that representatives can address these questions to several students at one time.

Materials

Worksheet: *Community Health Volunteers* (p. 494)

Worksheet   Name _____

COMMUNITY HEALTH VOLUNTEERS

Directions: Talk to various representatives from health agencies in your community. Use this worksheet to record your findings. For each agency, ask if they do or do not use volunteers. If they do use volunteers, try to find out what kinds of jobs the volunteers do for the organization.

Name of agency or organization	Use volunteers?	Jobs that volunteers do for the agency or organization
1. American Cancer Society	(YES) NO	Work on committees / Present programs / Raise money
2. March of Dimes	(YES) NO	Help run the organization / Organize walk-a-thons / Present programs / Stuff envelopes
3. American Lung Association	(YES) NO	Serve on committees / Promote school programs / Help raise money
4. American Heart Association	(YES) NO	Serve on Advisory committees / Present programs at schools
5. Al-Anon	(YES) NO	Help counsel others / Help organize functions
6. American Red Cross	(YES) NO	Work in blood donor centers / Give talks and courses about first aid

3. Health Volunteers Mural

After the health fair ask the students to participate in making a large wall chart entitled *Health Volunteers in Our Community*. Have students use their completed worksheets to make a chart of all the organizations and agencies that they surveyed at the health fair. Have small groups of students contact other agencies or organizations not at the fair to add to the wall chart. Groups should fill in the chart as they contact a new agency or organization about the use of volunteers. When the chart is finished, ask the students if they think individual participation in community health activities is important and why. Ask, "What would happen if no one volunteered to do things for the community? Are there any activities you may be interested in doing for the community?"

Materials

Wall chart: *Health Volunteers in Our Community*

Butcher paper

Felt pens or crayons

Rulers

Worksheets: *Community Health Volunteers* (completed by students) (p. 492); *Community Health Agencies and Organizations* (p. 494)

Evaluation. Getting Involved

Tell the students to imagine that a friend has just said, "My mom thinks I should go on a Walk-A-Thon for the March of Dimes—Birth Defects Foundation. It sure sounds like a dumb idea to me." Ask them to respond to their friend. In their response they should tell about individual participation in health activities in the community. These responses can be written or taped on a cassette recorder.

Materials

Optional: Cassette recorder and tape

Community health

Worksheet   Name _____

COMMUNITY HEALTH
VOLUNTEERS

    Directions: Talk to various representatives from health agencies in your community.
                Use this worksheet to record your findings. For each agency, ask if
                they do or do not use volunteers. If they do use volunteers, try to
                find out what kinds of jobs the volunteers do for the organization.

Name of agency or organization	Use volunteers?	Jobs that volunteers do for the agency or organization
1. _____	YES NO	_____
2. _____	YES NO	_____
3. _____	YES NO	_____
4. _____	YES NO	_____
5. _____	YES NO	_____
6. _____	YES NO	_____

Worksheet   Name _____

COMMUNITY HEALTH AGENCIES AND ORGANIZATIONS

Directions: The following is a list of several agencies that may or may not be in your community. Try to find the local chapter in your community. Look in the telephone book for local chapters. Check off those which are located in your community.

☑ Means we have a local chapter in our community

- ☐ A1-Anon
- ☐ Alcoholics Anonymous
- ☐ Allergy Foundation of America
- ☐ American Association for Rehabilitation Therapy
- ☐ American Cancer Society
- ☐ American Diabetes Association, Inc.
- ☐ American Foundation for the Blind, Inc.
- ☐ American Geriatrics Society, Inc.
- ☐ American Hearing Society
- ☐ American Heart Association
- ☐ American Institute of Family Relations, Inc.
- ☐ American Lung Association
- ☐ American Parkinson Disease Association
- ☐ American Red Cross
- ☐ Arthritis Foundation
- ☐ Cystic Fibrosis Foundation
- ☐ Epilepsy Foundation
- ☐ Gray Panthers
- ☐ Leukemia Society
- ☐ March of Dimes—Birth Defects Foundation
- ☐ Medic Alert Foundation
- ☐ Muscular Dystrophy Association
- ☐ The Myasthenia Gravis Foundation, Inc.
- ☐ Association for Gifted Children
- ☐ Association for Mental Health
- ☐ Association for Retarded Children
- ☐ Child Safety Council
- ☐ Council on the Aging
- ☐ Council on Alcoholism, Inc.
- ☐ Easter Seal Society for Crippled Children and Adults
- ☐ Hemophilia Foundation
- ☐ Kidney Foundation
- ☐ Multiple Sclerosis Society
- ☐ Society to Prevent Blindness
- ☐ Tay-Sachs and Allied Diseases Association, Inc.
- ☐ Planned Parenthood Federation
- ☐ Sickle Cell Disease Foundation of Greater New York
- ☐ United Cerebral Palsy Association, Inc.
- ☐ United Parkinson's Foundation

Community health

Appendixes

I n all areas of education, resources and materials are important additions to those provided by a school. Textbooks, study prints, films, filmstrips, transparencies, and posters are tools common to all teaching areas. Materials in health education present a mixed bag of blessings and problems. Since so many different kinds of agencies, organizations, and companies are interested in the health of today's youth, many free and inexpensive materials are available to the teacher. The problem is that sometimes materials are not appropriate or are factually incorrect or biased. This is not true of all materials, but it is important that you evaluate materials carefully before using them. The following are some suggestions for evaluating free materials:

1. Is the information factually correct?
2. Who is the author? Does the author have acceptable credentials in the health field?
3. Is it intended for teachers or students?
4. Is it appropriate for the specific age group?
5. Is it a high-quality item? Is it readable? Colorful? Interesting for student use?
6. Does it meet a specific teaching need, or will it just be a filler?
7. Does the item contain sensitive or controversial material? If so, should it be reviewed by other qualified school or community people before use?

Most materials do have a cost. With commercial vendors and textbook publishers there is no discount because selling educational materials is their business. Often, however, voluntary agencies, industry-sponsored sources, and professional organizations offer inexpensive or free materials to teachers. When contacting any of the organizations or companies, ask that a catalogue of their materials be sent. This catalogue will have more detailed descriptions of the specific items available and the current costs.

Remember to:

1. Plan ahead. Local agencies often loan films and other materials to teachers. It is important to give them plenty of advance notification to get the film on the day you desire. Additionally, it is essential to return a film on time so that they can allow others to use it.
2. Contact agencies on official school stationery. Be professional in your letter, and ask what services they can provide. Do not ask them to send you everything they have. Only ask for materials that you have real use for.
3. Do not stockpile materials. Order them only as the need arises.
4. Find out what you and your students can do for the agency in return, and *do* it.

SELECTED HEALTH EDUCATION CURRICULUM PROJECTS

Included within is a descriptive listing of a few health education programs found in various parts of the United States. They by no means represent all programs that exist. In some cases the programs require a commitment by the district or school. This means that the district or school needs to pay for materials and often teacher training to effectively use the program. It will be necessary to contact the organization responsible to find out the specific methods for implementing the program.

Know Your Body

Know Your Body (KYB) of the American Health Foundation is a teacher-delivered, behavior-oriented health education program for grades 1 to 8. With a focus on self-responsibility for health, decision-making skills, nutrition, exercise, and substance abuse prevention, the program is based on the premise that disease can be prevented and health promoted within the framework of a lifestyle-based school health education program.

A National Institutes of Health (NIH)-funded longitudinal evaluation of the fourth- to eighth-grade curriculum among 4000 children in the Bronx and Westchester County, New York, currently is underway. Early data analyses reveal significant improvements in health-related knowledge, attitudes, and behaviors, as well as in reducing the prevalence of obesity, high-blood pressure, and high blood cholesterol levels. In addition to the previously mentioned areas, KYB is found in Miami, Washington, D.C., and Chicago. A 3-year grant from the W.K. Kellogg Foundation supported introduction of KYB to first- to third-grade students in two Manhattan schools.

Contact
Know Your Body
American Health Foundation
320 E. 43rd St.
New York, NY 10017
212/953-1900

Growing Healthy

The *Growing Healthy* program for grades K to 7 is a planned sequential curriculum with a variety of teaching methods, a teacher training program, and strategies for eliciting community support for school health education. *Growing Healthy* involves students, teachers, educational administrators, other school staff, community health personnel, and the families of participating students. Through group and individual activities, children learn about their health lives by learning about their body systems. At each grade level a 9- to 13-week unit emphasizes the relationships between one's own health choices and the functioning of the system being studied. Access to a variety of stimulating resources, including audiovisual aids, models, guest speakers, and reading materials, is provided abundantly. *Growing Healthy* is designed to integrate with the lives and personality development of children by providing situations in which they may assume responsibility, research ideas, share knowledge, discuss values, make decisions, and create activities to illustrate their comprehension and internalization of concepts, attitudes, and feelings. Additionally, the curricula integrate with other school subjects such as reading, writing, arithmetic, physical education, science, and the creative arts. As teachers become familiar with the subject matter during training, they simultaneously learn teaching methods. Instead of the traditional classroom approach, the teacher uses a learning center approach, which allows children to move around the room, explore resources, and work together in groups. During the specialized team training, teachers receive packets of materials that help them develop and explain health-related concepts to students.

Contact
National Center for Health Education
30 East 29th Street
New York, NY 10016
(212) 689-1886

INTO ADOLESCENCE—CONTEMPORARY HEALTH SERIES

The Contemporary Health Series is actually two sets of modules that have been designed to provide educators with lessons challenging students to take personal responsibility for their health. The long range goals for the Contemporary Health Series are as follows:

Cognitive—Students will recognize the function of the existing body of knowledge pertaining to health and family life education.

Affective—Students will be able to experience personal growth in the development of a positive self concept and the ability to interact with others.

Practice—Students will gain skill in acting on personal decisions that relate to health-related life choices.

Within the Contemporary Health Series, there are two curricular subseries: *Into Adolescence* for middle school teachers and *Entering Adulthood* for high school teachers. The *Into Adolescence* subseries includes six different modules each focusing on a different health and family life topic. Modules titles are as follows:

Living in a Family
Learning About AIDS
A Time of Change (puberty)
Choosing Abstinence
Enhancing Self-Esteem
Learning About Reproduction and Birth

Contact

Network Publications/ETR Associates
P.O. Box 1830
Santa Cruz, CA 95601-1830
(408) 438-4080

WHERE DO I FIND THE MOST CURRENT HEALTH INFORMATION? WHAT IS HAPPENING WITH COMPUTERS IN HEALTH EDUCATION?

These and other questions can be answered by the staff of the National Health Information Clearinghouse (NHIC). This clearinghouse is a service run by the Office of Disease Prevention and Health Promotion of the U.S. Public Health Service. NHIC serves as a central source of information for health questions in all areas. Referrals are made to other organizations equipped to answer questions on specific health topics. If you have questions about where to get health information, resource guides for health education, or computer programs for use in the schools, contact the NHIC:

PO Box 1133
Washington, D.C. 20013
800/336-4797
800/522-2590 (in Virginia)

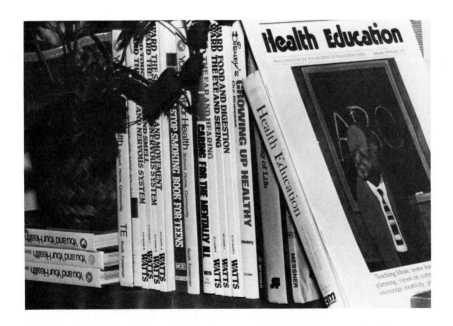

TABLE 1. Professional health education organizations

Organizations	Type of materials	Health topics	Levels	Comments
American Alliance for Health, Physical Education, Recreation, and Dance (AAHPERD) 1900 Association Dr. Reston, VA 22091 703/476-3400	Films Books for teachers Test manuals Publications for teachers and students Program and kits Textbooks: *Basic Stuff Series I and II*, K-12	Disease prevention and control Drug use and abuse Environmental health Growth and development Family life Mental and emotional health Nutrition Personal health Safety	P K,P,I,M M P P K,P,I,M I	
American Dental Association (ADA) Order Section 211 East Chicago Ave. Chicago, IL 60611 312/440-2500	Program Package for preschool to twelfth grade: *Learning About Your Oral Health* Films Kits Pamphlets and booklets Miniposters Badges	Consumer health Drugs, alcohol and tobacco Environmental health Growth and development Health careers Nutrition Personal health (dental) Safety and first aid	I,M I,M M K,P,I,M K,P,I,M K,P,I,M K,P,I,M K,P,I,M	
American Diabetes Association, Inc. (national headquarters) 600 Fifth Ave. New York, NY 10020 212/541-4310	Pamphlets	Disease prevention and control	M	
American Digestive Disease Society 7720 Wisconsin Ave. Bethesda, MD 20814 301/652-9293	Pamphlets	Disease prevention and control	I	

Organization	Materials	Topics	Level
American Hospital Association Media Center 840 N. Lake Shore Dr. Chicago, IL 60611 312/280-6000	Educational package programs Films Videocassettes Booklets and pamphlets Books Slides Posters	Alcohol Growth and development Health careers Mental and emotional health Nutrition Personal health Safety Smoking	General and adult
American Insurance Association Engineering and Safety Service 85 John St. New York, NY 10038 212/669-0400	Pamphlets Films	Safety and first aid	General and adult
American Optometric Association 240 N. Lindbergh St. Louis, MO 63141 314/991-4100	Pamphlets and leaflets Program packages Films	Consumer health — M Environmental health — M Personal health — I,M Safety and first aid — K,P,M Smoking — I,M	
American Pharmaceutical Association 2215 Constitution Ave. N.W. Washington, D.C. 20037 202/628-4410	Pamphlets	Drugs, alcohol, and tobacco — M Health careers — M	

Continued.

Key: K = Kindergarten, P = Primary, I = Intermediate, M = Middle School.
Modified from unpublished documents developed at the National Center for Health Education.
*This organization's *primary* interest is health education.

TABLE 1. Professional health education organization—cont'd

Organizations	Type of materials	Health topics	Levels	Comments
*American Public Health Association, School Health Education and Services Section (SHES/APHA) 1015 15th St. N.W. Washington, D.C. 20037 202/789-5600	Printed materials	General health education		SHES/APHA has a primary interest in health education in the schools.
*American School Health Association (ASHA) 1521 S. Water St. PO Box 708 Kent, OH 44240 216/678-1601	Professional journal Pamphlets and booklets Books and texts Curriculum guides Films Books (teacher resources)	Community health Disease prevention and control Drug use and abuse Family life Health careers Mental and emotional health Growth and development Personal health	K,P,I,M	Publishes *Journal of School Health*
*Association for the Advancement of Health Education (AAHE) 1900 Association Dr. Reston, VA 22091 703/476-3440	Professional journal Films Reprints Books	Alcohol Community health Dental health Disease prevention and control Drug use and abuse Mental and emotional health	M M M M	An association of the American Alliance for Health, Physical Education, Recreation, and Dance, and publisher of the journal, *Health Education*
*National Center for Health Education 30 E. 29th St. New York, NY 10016 800/232-2330	News and service magazine Pamphlets Resource guides Comprehensive School Health Program	General health education Growing Healthy	K,P,I,M	Works nationally, state-wide, and locally to promote health education in schools and workplace
*Society for Public Health Education, Inc. 703 Market St., Suite 535 San Francisco, CA 94103 415/546-7601	Professional journal	General health education		Largely concerned with community health education and publisher of *Health Education Quarterly*

TABLE 2. Governmental agencies

Agency	Type of materials	Health topics	Levels
Environmental Protection Agency Forms and Publications Center Research Triangle Park, NC 27711 919/541-2111	Printed materials	Environmental health	General and adult
High Blood Pressure Information Center 1501 Wilson Blvd. Arlington, VA 22209 703/558-4880	Booklets	Disease prevention and control	General and adult
National Archives and Records Service General Services Administration National Audiovisual Center Washington, D.C. 20409 301/763-1896	Information lists Catalogues	Consumer health Drug use and abuse Environmental health Health careers Safety and first aid	General and adult
National Clearinghouse on Drug Abuse Information Room 10A56, Parklawn Building 5600 Fishers Lane Rockville, MD 20857 301/443-6500	Pamphlets Films	Drug use and abuse	General and adult
National Health Information Clearinghouse PO Box 1133 Washington, D.C. 20013 800/336-5797	Publications Pamphlets Answers specific questions on telephone	Alcohol and smoking Consumer health Disease prevention and control Drug use and abuse Family life Mental health Physical fitness Personal health Safety	General and adult
National Heart, Lung and Blood Institute 9000 Rockville Pike National Institutes of Health Bldg. 31/4 A24 Bethesda, MD 20205 301/496-1051	Printed materials	Disease prevention and control Nutrition	General and adult
National Highway Traffic Safety Administration U.S. Department of Transportation Washington, D.C. 20590 202/426-1828	Printed materials	Alcohol Safety	K, P, I, M General and adult

Key: K = Kindergarten, P = Primary, I = Intermediate, M = Middle School.   *Continued.*

TABLE 2. Governmental agencies—cont'd

Agency	Type of materials	Health topics	Levels
National Institute of Alcohol Abuse and Alcoholism National Institutes of Mental Health 5600 Fishers Lane Rockville, MD 20857 301/468-2600	Pamphlets Reprints	Alcohol	General and adult
National Institute of Dental Research National Institutes of Health Bldg. 31/2 C34 Bethesda, MD 20205 301/496-4261	Pamphlets	Nutrition Personal health	M M General and adult
Office on Smoking and Health Room 1-10, Park Building 5600 Fishers Lane Rockville, MD 20857 301/443-1690	Technical information center	Smoking	General and adult
Public Documents Distribution Center Department 20 Pueblo, CO 81009	Pamphlets		General and adult
Public Health Service Environmental Health Service U.S. Department of Health, Education, and Welfare Rockville, MD 20857 301/881-1870	Pamphlets Reprints	Environmental health	General and adult

Key: K = Kindergarten, P = Primary, I = Intermediate, M = Middle School.

TABLE 2. Governmental agencies—cont'd

Agency	Type of materials	Health topics	Levels
Superintendent of Documents U.S. Government Printing Office Washington, D.C. 20402 202/783-3238	Pamphlets Posters	Alcohol Community health Disease prevention and control Drug use and abuse Environmental health Growth and development Nutrition Personal health (dental) Safety and first aid Smoking	M I,M I,M I M P,I K,P,I,M
U.S. Center for Health Promotion and Education Centers for Disease Control 1600 Clifton Atlanta, GA 30333 404/633-3311	Printed materials	General health education	General and adult Guidelines about AIDS education
U.S. Office of Disease Prevention Health Information and Promotion Hubert Humphrey Building 200 Independence Ave. S.W. Washington, D.C. 20201 202/655-4000	Printed materials	General health education	General and adult Developing health objectives for the nation for the year 2000.

TABLE 3. Voluntary and nonprofit health agencies

Agency	Type of materials	Health topics	Levels	Comments
Agency for Instructional Television 1111 W. 17th St. Bloomington, IN 47401 812/339-2203	Films Videocassettes Computer Software	Mental and emotional health Safety Social health	General and adult	Contact local chapter
American Cancer Society, Inc. (national headquarters) 3340 Peachtree Rd. NE Atlanta, GA 30026 404/320-3333	Program packages Other instructional kits Films and guides Pamphlets Posters Computer Software	Community health Consumer health Disease prevention and control Drugs, alcohol, and tobacco Family life Growth and development Mental and emotional health Nutrition Personal health	K,P,I,M M P,I,M P,I,M K,P,I K,P,I,M K,P,I,M I K,P,I,M	
American Heart Association (national headquarters) The National Center 7320 Greenville Ave. Dallas, TX 75231 214/750-5300	Program packages Brochures Pamphlets Films and filmstrips Cassettes Games Posters Photographic slides	Consumer health Disease prevention and control Drug use and abuse First aid Growth and development Nutrition Personal health	M M K,P,I J K,P,I,M K,P,I,M K,P,I	Contact local chapter
American Lung Association (national headquarters) 1740 Broadway New York, NY 10019 212/245-8000	Program packages Films Literature and periodicals Posters Buttons and stickers Slides and cassettes	Community health Disease prevention and control Growth and development Environmental health	M P M	Contact local affiliate

Organization	Materials	Topics	Grade level	Notes
American Red Cross National Headquarters 17th and E Sts. N.W. Washington, D.C. 20006 202/737-8300	Educational series on blood and circulatory system Films and filmstrips Pamphlets and leaflets Textbooks Posters	Community health Consumer health Family life Growth and development Mental and emotional health Personal health Safety and first aid	K,P M I,M K,P,I,M P,I I,J K,P,I,M	Contact local chapter
Arthritis Foundation (national headquarters) 3400 Peachtree Rd. N.E., suite 1101 Atlanta, GA 30326 404/266-0795	Pamphlets Reprints	Disease prevention and control	P,I,M	
Asthma and Allergy Foundation of America 9604 Wisconsin Ave., suite 100 Bethesda, MD 20814 301/493-6552	Pamphlets Films	Disease prevention and control Growth and development	General and adult	
Cystic Fibrosis Foundation (national headquarters) 6000 Executive Blvd., suite 309 Rockville, MD 20852 301/881-9130	Leaflets and pamphlets Films	Disease prevention and control Growth and development	General and adult	
Epilepsy Foundation of America 1828 L St. N.W., suite 406 Washington, D.C. 20036 202/293-2930	Pamphlets Paperback books Films Cassettes Slides	Disease prevention and control	General and adult	
Health Education Service, Inc. PO Box 7126 Albany, NY 12224 518/392-3951	Pamphlets Posters Videotapes	Family life Personal health (dental) Safety and first aid	M K,P I	Some materials available in Spanish

Key: K = Kindergarten, P = Primary, I = Intermediate, M = Middle School.

Continued.

TABLE 3. Voluntary and nonprofit health agencies—cont'd

Agency	Type of materials	Health topics	Levels	Comments
March of Dimes—Birth Defects Foundation 1275 Mamaroneck Ave. PO Box 2000 White Plains, NY 10602 914/428-7100	Program packages Films and filmstrips Pamphlets	Consumer health Disease prevention and control Drug use and abuse First Aid Growth and development Nutrition Personal health	M M K,P,I J K,P,I,M K,P,I,M K,P,I	Contact local office
Muscular Dystrophy Association (national headquarters) 810 Seventh Ave., 27th floor New York, NY 10019 212/586-0808	Pamphlets Films	Disease prevention and control	P	
National Congress of Parents and Teachers (NCPT) 700 N. Rush St. Chicago, IL 60611 312/787-0977	Program package Health education curricula Pamphlets	Consumer health Community health Disease prevention and control Drug use and abuse Environmental health Family life Growth and development Mental and emotional health Nutrition Personal health Safety and first aid	General and adult	
National Council on Alcoholism, Inc. Publications Department 733 Third Ave., suite 1405 New York, NY 10017 212/986-4433	Pamphlets Books	Alcohol	General and adult	

Source	Materials	Subject areas	Levels	Notes
National Easter Seal Society for Crippled Children and Adults 2023 W. Ogden Ave. Chicago, IL 60612 312/243-8400	Pamphlets	Dental health Disease prevention and control Growth and development Safety	General and adult	
National Health Council 70 W. 40th St. New York, NY 10018 212/869-8100	Pamphlets	Health careers	General and adult	
National Safety Council 425 N. Michigan Ave. Chicago, IL 60611 312/527-4800	Films Pamphlets Posters	Safety	General and adult	
National Society to Prevent Blindness (NSPB) (national headquarters) 79 Madison Ave. New York, NY 10016 212/684-3505	Pamphlet Films Charts	Disease prevention and control Growth and development Safety and first aid	P,I,M P,I,M P,I,M	Contact local affiliate
Network Publications/ETR Associates P.O. Box 1830 Santa Cruz, CA 95601-1830 (408) 438-4080	Pamphlets Books Curricula Videos	Family life Disease prevention and control (AIDS) Drug use and abuse Growth and development Mental and emotional health	P,I,M General and adult	Some items in Spanish Teacher training available

Continued.

TABLE 3. Voluntary and nonprofit health agencies—cont'd

Agency	Type of materials	Health topics	Levels	Comments
Public Affairs Committee, Inc. 381 Park Ave. S. New York, NY 10016 212/683-4331	Pamphlets Filmstrips	Alcohol Community health Dental health Disease prevention and control Drug use and abuse Family life Growth and development Health careers Mental health Nutrition Personal health Safety and first aid Smoking	General and adult	
United Cerebral Palsy Association, Inc. (national headquarters) 66 E. 34th St. New York, NY 10016 212/677-7400	Pamphlets	Disease prevention and control	General and adult	Contact local office
Wisconsin Clearinghouse for Alcohol and Other Drug Information 1954 E. Washington Ave. Madison, WI 53704-5271 608/263-2797	Pamphlets and booklets Fact sheets Posters	Drug use and abuse Family life Mental and emotional health Safety and first aid	P,I,M P,I,M P,I,M M	

Key: K = Kindergarten, P = Primary, I = Intermediate, M = Middle School

TABLE 4. Industry-sponsored sources

Source	Type of materials	Health topics	Levels	Comments
Aetna Life & Casualty Public Relations Department 151 Farmington Ave. Hartford, CT 06115 203/273-0123	Pamphlets Films	Alcohol Personal health Safety	General and adult	
American Automobile Association (AAA) Traffic Engineering and Safety Department 8111 Gatehouse Rd. Falls Church, VA 22047 703/222-6541	Films Slides Posters and guides Booklets	Alcohol Traffic safety	K,P,I,M K,P,I,M	Free materials; contact local offices
The Life Cycle Center Kimberly-Clark Corp. PO Box 551 Neenah, WI 54956 414/721-2000	Booklets and pamphlets Instructional kits Wall charts Filmstrips and cassettes Films (16mm)	Community health Disease prevention and control Emotional health Family life Growth and development Personal health	M I,M M M I,M I,M	
Metropolitan Life Insurance Health and Safety Education Division 1 Madison Ave. New York, NY 10010 212/578-2211	Pamphlet Films Wall cards Posters	Dental health Disease prevention and control Growth and development Mental health Personal health Safety and first aid	General and adult	Conducts "Healthy Me" grant program; information about successful local programs is available
National Dairy Council 6300 N. River Rd. Rosemont, IL 60018 312/696-1020	Printed materials Films Slides and transparencies Computer software Multimedia packages Programs and kits Pamphlets Posters and wall charts	Disease prevention and control Nutrition Personal health (dental) Smoking	K,P,I,M	Contact local affiliate

Continued.

Key: K = Kindergarten, P = Primary, I = Intermediate, M = Middle School

TABLE 4. Industry-sponsored sources—cont'd

Agency	Type of materials	Health topics	Levels	Comments
Prudential Insurance Co. of America Public Relations Department PO Box 36 Newark, NJ 07101 201/877-6000	Pamphlets Films	Disease prevention and control Drug use and abuse Growth and development Nutrition Personal health Safety and first aid	General and adult	
Shell Film Library 5000 Park St. N. St. Petersburg, FL 33709 813/541-5763 (Loan) 813/541-7571 (Purchase)	Films Videocassettes	Environmental health	M	Films also may be leased.
Tambrand, Inc. 5 Dakota Dr. Lake Success, NY 11042 516/437-8800	Audiovisual teaching aid Pamphlets Anatomical charts	Community health Family life Growth and development	M M M	
Tupperware Educational Services Department EFC 80 PO Box 2353 Orlando, FL 32802 305/847-3111	Educational kits Filmstrips	Consumer health Emotional health Growth and development Nutrition	P,I K,P P K,P,I	Some available in Spanish

Key: K = Kindergarten, P = Primary, I = Intermediate, M = Middle School

Glossary

affective domain relates to the values, beliefs, interests, attitudes, emotions, and feelings of individuals

affective objectives statements of teaching and learning purposes concerned with favorably influencing attitudes, values, or interests

AIDS (acquired immunodeficiency syndrome) an infection caused by a virus (HIV) transmitted through specific means, principally sexual intercourse, but also through sharing needles, syringes and other drug abuse paraphernalia, from an infected woman to her fetus or newborn infant, and by transfusion, specially in the case of hemophiliacs

anecdotal record a type of cumulative individual record that emphasizes episodes of behavior important in the character or personality

child abuse any act of either commission or omission that endangers or hinders a child's physical or emotional growth and development

cognitive domain relates to the ability to deal with knowledge and factual information from an intellectual perspective

community health council cooperative body representative of all community health-interested organizations and agencies

competency ability to perform at some predetermined acceptable level of expertise, usually less than mastery

comprehensive school health program the planned coordinated provision of health services, a healthful environment, and health instruction for all children in a school, where each of the components complements and is integrated with the others in the total scope of the body of knowledge unique to health education

conceptual approach a curriculum organizational plan that employs generalizations or concepts as the framework of its scope

congenital a physical defect or abnormality existing at birth or before but not due to heredity, e.g.

cerebral palsy, blindness or deafness of an infant whose mother suffered from measles (rubella) during her pregnancy

content the subject matter of health education; *see also* process

cumulative health folder a form used by school health service professionals to maintain records of screening tests, medical examinations, immunizations, illnesses or disabilities, anecdotal records of health-related behaviors that threaten a student's learning ability, and any other information relevent to the education and well-being of a schoolchild throughout his or her public school education

direct health teaching instruction given during regularly scheduled periods, having an organized, planned curriculum in equal status with all other basic studies

disease prevention deliberate actions planned and taken for the purpose of maintaining health, protecting against disease, early diagnosis and treatment of suspected disease, and rehabilitating disabled persons to the degree possible

elementary school usually refers to kindergarten to grade 6 or grade 8; in this text, refers to kindergarten to grade 8

evaluation a means of making informed decisions about the quality of a product or a performance; may be ongoing, or *formative,* as a means of assessing progress, or *summative* as a means of determining total growth or change as a total outcome of some specified treatment or program; includes but is not limited to quantitative measurement

experiential teaching the provision of activities that are realistic, involve multiple senses, and require the learner to participate fully, affectively, physically, and cognitively; sometimes called hands-on learning (the student learns by doing)

face validity a quality of test design based on the fact that the items do match the subject matter of concern

footcandle the amount of light on a surface that can be seen at a distance of 1 foot from a lighted standard candle

follow-through procedures procedures used to check on the outcome of a referral of a child for further diagnosis or treatment of a health problem

free-response test one in which the student uses his or her own words to respond in writing to a relatively small number of questions

general objectives broad abstract statements expressing educational goals for several years; or to serve as guidelines for the more specific objectives of a given course of study

handicapping conditions any condition that limits a child's mobility, strength, or well-being to the extent that special teaching may be required; includes mental retardation, speech impairment, visual impairment, hearing impairment, learning disability, emotional disturbance, orthopedic handicap, deaf-blindness, or health impairments associated with other conditions such as autism

health a quality of life involving dynamic interaction and interdependence of the physical, social, and mental and emotional dimensions of an individual's well-being

health attitudes relatively lasting clusters of feelings, beliefs, and behavior tendencies directed toward specific objects, persons, or situations related to health

health behavior actions customarily taken by an individual that have an impact on personal and community wellbeing

health belief a health-related statement or sense, declared or implied intellectually or emotionally, and accepted as being true by an individual or group; sometimes referred to as the conventional wisdom

health counseling procedures by which teachers, nurses, and physicians interpret a problem to students and their parents as a means of helping them find a solution

health education systematically organized activities designed to aid students in gaining the knowledge, skills, understanding, attitudes, and behavior patterns necessary for living healthfully; also health instruction, as a term used interchangeably in this book

health education goals long-range plans specified as the desired overall outcome of instruction

health guidance general assistance given by school personnel (such as nurses and teachers) to students and their parents to help them solve health problems that hinder a child's ability to learn

health habit a health practice that has become a routine activity

health knowledge authoritative concepts, generalizations, and supporting factual data deemed representative of the discipline of health education

health promotion any combination of health instruction and community organizations efforts supportive of individual or group behaviors conducive to improvement of their health status

health services all the efforts of the school to conserve, protect, and improve the health of the school population; includes appraisal of student health, prevention and control of disease, prevention or correction of physical defects, health guidance and supervision, and emergency care

healthful conducive to the maintenance or promotion of an individual's wellbeing

healthful school environment the quality of the physical, social, and emotional dimensions of a school; provided through procedures to maintain a safe and sanitary environment that promotes the health of both students and school personnel

healthy an optimum state or quality of life

hereditary a disease or tendency to certain diseases transmitted from parents to offspring, and carried by the genes, e.g. cystic fibrosis, sickle cell anemia, hemophilia

holistic health that state of being in which a person's body, mind, and spirit are in balance, functioning with utmost capacity or potential (high-level wellness), and in tune with natural and social environments, as well as with the cosmos (the spiritual environment)

hygiene personal health care, especially techniques and standards of grooming and cleanliness

initiating activity procedures to set the stage for what is to follow; may be done by recalling known related experiences, materials, or problems before entering into a new lesson

instructional objective an operational or enabling objective that describes what the learner should be able to do after a lesson that she or he could not have done before

integration in curriculum means by which a subject area is introduced and treated in a given educational situation so that subject areas are not treated separately, but logically as they relate to a broad unit of study

intermediate level in this text, grades 4 to 6

middle school in this text, a school with grades 7 and 8; also called junior high school; other possible combinations of grades found in schools called junior highs, middle schools, or intermediate schools: grades 7 to 9, almost always called junior high schools; grades 6 to 8, often called middle schools or intermediate schools; and grades 5 to 8, also called middle or intermediate schools

learning opportunity a situation in which relevant knowledge and activities are provided to stimulate the learner to become actively involved in the development of specified knowledge and skills

life style decisions made and resulting actions taken by individuals that typically affect their health

mandates laws requiring that certain actions be carried out in prescribed ways

measurable objective one whose achievement can be assessed in the classroom by means of an evaluation procedure exactly matching the objective's expressed intent

measurement quantitative description of student learning or progress; status determination

middle school see junior high school

mock-up a simplified and clarified working model of part or all of a real device, for example, driver-training devices and the head and torso used in CPR practice

morbidity statistics reported incidence of specified diseases and other health problems

need (1) the degree to which the present condition of an individual differs from some acceptable norm (2) the natural urge to maintain a balance between internal drives and external conditions (physiological, psychological, and integrative needs) (3) felt needs: interests and concerns arising from intense desire to know about something or how to solve some problem

negligence failure to do something that a reasonable person would do, or doing something that a reasonable and prudent person would not do

norms average scores on a standardized test based on data obtained through its application to a population of students of a specified grade level or age

organizing elements the range of subject areas or health topics considered to structure the body of knowledge of health education (body systems, health problems, content areas, topics, and generalizations or concepts).

organizing threads continuing curriculum emphases, health concepts, values, and problem-solving skills that provide the basis for continuity and integration

permissive legislation laws that establish the right to carry out a specified action, without requiring that it be done

primary level the early elementary school years, specifically kindergarten to grade 3

problem-solving method a logical process by means of which data are gathered and reasonable hypotheses are formulated and tested, until the best possible solution is discovered to a given health problem

process all the cognitive operations applied in the use of the subject matter of health education; see also content

psychomotor objectives those describing physical activities that can be practiced observably and demonstrated directly; for example, in health education, first aid techniques and toothbrushing skills

reliability the consistency and stability with which a test measures whatever it is measuring; an essential aspect of validity

resource persons parents, health providers, and other concerned adults who voluntarily assist teachers and schools in the promotion of the school health program; may include health services, instruction, advisement, fund raising, and other appropriate activities

risk factors characteristics or patterns of health behaviors that increase a person's risk of disease. These are either modifiable (e.g., age, sex) or unmodifiable, e.g. cigarette smoking, overweight)

school health committee a representative group of individuals drawn from school administration, faculty, staff, community, and students; a fact-finding, recommending, advisory body

school health education instruction designed to improve health-related knowledge, attitudes, and behavior

scope   the entire range of organizing elements (subject matter categories) considered within health education curriculum plan

screening tests   preliminary appraisal techniques used by teachers or school nurses to identify children who appear to need diagnostic tests carried out by medical specialists

self care   the active involvement of lay persons on their own behalf in health promotion and disease prevention procedures or activities

semantic differential test   an instrument based on the scales developed by Osgood, Suci, and Tannenbaum* as a means of measuring attitudes toward specific concepts

sequence   a plan for the ordering of organizing elements either vertically (year to year) or horizontally (day to day and week to week) for any one course of study

standardized test   one whose validity and reliability have been established by means of careful statistical and other procedures; norms provided as well

*Osgood, C.E., Suci, G.J., and Tannenbaum, P.H.: The measurement of meaning, Urbana, Ill., 1957, University of Illinois Press.

structured-answer test   an objectively scorable instrument by means of which the student indicates an answer to each item by checking or circling the best or correct choice among those alternatives offered

taxonomy of educational objectives   a scheme classifying educational objectives according to six levels of cognition, from lowest to highest in complexity, where the ability to demonstrate skill in each presupposes and depends on achievement of those preceding it in the hierarchy

teaching method   a process that involves the reasoned ordering or balancing of the elements of an educational function, that is, purposes, nature of the learner, materials of instruction, and total teaching and learning situation

teaching techniques   procedures or activities used by teachers for facilitating practice of instructional objectives, for example, field trips, role playing, lectures, and debates

tort law   civil liability laws governing torts (acts or failures to act by which a person injures another person or his or her property or reputation either directly or indirectly)

validity   the extent to which a test correlates with some criterion external to the test itself; that is, does it measure what it claims to measure?

values   preferences for ideas, things, or behaviors that are shared and transmitted within a community

Bibliography

GENERAL REFERENCES

Anderson, C.L., and Creswell, W.H., Jr.: School health practice, ed. 8, St. Louis, 1984, The C.V. Mosby Co.

Anspaugh, V., Ezell, G., and Goodman, K.: Teaching today's health, Columbus, 1987, O.Merrill.

Bradley, B.: School: The parent factor. Parents 63: 111, 1988.

Burt, J.J., Meeks, L.B., and Pottebaum, S.M.: Toward a healthy lifestyle through elementary health education, Belmont, Calif., 1980, Wadsworth, Inc.

Cornacchia, H., Olsen, L., Nickerson, C.: Health in elementary schools, ed. 7, St. Louis, 1988, The C.V. Mosby Co.

Dorman, S.M. and Foulk, D.F.: School Health Education and Advisory Councils, The Education Digest, 53: 21, 1988.

Eng. R., and Wantz, M.: Teaching health education in the elementary school, Boston, 1978, Houghton Mifflin Co.

Evans, D.: A school health education program for children with asthma aged 8-11 years. Health Education Quarterly, 14: 267, 1987.

Fodor, J.T., and Dalis, G.T.: Health instruction: theory and application, ed. 4 (in press), Philadelphia, 1989, Lea & Febiger.

Green, L.W.: Health education planning—a diagnostic approach, Palo Alto, Calif., 1980, Mayfield Publishing Co.

Greene, W.H., Jenne, F.H., and Legos, P.M.: Health education in the elementary school, New York, 1978, Macmillan, Inc.

Joint Committee on Health Problems in Education: Health Education, ed. 5, Washington, D.C., 1961, National Education Association and American Medical Association.

Kime, R., Schlaadt, R., and Tritsch, L.: Health education—an action approach, Englewood Cliffs, N.J., 1977, Prentice-Hall, Inc.

McGrath, R.E.: Developing concepts of health in early childhood, Buffalo, N.Y., 1977, DOK Publishing.

Newton, J. (ed.): School health: For health professionals. Elk Grove Village, IL., 1987, American Academy of Pediatrics.

Pollock, M.B.: Planning and implementing health education in schools, Palo Alto, 1987, Mayfield Publishing.

Read, D.A., and Green, W.H.: Creative teaching in health, ed. 3, New York, 1980, Macmillan, Inc.

Schaller, W.E.: The school health program, ed. 5, Philadelphia, 1981, W.B. Saunders Co.

Wheatley, G.M., and Hallock, G.T.: Health observation of school children, ed. 3, New York, 1965, McGraw-Hill Book Co.

PERSONAL HEALTH AND FITNESS

Barnes, K.E.: Preschool screening: the measurement and prediction of children-at-risk, Springfield, Ill., 1982, Charles C Thomas, Publisher.

Cornacchia, H.J., and Barrett, S.: Consumer health: A guide to intelligent decisions, St. Louis, 1984, The C.V. Mosby Co.

Crawford, J.H.: Sources of dental health teaching aids, J. Sch. Health **52**:54, 1982.

Dental care questions and answers, New York, 1982, Metropolitan Life Insurance Co.

Eng, A., and others: Increasing students' knowledge of cancer and cardiovascular disease prevention through a risk factor education program, J. Sch. Health **49**:505, 1979.

Fassbender, W.: You and your health, ed. 2, New York, 1980, John Wiley & Sons, Inc.

Lice aren't nice, Young Children, **42**:46, 1987.

Lynch, A.: Redesigning school health services, New York, 1983, Human Sciences Press, Inc.

McDermott, R.J., and Marty, P.J.: Making screening testing educational for elementary pupils: a pre-professional exercise. Health Educ. **12**(3):40, 1981.

McGrath, R.E.: Developing concepts of health in early childhood, Buffalo, N.Y., 1977, DOK Publishing.

Miller, C.A., et al. Monitoring children's health, key indicators, Washington D.C., 198?, American Public Health Association.

Rowan, C.T., and Mazie, D.M.: The mounting menace of steroids. Reader's Digest, **132**:133, 1988.

Sunglass savvy. Good Housekeeping, **206**:110, 1988.

Sunscreens. Consumer Reports, **54**:370, 1988.

Watson, M.L.: The relationship between dietary factors and dental caries, J. Sch. Health **52**:39, 1982.

Wynder, E.L., Hertzberg, S., and Parker, E., editors: The book of health, New York, 1981, Franklin Watts, Inc.

MENTAL AND EMOTIONAL HEALTH

Chance, P. and Fischman, J.: The magic of childhood. Psychology Today, **21**:48, 198?.

de la Sota, A., Lewis, M.A., and Lewis, C.E.: Actions for health: decision making and self-reliance activities for healthful living, grades 1-6, Reading, Mass., 1980, Addison-Wesley Publishing Co., Inc.

Earle, P.T., Rogers, C.S., and Wall, J.G.: Child development: an observation manual, Englewood Cliffs, N.J., 1982, Prentice-Hall, Inc.

Kagan, J.: Biological basis of childhood shyness. Science, **240**:167, 1988.

Lezine, K.: When your child needs help. **62**:126, 1987.

Marks J.: "We have a problem." Parents **63**:56, 1988.

Miller, D.F., and Wiltse, J.: Mental health and the teacher, J. Sch. Health **49**:374, 1979.

Ostrower, E.G.: A counseling approach to alcohol education in middle schools, School Counselor, **34**:209, 1987.

Rubin, L.D., and Price, J.H.: Divorce and its effects on children, J. Sch. Health **49**:552, 1979.

Shamsie, C.J., editor: New directions in children's mental health, Cambridge, 1979, Harvard University Press.

Thatcher, R.W.: Growth sprints mirror mental milestones. Psychology Today, **21**:13, 1987.

Timmreck, T.C.: Will the real cause of classroom discipline problems please stand up! J. Sch. Health **48**:491, 1978

FAMILY LIFE

Barlow, D.: Sexually transmitted diseases: the facts, New York, 1979, Oxford University Press.

Dickman, I.R.: Winning the battle for sex education, New York, 1982, Sex Information and Education Council of the U.S.

Riggs, R.S., and Taylor, R.M.: Incest: the school's role, J. Sch. Health **52**:365, 1982.

Roberts, F.: Sex education in schools. Parents **62**:50, 1987.

Silverstein, C.D., and Buck, D.M.: Parental preferences regarding sex education topics for sixth graders. Adolescence. **21**:970, 198?.

Taussig, W.C.: Sixth grade children's questions regarding sex, J. Sch. Health **52**:412, 1982.

Wurtele, S.K., and Miller-Perrin, C.L.: Sexual abuse prevention: Are school programs harmful? The Education Digest **53**:52, 1988.

Yarber, W.L.: Answering questions about sex, Sci. Teacher **44**:20, 1977.

NUTRITION

Cassery, A.R.: Anorexia and bulimia-the maladjusting coping strategies of the 80's. Psychology in the Schools. **24**:45, 198?.

Calloway, D.H., and Carpenter, K.O.: Nutrition and health, Philadelphia, 1981, W.B. Saunders Co.

Chaney, M.S., and Ross, M.L.: Nutrition, ed. 8, Boston, 1981, Houghton Mifflin Co.

Deutsch, R.M.: The nuts among the berries, rev. ed., New York, 1968, Ballantine Books, Inc.

Deutsch, R.M.: The new nuts among the berries. Palo Alto, Calif., 1977, Bull Publishing Co.

Frankle, R.T.: It's never too early for nutrition education, J. Sch. Health **50**:387, 1980.

Glines, D. and Ripp, D.: Allergies and problem students. Health Education **19**:34, 1988.

Guthrie, H.A.: Introductory nutrition, ed. 5, St. Louis, 1983, The C.V. Mosby Co.

Meyers, L.D., and Jansen, G.R.: A nutrient approach in the fifth grade, J. Nutr. Educ. **9**(3):127, 1977.

Moomaw, M.S.: Involving students in nutrition education, J. Sch. Health **48**:121, 1978.

Poolton, M.A.: What can we do about food habits? J. Sch. Health **48**:646, 1978.

Rapp, D.: Recognize and manage your allergies. New Canaan, CT., 1987, Keats Publishing Co.

Scarpa, I.S., Kiefer, H.C., and Tatum, R.: Sourcebook on food and nutrition, ed. 3, Chicago, 1982, Marquis Professional Publications.

Smith, M.K., and Phillips, J.: Curriculum guides for nutrition education, J. Sch. Health **50**:371, 1980.

DISEASE PREVENTION AND CONTROL

Acne: new approaches to an old problem, Consumer Reports **46**:472, 1981.

Benenson, A.S., editor: Control of communicable diseases in man, ed. 14, Washington, D.C., 1985, American Public Health Association.

Fields, W.T.: Dental myths: a baker's dozen, J. Sch. Health **52**:33, 1982.

Immunization: protection against childhood diseases, no. FL565, New York, fall 1980, Public Affairs Committee. (Pamphlet.)

McCann-Sanford, T., and others: Knowledge of upper respiratory tract infection in elementary school children, J. Sch. Health **52**:525, 1982.

The report of the Committee on Infectious Diseases, ed. 19, Evanston, Ill., 1982, American Academy of Pediatrics.

Tevis, B.W.: Teaching ideas in cardiovascular health, J. Sch. Health **48**:92, 1978.

ACCIDENT PREVENTION AND SAFETY

Accident facts, Chicago, 1987, National Safety Council.

Benson, J. and Anderson, J.: Respond: Teaching children self-protection. Seattle, 1985, Special Child Publications.

Carney, C.L.: Summer safety and first aid. Parents **62**:96, 1987.

Holcomb, B.: Child safety is up to you. Parents **63**:68, 198?.

Loomis, C.: Safety for latchkey children. Parents **62**:13, 1987.

Miller, D.F.: Safety: an introduction, Englewood Cliffs, N.J., 1982, Prentice-Hall, Inc.

Mroz, J.H.: Safety in everyday living, Dubuque, 1978, William C. Brown Co., Publishers.

Strasser, M.K., and others: Fundamentals of safety education, ed. 3, New York, 1981, Macmillan, Inc.

10 steps to a safer new year. Science Teacher **54**:25, 1987.

CONSUMER HEALTH

Cornacchia, H.J., and Barrett, S.: Consumer health: a guide to intelligent decisions, ed. 3, St. Louis, 1984, The C.V. Mosby Co.

Editors of Consumer Reports: The medicine show, Mt. Vernon, N.Y., 1980, Consumers Union.

Schaller, W.E., and Carroll, C.R.: Health quackery and the consumer, Philadelphia, 1976, W.B. Saunders Co.

Shipley, R.R., and Plinsky, C.G.: Consumer health: protecting your health and money, New York, 1980, Harper & Row, Publishers, Inc.

USE AND ABUSE OF DRUGS

Brecher, E.M., and Editors or Consumer Reports: Licit and illicit drugs, Boston, 1972, Little, Brown & Co.

Caffeine: how to consume less, Consumer Reports **46**:597, 1981.

Caffeine: what it does, Consumer Reports **46**:595, 1981.

Carroll, C.R.: Drugs in modern society. Dubuque, 1985, W.C. Brown.

Cornacchia, H.J., Smith, D.E., and Bentel, D.J.: Drugs in the classroom: a conceptual model for school programs, ed. 2, St. Louis, 1978, The C.V. Mosby Co.

Dennison, D., Prevet, T., and Affleck, M.: Alcohol and behavior: an activated education approach, St. Louis, 1980, The C.V. Mosby Co.

Erb, L., and Anderson, B.D.: The fetal alcohol syndrome (FAS), Clin. Pediatr. **17**:644, 1978.

Hafen, B.Q.: Addictive behavior: Drug and Alcohol abuse. 1982, Morton Publishing.

Is Bayer better? Consumer Reports **47**:347, 1982.

Jones-Witters, P., and Witters, W.L.: Drugs and society: a biological perspective, Belmont, Calif., 1983, Wadsworth, Inc.

Kids can be drink and drug free. Parents **62**:22, 1987.

Kinney, J., and Leaton, G.: Understanding alcohol, St. Louis, 1982, The C.V. Mosby Co.

Kupfer, A.: What to do about drugs. Fortune **117**:39, 1988.

Newman, S.: It won't happen to me, True stories of teen alcohol and drug abuse. New York, 1987, Putnam Publishing Group.

Petsonk, C.A., and McAlister, A.L.: "Angel dust": an overview of abuse patterns and prevention strategies, J. Sch. Health **49**:565, 1979.

Ray, O. and Ksir, C.: Drugs, society, and human behavior. St. Louis, 1987, The C.V. Mosby Co.

Seffrin, J.R., and Randall, B.G.: Tobacco use and oral health, J. Sch. Health **52**:59, 1982.

Silverman, H.M., and Simon, G.I.: The pill book, New York, 1980, Bantam Books, Inc.

Werch, C.E., McNab, W.L., Defreitas, B., and Bertschy, M.L.: Motivations and strategies for quitting and preventing tobacco and alcohol use. J. Sch. Health **58**:156, 1988.

Witters, W., and Venturelli, P.: Drugs and society, ed. 2, Boston, 1988, Jones and Bartlett.

ENVIRONMENTAL HEALTH

American Thoracic Society: Your health and air pollution, New York, 1980, American Lung Association.

As you live and breathe, New York, 1980, American Lung Association.

Dubos, R.: Man, medicine, and environment, New York, 1968, Praeger Publishers.

Miller, G.T., Jr.: Living in the environment: concepts, problems, and alternatives, ed. 3, Belmont, Calif., 1982, Wadsworth, Inc.

Pollution primer, New York, 1978, American Lung Association

Shakman, R.A.: Where you live may be hazardous to your health: a health index to over 200 American communities, New York, 1979, Stein & Day Publishers.

Smolensky, J.: Principles of community health, ed. 5, Philadelphia, 1982, W.B. Saunders Co.

Willgoose, C.E.: Environmental health: committee for survival, Philadelphia, 1979, W.B. Saunders Co.

COMMUNITY HEALTH

Halleron, T., and Pisaneschi, J. (editors): Aids Information Resources Directory, New York, American Foundation for AIDS Research, April, 1988.

Green, L.C., and Anderson, C.L.: Community health, ed. 5, St. Louis, 1986, The C.V. Mosby Co.

Boosting children's health with vaccinations. Consumers Research **70**:20, 1987.

Smolensky, J.: Principles of community health, ed. 5, Philadelphia, 1982, W.B. Saunders Co.

Shirreffs, J.H.: Community health, Contemporary perspectives. Englewood Cliffs, NJ., 1982, Prentice-Hall.

Watch out for the tick attack. Consumer Reports **54**:382, 1988.

Index

A

Abuse
  of children, 27, 29
  of drugs; *see* Drug use and abuse
Accident prevention and safety, 49-50, 87
  on field trips, 133-134
  and fires, 49-50
  and first aid; *see* First Aid
  at home, 468-474
  intermediate level education on, 320
  middle school level education on, 419-420
  Mr. Yuk symbol in, 246
  primary level education on, 243-245
  scope and sequence plan on, 227
  teaching activity ideas on
    intermediate level, 364-370
    middle school level, 468-474
    primary school level, 279-287
Advertisements and consumer health education, 420; *see also* Consumer health education
Affective objectives, 109-110
AIDS prevention education, 63, 65, 76, 207-213, 224, 361-363
  AIDS content specifics for teachers, 211-213
  CDC recommendations regarding school programs in, 211
  learning activity idea for intermediate level, 417-418
Air pollution, 324
Alcohol use, 323; *see also* Drug use and abuse
  abstinence from, and disease prevention, 461-463
  laws regulating, 322-323, 379-382, 383
  peer pressure in, 479-482
Anecdotal health record entries, 38
Anger, handling of, 313, 335-341
Anorexia nervosa, 415
Artificial respiration, 364-370, 419
Attitudes
  and beliefs of children about health, 14, 69
  definition of, 151
  evaluation of, 151-152
  measurement of, 153
  semantic differential testing of, 153-154
Audiovisual aids in health education, 136-139
  evaluation of, 155-156

B

Behavioral objectives; *see* Measurable objectives
Beliefs fundamental to school health programs, 17
Bicycles, safety rules on, 320
Binary choice test, 183-185
Bloom Taxonomy of Educational Objectives, 108, 123
Board of health, responsibilities of, for health in schools, 39
Body systems
  age-related changes in student questions on, 71
  health education approach based on, 71
Booklets for health teaching, evaluation of, 163
Breakfast programs in schools, 48
Buzz sessions, 131

C

Cancer, in relation to lifestyle, 460, 465-466
Cardiopulmonary resuscitation, 124, 321
Cardiovascular diseases
  and lifestyle, 35, 460-467
  prevention of, 354-363
Careers, health related, 425
  intermediate education on, 395-400
  middle school education on, 425, 475-477
  primary school education on, 247, 288-292
Chickenpox, 41
Child abuse, 27-29
  and mandatory report laws, 27
  prevention of, 240
Classroom environment, emotional aspects of, 73; *see also* Environmental health
Classroom tests; *see* Tests
Cognitive objectives, 108-109
Cold, common, 41
Committee on health, school, 61-62
Communicable disease, classroom defense against, 17
Community health council, functions of, 24
Community health education, 193, 224, 325
  on career opportunities in, 303, 305
  intermediate school level education for, 325

Community health education—cont'd
  middle school level education for, 425-426
  primary school level education for, 247
  scope and sequence plan for, 229
  and services provided by health workers, 303-308
  teaching activity ideas for
    intermediate school level, 395-401
    middle school level, 491-494
    primary school level, 303-308
  on voluntary participation in community health activities, 325, 491-495
Community health resources
  governmental health agencies, materials available from, 52-53t
  industrial organizations as sources of teaching aids in, 60
  official health agencies as, services of; *see* Governmental agencies
  parent-teacher groups as, school health promotion projects for, 61
  private physicians and dentists as resource people in schools, 54
  professional health organizations as, services of, 54
  service clubs as, specific health problem concerns and services for, 60
  voluntary health agencies as; *see* Voluntary and nonprofit health agencies
  youth groups as, health promotion activities of, 60
Competency
  definition of, G-1
  as goal of health education, 99-100
Completion tests, 182
Comprehension as instructional objective, 103, 108, 124
Comprehensive school health education, 17-64
Conceptual approach to curriculum design, 88-90
Conjunctivitis, 41
Connecticut Survey of health interests, 15, 72
Consumer health education, 245, 320-322
  on advertisements directed at children, 245

Consumer health education—cont'd
  on advertising appeals, 371-378
  on food products, 245
  on health helpers, 245-247, 288-292
  on health quackery, 322
  scope and sequence plan for, 228
  on selection of health advisers, 475-478
  teaching activity ideas
    intermediate level, 371-378
    middle school level, 475-478
    primary level, 288-292
Content
  appropriate for intermediate-level students
    accident prevention and safety, 320
    community health, 325
    consumer health, 320-322
    disease prevention and control, 318-320
    environmental health 324-325
    family life, 314-316
    mental and emotional health, 313-314
    nutrition, 316-318
    personal health and fitness, 310-312
    use and abuse of drugs, 322
  appropriate for middle school level students
    accident prevention and safety, 419-420
    community health, 425-426
    consumer health, 420-421
    disease prevention and control, 415-418
    environmental health, 423-424
    family life, 411-412
    mental and emotional health, 408-411
    nutrition, 413-415
    personal health and fitness, 404-408
    use and abuse of drugs, 422-423
  appropriate for primary-level students
    accident prevention and safety, 279-287
    community health, 303-308
    consumer health, 288-292
    disease prevention and control, 271-278
    environmental health, 299-302
    family life, 262-266
    mental and emotional health, 258-261
    nutrition, 267-270
    personal health and fitness, 251-257
    use and abuse of drugs, 293-298
Controversy and criticism of health teaching, ways to avoid, 215-217
Council on health, community, 61
Counseling as tool of guidance, 38

CPR: see Cardiopulmonary resuscitation
Criteria for selection of appropriate teaching techniques, 127
Culminating activities in lesson plans, 140-141
Cumulative health folders, 36, G-1
Curriculum plans, written guides to
  body systems design of, 79
  community influences on, 74-76
  conceptual approach to, 82-84
  content areas of, 81; see also Content
  crisis-generated aspects of, 77
  cycle plan of, 85
  direct teaching of, 87-88, 93, 128-136
  essential information of, 78
  evaluation of, 157-158
  goals of 69, 97-99
  integration scheme for, 86, 93
  learner needs, determining, 70-74
  learning opportunity compared with lesson plan in, 91
  macroscopic and microscopic views of, 90-91
  measurable objectives, 103, 104-108
  relevant to development of, 110
  organizing elements of, 79-86
  packaged guides for, 91-92
  planning of, 69, 90, 117-118
  problem-focused, 61, 79-80
  process as subject matter of, 76
  scope and sequence of, 79, 86, 92, 117
  for sexuality education; see Sexuality education
  state laws concerning, 24-26
  teacher role in development of, 90-91
  topic design of, 82
Cycle plan for health curriculum, 85

D

Decision making, steps in, 314
Dental health
  annual examinations for, 45
  nutrition affecting, 44, 236-237
  preventive care for, 45
  teacher observation of, 29
  toothbrushing techniques promoting, 44
Denver Study of health interests, 71
Disease prevention and control, 242-243, 318-320
  and community health; see Community health
  immunization in, 9, 37, 43, 320; see also Immunization
  at intermediate education level, 318-320
  at middle school level, 415-418
  at primary school level, 242-243
  in schools
    as established by district and school board policies, 39

Disease prevention and control—cont'd
  in schools—cont'd
    teacher observations in, 17, 29-35
    scope and sequence plan on, 227
    teaching activity ideas for
      intermediate school level, 354-363
      middle school level, 460-467
      primary school level, 271-278
Diphtheria, 42
Distractors in multiple choice tests, 185-186
Domains of learning behaviors, 98
Drawings, student expressions of learning, 190
Drug use and abuse; 245, 322; see also Alcohol use; Smoking
  age-related changes in student questions on, 71
  AIDS-related injected-drug use problems, 211
  direct health teaching on, 87
  evaluation activities on, 189
  guidelines for education about, 217
  federal laws controlling, 322-323, 379-386
  function of district policy statements in avoiding conflicts about, 215-216
  hazardous legal substances, 293-297
  influence of federal drug abuse education guidelines on school programs and, 213
  intermediate education on, 322
  legal aspects of school locker search and, 213-214
  middle school education on, 422-423
  peer pressures in, 422-423, 479-485
  primary school level education on, 245
  scope and sequence plan on, 228
  teaching activity ideas on
    intermediate school level, 379-386
    middle school level, 479-485
    primary school level, 293-298
Dry toothbrushing technique, 45

E

Ears and hearing
  screening for disorders of, 33-35
  teacher observation of, 28-29, 32
Elementary school health instruction, advantages of, 5
Emergency care, first aid kits required for, 43
Emotional health; see Mental and emotional health
Enabling objectives, 91, 100
Environmental health
  intermediate level education on, 324-325

Environmental health—cont'd
  middle school level education on, 423-424
  and prevention of pollution, 324, 387
  primary level education on, 246-247
  of schools, 47-50
    accident prevention and safety in, 49
    acres required for, 47
    curriculum planning based on evaluation of, 73
    definition of, G-3
    in food service programs, 48
    heating and ventilation in, 47-48
    legislation concerning, 26
    lighting in, 47
    mental and emotional aspects of, 50
    in play areas, 47
  scope and sequence plan on, 229
  teaching activity ideas on
    intermediate, 387-394
    middle school, 486-490
    primary, 299-302
  and types of pollution, 324-325
Essay tests, 181
Evaluation procedures, 148-167
  compared with measurement, 148-149
  of curriculum plans, criteria for, 157-158
  definition of, 148
  goal of, 148
  of learners
    effects of evaluation procedures on, 156
    health behaviors of, 154
    health beliefs and attitudes of, 151
    health knowledge of, 151
    relationship to learning opportunities, 149
    relevance to instructional objective, 149
  in school program, purposes of, 148
  summative versus formative uses of, 148-149
  of teacher effectiveness
    approaches to, 158-160
    criteria applicable to, 160-161
    performance indicators for (PET), 159
  of teaching materials and resources, criteria for, 162-166
Excitement education, 135
Exercise, 234, 235, 405-407
  and disease prevention, 408, 416, 460-462
  and physical fitness, 312, 405-407, 432-434
  and pulse rate, 406, 432-433

F

Family life education, 223
  on changing composition of families, 262-266
  on growth and development in puberty, 315, 342-347
  intermediate level education on, 314-316
  middle school level education on, 411-413
  primary school level education of, 240
  on reproductive processes of, 446-454
  scope and sequence plan for, 226
  teaching activities for
    intermediate, 342-347
    middle school, 446-453
    primary school, 262-266
Feasibility of instructional objectives, 104-107
  evaluation of, 112
Films and filmstrips, 164
  essential previewing of, 164
  evaluation checklist for, 165
Fire prevention, 49
  practice drills for, 43, 49-50, 468-474
First aid, 43, 279-287, 364-370, 419-420
  for bleeding, 245
  for breathing problems, 419
  for burns, 245
  cardiopulmonary resuscitation in, 321
  intermediate level instruction on, 364-370
  legal aspects of, 26-27
  middle school level instruction on, 419-420
  for poisoning, 420
  primary level instruction on, 245
  in school and playground accidents, 26, 43
Fluoride, effects of use of, 44, 107, 109
Follow-through procedures, 36, G-2
Foods; see Nutrition
Foot candle, 47, G-2
Formative evaluation, 148-149
Friendships and emotional and mental health, 258, 314, 411

G

Goal statements for health teaching
  compared with operational objectives, 97-98
  competency statements as, 99
  function of, in curriculum design, 97
  national priorities in, 75
Governmental agencies
  on consumer protection, 52
  on environmental protection, 53
  teaching materials of, A-9 to A-11
Grades (grading)
  definitions of, 191

Grades (grading)—cont'd
  formative and summative uses of, 192
Growth and development of children
  and changes in health interests, 71
  characteristics of, 73, 107, 122
  and curriculum planning, 73, 117
  and lesson planning, 127-128
  in puberty, 315, 342-347
  and selection of teaching techniques, 122-123
Guidance and counseling, health related, 29

H

Habits, health related, G-2; see also Life style
Hands-on learning activities, 134-135
Head lice, 40
Health
  attitudes toward, 151
  definition of, 5, G-2
  and illness, children's beliefs about, 14, 256-257
Health behavior, definition of, 6
Health beliefs, 151
Health curriculum planning, sources of
  body of knowledge, as a curriculum source, 78
  community, as a curriculum source
    current health crises in, 77
    legislative and political factors in, 76
    local community health needs and concerns in, 76
    national health and education goals in, 75
    parental values and attitudes toward health instruction in, 76
    pressures shaping local curriculum decision in, 76-77
  learners as a primary source of data
    growth and development characteristics of, 73
    health concerns and problems of, 74
    needs and interests of, 70
Health education
  causes of misperceptions about, 9
  definitions of, 8
  goals of, 16
  as outcome, 8
  overall purposes of, 8
  as profession, 8
  settings of, 8
  special language of, 5-8
  special processes of, 8
  television, influence on, 4
  as total school health program, 8
Health instruction; see also Health teaching
  aims of, 16
  interrelationships among activities of total program in, 50

Health objectives for nation, priority areas of, 12t
Health practices, 6
Health records, confidentiality of, 38
Health status, determinants of, 4
Health teaching
  direct techniques in
    brainstorming, 130
    buzz sessions, 131
    discussion, 129
    experiential activities, 134-135
    field trips, 133
    lecture, 128
    lecture-discussion, 130
    panel discussion, 131
    role playing, 132-133
    values-related activities, 135-136
  as general education, 16, 18
  problem solving as the primary method of, 125
  responsibility for
    of family members, 12
    of school faculty and personnel, 13
    of significant community members and organizations, 13-14
  vicarious teaching techniques, 137-138
Healthful life style, 19
Healthful school environment, key elements of
  acreage required for school site and plant, 47
  for food service programs, 48
  heating and ventilation standards for, 47
  legislation concerning, 24-28
  mental and emotional aspects of, 50
  play areas, provision of, 47
  recommended lighting in classrooms, 47
  safety and fire prevention procedures and equipment for, 49
  school personnel, health of, 50
Healthy versus healthful, meanings of, 5-6
Healthy People, Surgeon-General's Report, 80
Hearing; see Ears and hearing
Hepatitis, 41
HIV; see AIDS prevention education
Holistic view of health, 5
Horizontal sequence of curriculum organizing elements, 84-85, 88-89
Hygiene, study of, 5

I
Identification of learner needs, 70-74
Immunization
  required for school entry, 36-37
  state laws regarding, 43
Impetigo, 40
Industry-supported sources, 54, 60
  teaching materials of, A-17 to A-18
Influenza, 40

L
Land pollution, 324
Learning
  as behavioral change, 120
  as conceptualizing, 119
  function of the senses in perceiving, 119
  role of past experience in interpreting perceptions, 120
  social learning theory of, 120-121
Learning activities, criteria of worth of, 124
Legal aspects
  civil liability, 26-27, G-5
  of communicable disease control, 38, 43
  of confidentiality of health records, 38
  of consumer protection, 420-421
  of drug use and abuse, 322-323
  of first aid and treatment, 43
  mandatory laws, 26
  of negligence, 26
  of reporting child abuse, 27
  of sexuality education, 217
  of special education for handicapped children, 46
  state legislation on health education, 24-26
  tort laws, 26
Legislation; see Legal aspects
Lesson plan; see also Teaching activities
  compared with learning opportunity, 91, 140-141
  components of, 139-140
  culminating activities for, 140
  initiating activities for, 139
  measurable objective of, 139
  model for developing, 143
  as process versus content-oriented, 118
Liability laws, 26
Life cycle, changes of family roles in, 316
Life style
  definition of, 6-7, 10
  and disease prevention
    in intermediate level education, 319, 354-363
    in middle school level education, 416, 460-471
    in primary level education, 233
  and individual health problem solving patterns, 51
  influence of friends and family on, 329-334; see also Peer pressure
  and personal health and fitness, 251-257, 430-438
Lighting of classrooms, 47
Likert scales, 154

M
Mandated versus permissive legislation, 26

Mandatory legislation, 24-26
  on child abuse reporting, 27
Matching item tests, 182
Meals; see also Nutrition
  food choices for, 348-353
  served in schools, 48, 295-298
Measles, German, 42
Measurable objectives
  advantages in use of, 110
  definition of, 101-102
  and lesson planning, 104-105
Medical examination of school children, 30
Mental and emotional health, 223
  of abused children, 27, 29
  and coping with feelings, 409-410
  and friendship, 258-261
  intermediate school level education on, 313-314
  middle school level education on, 408-411
  primary school level education on, 238-239
  of school environment, 50
  scope and sequence plan for, 225
  teaching activity ideas
    for intermediate school level, 335-341
    for middle school level, 408-411
    for primary school level, 258-261
Mr. Yuk stickers, 246
Morals in sexuality education, 205, 217
Motivation of learners, evaluation procedures effects on, 156
Mouth to mouth respiration, training in, 364-370
Multiple choice tests, 185-186
Mumps, 41

N
National Congress of Parents and Teachers, 60-61
National health goals, 11
National Health Information Clearinghouse (NHIC), A-5
National health problems, priority areas of, 11
Negligence, definition of, 26
Noise pollution, prevention of, 387-393
Norm-referenced tests, 173
Nutrients, classes of, 317; see also Nutrition
Nutrition, 223
  and calorie intake and body weight, 454-459
  and characteristics of different foods, 267-270
  and consumer health education on foods, 371-378
  and dental health, 46, 236-237
  and disease prevention, 461
  evaluation activities on, 190
  and food choices for meals and snacks, 241-242
  and food diary records, 348-351
  and food groups, 241-242, 414

Nutrition—cont'd
  influence of friends and family on, 241
  and ingredient labels on packaged foods, 321
  intermediate level education on, 316-318
  middle school level education on, 413-415
  and nutritional value of foods, 348
  and personal health and fitness, 198
  primary level education on, 240-241
  and school food services, 48
  scope and sequence plan on, 226
  teaching activity ideas for
    intermediate level, 328-402
    middle school level, 454-459
    primary school level, 267-270
  thinking tasks related to, 123-124

O
Objectives, instructional
  afffective, 109-110
  behavioral, 102-103
  behavioral terms used in, 108-109
  criteria for development of, 104-108
  as facilitating evaluation, 110-111
  feasibility aspects of, 107
  function of, in curriculum development, 97
  general versus specific, functions of, 100
  and lesson planning, 139
  life-long application and worth of, 106
  major components of, 101
  measurable, 101-102
  operational model of, 103-104
  programmed instruction model of, 102-103
  psychomotor, compared to action goal, 99
  rating scale for, 111
  relationship to goals, 100
  taxonomy model of, 103
Observation of children in school
  appearance and behavior, 29
  and child abuse detection, 27
  and disease detection, 28
  ears and hearing, 28-29, 32
  eyes and vision, 29-30
Operational objective, 103, 104-108
Organizing elements, 79, 92, G-4
  content areas as, 81
  sequence of, 84, 92

P
Paideia proposal, 10
Parent-teacher groups, 60-61
  on sexuality education, 217
Pathogens, 318-319
Pediculosis, 40
Peer pressure, 329-334, 376
  on drug use behaviors, 479-485
  in intermediate school, 329
  in middle school, 411

Permissive legislation, 26, G-4
Personal health and fitness, 223
  and dental health care, 235
  and disease prevention, 233
  and health-promoting habits, 252-257, 430-438
  influence of family and friends on establishing, 291, 324-334
  intermediate education on, 310-312
  middle school education on, 404-408
  and nutrition, 198
  primary school education on, 233-238
  teaching activity ideas
    intermediate level, 329-334
    middle school level, 430-438
    primary school level, 251-257
Pertussis, 42
Philosophy of health education, 157
Physical appearance of children
  of abused children, 27-29
  teacher observation of, 28, 29, 30, 32
Physicians, 396-399; see also Careers, health related
  professional organizations of, 54, A-6 to A-8
  as resource persons for health education programs, 54
Piaget, theory of, 5, 14, 73, 117
Pinworm disease, 41
Pollution, environmental
  prevention of, 233-247, 324-325, 387-394
  primary school level education on, 298-302
  types of, 324-325
Problem solving and process-focused instruction, 118
Problem solving method, steps in applying, 125-126
Professional organizations, health-related, 54
  teaching materials of, A-6 to A-8
Puberty, growth and development in, 315

R
Referral procedures, 36
Reliability of tests, defined, G-4
Reproductive processes, 315-316, 446-454; see also Sexuality education
Responsibility, definition of, 26
Ringworm, 40
Risk factor, definition of, 7-8
Role playing, 132-133
Rubella, 42
Rubeola, 40

S
Safety
  and accident prevention, 243-245
  control of hazards in the home, 468-474
Sanitation in schools, 47
  in food services, 48-49

Scabies, 40
Scarlet fever, 92
School Health Education Study, 85
  scope and sequence chart of, 88-89
School health program
  as accepted responsibility of schools, 16-18
  components of, 8
  dental services provided in, 46
  emergency care of children in school, 43
  environmental health, provisions for, 47-50
  food service programs in, 48
  health committee, functions of, 61
  health records, maintenance of, 36-38
    confidentiality of, 36
    model form for data storage, 37
  instruction, provisions for, 50-51
  key role of teachers in provision of, 16-18
  legal aspects of, 24-27
  legislation affecting teachers, tort laws, 26
  patterns of organization for, 62
  policy decisions, weight on, 38-39
  principal components of, 8, 23
  public health laws affecting, 24
  screening programs provided in, 30-31
School health services, procedures of
  care of handicapped, 46
  communicable disease, control of, 38
    policies needed for, 38-39
    procedures for, 38
    signs and symptoms of, 40-42t
  dental health program, 44-46
    basic activities of, 46
    techniques promoting oral health, instruction in, 44-45
  emergency care, 43; see also First aid
  follow-through, procedures of, 36, 38
  health appraisals, 30-35
  health guidance, methods of, 38
  health records, maintenance of, 36
  principles of special education requirements, 46
  referral procedures, 36
  and specified handicapping conditions, 46
  teacher-nurse conference, significance of, 36
  teacher observation, purposes of, 28
    child abuse, evidence of, 27, 240
    ill health or disability, signs of, 29
Scope
  of health education
    definition of, 79
    organizing elements commonly used in describing, 79-84
      body systems design, 79
      conceptual approach, 82

Scope—cont'd
 of health education—cont'd
  organizing elements commonly
    used in describing—cont'd
   health content area design, 81
   health problems design, 80
   health topic design, 82
  and sequence
   charts of, 85, 88-89
   decisions determining, 84-85
   of organizing elements, 79, 117
Screening tests, 30-35
Self-care, definition of, 7
Self-esteem of children and teaching
    techniques, 122
Self-reliance, 16, 17, 19
 methods of teaching, 8
Self-report instruments, 153-155
Self-responsibility, 19
Semantic differential test of meaning,
    153
Sequence of health instruction
 cycle plan sequence, 85
 horizontal versus vertical se-
    quence, 92, 117
 spiral plan sequence, 86
Sexuality education
 age-related changes in student in-
    terest in, 71
 and AIDS prevention education,
    207, 211-213
 AIDS-related specific concepts for
    teachers, 211
 classroom atmosphere for, 210
 community guidelines on, 205-206,
    211
 controversy and criticism related,
    204-218
 curriculum advisory committee on,
    215-216
 laws concerning, 217
 minority views affecting, 214-215
 necessity of selecting qualified
    guest speakers for, 210
 parent notification of, 217
 parent's role in, 204, 206-207
 personal biases affecting, 210
 problems in teaching, ways to
    avoid, 207, 208-209
 puberty, changes of, 315
 questionable terminology used in,
    209
 school board policies on, 215-216
 and sexual activity of learners, 207,
    211
 teacher problems with, 207, 208-210
 use of trained personnel for, 217
 values and morals approaches in,
    205-206
SHES; see School Health Education
    Study
Short answer tests, 182
Skill training
 affective, 109-110
 cognitive, 118-123
 psychomotor, 124
Sleep and personal health and fit-
    ness, 380, 405

Smokeless tobacco, use of, by chil-
    dren, 11
Smoking
 content on
  for intermediate school level ed-
    ucation, 319-323
  for middle school level educa-
    tion, 423
  for primary school level educa-
    tion, 247
 evaluation activity for, 190
 intermediate level education on,
    322
 and laws regulating purchase and
    use of cigarettes, 323, 384
 as lifestyle risk factor, 7, 11, 12
 middle school level education on,
    422-423
 as motivated by role model adult
    behavior, 13, 17
 peer pressure in, 329-332
 and personal health and fitness, ef-
    fects on, 311
 and prevention education timing,
    11
Snellen Vision Test, 30-32
Social Learning Theory (SLT), 121-
    122
Special education programs for hand-
    icapped children, 46-47
Specific versus general objectives,
    functions of, 100-101
State policies
 on child abuse, 27
 on health education, 26
 on sexuality education, 217
Stress management, 313
 coping strategies for, 409-410, 439-
    445
 and disease prevention, 416, 461
 and mental and emotional health,
    409, 439-446
 Students Speak, 71-72; see also
    Trucano, Lucille
Summative evaluation, 148-149
Swimming, safety rules for, 320

T
Teachers
 as role models, 13
 evaluation of, 112, 158-162
 health of, 50
 in conference with school nurse,
    335-336
 in curriculum development, 90
 in parent-teacher groups, 60-61
 in sexuality education
  on curriculum advisory group of,
    215
  training needed by, 217
 observation of children by, 17, 28-
    29
 role of, in elementary schools, 16-
    18
 tests written by, 173, 174, 197
  evaluation of, 188
 tort laws affecting, 26-27

Teaching activities—cont'd
Teaching activities; see also Lesson
    plan
 on accident prevention and safety
  intermediate level, 364-370
  middle school level, 468-474
  primary level, 279-287
 on community health
  intermediate level, 395-401
  middle school level, 491-494
  primary school level, 303-308
 on consumer health
  intermediate level, 371-378
  middle school level, 475-478
  primary school level, 288-292
 as critical element in teaching pro-
    cess, 117
 on disease prevention and control
  intermediate level, 354-363
  middle school level, 460-467
  primary school level, 271-278
 on drug use and abuse
  intermediate school level, 379-386
  middle school level, 479-485
  primary school level, 293-298
 on environmental health
  intermediate level, 387-394
  middle school level, 486-490
  primary school level, 299-302
 on family life
  intermediate school level, 342-
    347
  middle school level, 446-453
  primary school level, 262-266
 on mental and emotional health
  intermediate school level, 335-
    341
  middle school level, 439-445
  primary school level, 258-261
 on nutrition
  intermediate school level, 348-
    353
  middle school level, 454-459
  primary school level, 267-270
 on personal health and fitness
  intermediate school level, 329-
    334
  middle school level, 430-438
  primary school level, 251-257
Teaching activity ideas; see also Les-
    son plan
 for intermediate level students,
    329-401
 for middle school level students,
    430-494
 for primary school level students,
    251-308
Teaching techniques based on social
    learning theory
 modeling, 121
 self-monitoring, 122
 self-rewarding, 122
 skill training, 121
Television
 and consumer education regarding
    advertisements, 420
 as health instruction tool, 4, 136

Television—cont'd
  influence of, on health behavior, 13
Tests
  achievement, 175
  categories of, 177
  classroom, 174
  construction of, 175
  as criterion-referenced assessment of
    health actions, 191
  evaluation activities, 189-191
  free response
    essay, 180-181
    short answer and completion, 182-
      183
  free response vs structured response
    mode, 177
  item preparation, guidelines for, 184
  matching item, 187
  as means of assessing affective ob-
    jectives, 191
  as measures of learning status,
    173
  multiple choice, 185-186
  planning of, 175
  standardized, 187
  terminology of, 173
  true-false, 183-185
Tetanus, 42
Textbooks
  in direct health teaching, 84, 87,
    90

Textbooks—cont'd
  evaluation of, 162
  in evaluation activities, 190
  in values clarification, 135
Thinking tasks versus recitation in
    health education, 123-124
Topic design of health curriculum, 82
Tort laws, 26-27, G-5
Traffic safety in school area, 49
Transportation of children for emergen-
    cy care, 44
Trucano, Lucille, 10
True-false tests, 183-185

U

U.S. Centers for Disease Control, rec-
    ommendations regarding
    AIDS education, 211-212

V

Vaccine; see Immunization
Validity of tests, 173, 187
  face, G-2
Values
  basic to sexuality education, 206
  clarification of, 205
  definition of, 152, 205, G-5
  evaluation of, 152-153
  implicit in affective objectives, 109-
    110
Ventilation and heating of classrooms,
    47-48

Vertical sequence of curriculum orga-
    nizing elements, 84-85, 88-89
Vicarious teaching techniques, 128,
    136-139
Vision
  screening tests for, 30-32
  teacher observation of, 29
Visual aids in health teaching, 136-139
Voluntary and nonprofit health agen-
    cies, 55-57t
  participation in, 491-494
  teaching materials of, A-12 to A-16

W

Water, pollution of, 387
Weight
  and calorie intake, 407, 454-459
  normal as disease prevention, 416
Wellness
  compared with illness, 256-257, 271-
    278
  high level, 5
  promotion and maintenance of, as
    goal of health education, 16,
    28
Whooping cough, 42
Wounds, first aid for, 281-287

Y

Youth groups, health education poten-
    tial of, 60